THE
ENCYCLOPEDIA
OF
AGING
AND
THE ELDERLY

THE
ENCYCLOPEDIA
OF
AGING
AND
THE ELDERLY

F. Hampton Roy, M.D.
and
Charles Russell, Ph.D.

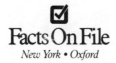

Facts On File
New York • Oxford

The Encyclopedia of Aging and the Elderly

Copyright © 1992 by F. Hampton Roy and Charles Russell

All rights reserved. No part of this book may be reproduced or utilized in any form
or by any means, electronic or mechanical, including photocopying, recording, or
by any information storage or retrieval systems, without permission in writing from
the publisher. For information contact:

Facts On File, Inc.	Facts On File Limited
460 Park Avenue South	Collins Street
New York, NY 10016	Oxford OX4 1XJ
USA	United Kingdom

Library of Congress Cataloging-in-Publication Data
Roy, Frederick Hampton.
　　The encyclopedia of aging and the elderly / F. Hampton Roy and Charles Russell.
　　　　p.　cm.
　　Includes bibliographical references and index.
　　ISBN 0-8160-1869-3
　　1. Gerontology—Encyclopedias.　2. Geriatrics—Encyclopedias.
3. Aging—Encyclopedias.　4. Aged—Encyclopedias.　I. Russell,
Charles H.　II. Title.
HQ1061.R69　1992
305.26′03—dc20   91-23435
　　　　　　　　　　　　　　　　　　　　　　　　　　　　　　CIP

A British CIP catalogue record for this book is available from the British Library.

Facts On File books are available at special discounts when purchased in bulk
quantities for businesses, associations, institutions or sales promotions. Please call
our Special Sales Department in New York at 212/683-2244 (dial 800/322-8755
except in NY, AK or HI) or in Oxford at 865/728399.

Composition by the Maple-Vail Book Manufacturing Group
Manufactured by Hamilton Printing Company
Printed in the United States of America.

10 9 8 7 6 5 4 3 2 1

This book is printed on acid-free paper.

CONTENTS

PREFACE

The growth of the older population is one of the most spectacular phenomena of present American history. Already there are more than 30 million Americans over age 65, and this number will double early in the next century. If we select age 50 as the start of later life, our older population, which now stands at about 65 million, will expand to more than 100 million before today's infants reach midlife. America has never witnessed anything like it— call our era "The Aging Boom."

Even more interesting, the Baby Boom generation, which has made up the bulk of the youth component of our population since the early 1960s, is about to move from adulthood to age. Born between 1946 and 1964, the vanguard of this age *cohort* (to use the technical word designating a part of the population born during the same time period) will reach age 50 in 1996. Considering that many members of this generation reached adulthood during the youth rebellion of the 1960s and its aftermath, how will they live their senior years? Will the Baby Boomers manage to live a satisfying and well filled old age? One might hope so, but the answer rests, as it does for us all, less on hope than on the Baby Boomer's understanding of age.

At the threshold of the Aging Boom, Americans have an unhappy aversion to age—we remain a youth-oriented culture. Public opinion polls show that the majority of our population thinks of the elderly as deprived, and old age as a time of life when poverty, ill health, boredom, and loneliness prevail. This opinion is wrong, but it's what we think.

Today we desperately need solid information about age so that we may achieve the fullest potential of the senior years. The present volume is dedicated to the task of filling the gap in America's understanding, of reversing the common opinion, by opening America to the rich possibilities of age. Written jointly by Hampton Roy, M.D., a physician, and Charles Russell, Ph.D., a social gerontologist, this encyclopedia is unique because it presents a medical and social/psychological perspective on age. From it the reader will learn the major elements of geriatric medicine that provide a key to health in later life, and the central facts about how older people live, feel, and think. The subjects of mental health, sexuality, the challenges of age, age in philosophy and literature, all these and many other topics that appear in this book show the way to a vital life in the senior years. Whether browsing here and there in a leisurely way or going through the volume systematically from beginning to end, the reader will come away vastly better informed about later life, and will, therefore, be more capable of living age to its fullest.

As the physician in this pair of authors I would like to acknowledge Kate Kelly, former editor at Facts On File, and Ray Powers, my agent, in their efforts to nurture the concept of this book. I am indebted to the many individuals who assisted with the preparation of this manuscript, including Renee Tindall, Anita Boyett, Kim Bridges, Anita Scott, Karen Montgomery, Mary Pennington, Sherry Mayer, Nora Rengers, Adrienne Hart, Auburn Steward, Alice Nicholson, Ruby Nichols, Cheryl Bridgers, Debbie Bentley, Louise Gear, and Mary Michelle Nichols.

As the gerontologist in this pair of authors, I wish to acknowledge the outstanding social, psychological, humanistic, and practical work that has gone on in this important discipline over the past 50 years, and especially to thank those who trained and influenced me in the subject of gerontology: Dr. James Birren, former dean and Brookdale Distinguished Scholar at the Ethel Percy Andrus Gerontology Center, University of Southern California, and now at UCLA; Dr. Howard Rosencranz, Emeritus Professor of Gerontology at the University of Connecticut; and Dr. Nancy Sheehan, Coordinator of the Travelers Center on Aging at the University of Connecticut; Inger Megaard Russell, RN and diplomate in hospital administration, who before she married me served as the associate director of a large nursing home in Norway. I should also like to thank the faculty of the University of Connecticut who introduced me to the field of sociology and taught me its meaning and methods: Professors Mark Abrahamson, Gerold Heiss, Kenneth Hadden, Myra Marx Ferree, and Floyd Dotson.

But, equally, it is essential to acknowledge the millions of Americans who have helped to create the vast potential of modern aging. Starting with the architects of the Social Security program, they include all those who have helped to define age as a vital and important period of life. Readers should refer to Appendix II for a list of organizations that have contributed to this progress, but here we mention the AARP, the National Council on Aging, the federal agencies that provide funds for aging programs, especially the National Institute on Aging, the insurers and businesses that have set up retirement and pension plans, the architects, developers, and contractors who have created the burgeoning retirement communities and housing projects for the elderly, and the financiers who have had the foresight to supply funds for these projects—a unique feature of the American approach to aging is that much of the initiative has come from private enterprise, quite unlike Europe where the government has been the major actor. And, most of all, the older population itself deserves recognition— it has been, and remains, a pioneer generation that is forging the way into a new world where Americans can live the last years of their lives as their very best years.

Hampton Roy, M.D.   Charles H. Russell, Ph.D.
Physician   Certified Gerontologist

INTRODUCTION

Dramatic differences in how people age raise questions about the biology of aging. Human life span can be extended only by identifying the basic processes of aging. Many factors, such as environment, preprogrammed genetics, cell depletion, organ exhaustion, and overall "wear and tear," rather than any single factor, seem to be involved.

All parts of the body are affected by aging. As the body ages the bones lose calcium. The bones become more brittle and heal more slowly. After age 60, degenerative arthritis often develops. The cartilage around the joints is often "worn" from years of use, and the lubricating fluid is often depleted. This makes for a slower-moving, stiffer person.

The brain shrinks as a person ages. Although the brain shrinks, intelligence doesn't seem to be affected. Most people maintain a high level of mental competence throughout life. A slight loss of memory usually occurs after age 50. The reflexes also become slower.

Hearing losses usually begin around age 30. Men are more likely than women to encounter hearing losses. The first loss is usually among the high notes (above 15,000 hertz). Many older people also have trouble distinguishing between speech and background noise.

The lens of the eye steadily hardens over the years, often making it difficult for people over 40 to focus on near objects. Older eyes are also prone to cataracts and glaucoma. Pupils become smaller with age, allowing in less light and limiting night vision.

As the body ages, it becomes flabbier. The amount of flab is determined by pinching the skin beneath the shoulder blade and measuring how thick it is. At age 20, the distance is usually 12 millimeters; at 30 it is about 14 millimeters. After 40 the distance remains about 16 millimeters.

As the body ages, the hair becomes thinner. At age 20, the diameter of a single hair is 101 microns. By age 70 the diameter has decreased to about 86 microns. Balding usually begins at the temples, producing a widow's peak that recedes with age. Next, the monk's spot, the circle on the back of the head, begins to lose hair. The two areas may eventually meet and leave a man bald. Although balding occurs mostly in men, women are also affected. Most women have thinning of the hair but very few actually become bald.

As the body ages, the heartbeat becomes weaker. The heart pumps less blood with each beat, so that the heart has to work harder to keep the body nourished. Indeed, cardiovascular disease is the leading cause of death among the elderly.

As a person ages the muscles weaken, causing the back to slump. The disks between the bones of spine deteriorate and move closer together causing a loss of height. At age 30, about 70 pounds of a man's 175 pounds are muscle. Over the next 40 years a man will lose 10 pounds of that muscle. His shoulders narrow. The muscle becomes weaker and stiffer with age. A man's strength peaks at about 30 years of age and then steadily diminishes. In women, the decrease of muscle strength begins in the twenties. Fat gradually replaces muscle in the female body.

As the body ages, the nails grow more slowly. At age 20 a person's nails will grow .94 millimeters a week. At age 70 the nails grow only about .60 millimeters a week.

Reaction time slows with age. The reason for the slowdown of the reaction time is the increased time required by the brain to process information, make decisions, and dispatch signals.

The skin wrinkles automatically with age. The skin loses water and its molecules bind to each other, making for a stiffer, less elastic skin structure. The skin spreads out and thins, causing it to be "baggy" on the body.

Stamina decreases with age. The weakening of the heart, lungs, and muscles means that there is less oxygen coming in, and this oxygen is slower to disperse to the muscles. For instance, a healthy 70-year-old person can run a marathon, but it will take him or her at least an hour longer than it took at age 30.

A man's basal metabolism slows down by 3 percent each decade. Muscle and tissue die and are replaced by accumulated fat. At age 20 a man who weighs 165 pounds will be 15 percent fat. At age 70 this man will weigh about 178 pounds with 30 percent of his weight being fat. In women, the number of calories necessary to maintain a weight decreases by ten percent each decade after 20.

These body changes are an inevitable part of aging. They occur so gradually that most people do not recognize the changes.

SOURCES: Krieger, L. "Why Do People Get Old." In *Aging,* Goldstein, E. C., ed. Vol. 3, Art. 18. Boca Raton, Fl.: Social Issues Resource Series, Inc., 1981.
Tierney, J. "The Aging Body." In *Aging,* Goldstein, E.C., ed. Vol. 2, Art. 24. Boca Raton, Fl.: Social Issues Resource Series, Inc., 1981.

A

AARP See AMERICAN ASSOCIATION OF RETIRED PERSONS.

accidents Although accidents rank behind a number of other leading causes of death among the elderly, they are of special concern because they represent the most avoidable of all killers. Older people are more likely than the young to make a poor recovery and to experience complications from an accidental injury, with correspondingly higher health-care costs as well as disability and death. Among teenagers and youths the death rate from accidents is high (64 per 100,000 people) because they tend to take more risks in such things as sports, high speed driving, and motorcycling. At age 65–74, long after the risk-taking behavior of young people has passed, the death rate from accidents is slightly lower (61 per 100,000), but after age 75 it increases nearly three times (166 per 100,000).

For 15- to 24-year-olds motor vehicle accidents rank first as a cause of accidental death (46 per 100,000), and they also rank first, though at a much lower level, for people age 65–74 (22 per 100,000). After age 75, falls become the main cause of accidental death (86 per 100,000), while automobile deaths stand at 30 per 100,000. As these figures show, the death rate from automobile accidents is greater after age 75 than at age 65–74, but this is due in part to the greater frailty of the 75+ age group. With respect to pedestrian deaths due to motor vehicles, older people rarely die from this cause (in a recent year about 2,000 such deaths occurred among the several million people who died over age 65), but experts observe that traffic lights may change too quickly to allow the old enough time to cross streets and intersections in safety.

In accidental injuries that occur when people are at work, the statistics run contrary to what one might expect—older people have a much lower accident rate at work than most younger age groups. At 65+ there is a .41 injury rate compared to 1.38 at 20–24, 1.15 at 25–34, .89 at 35–44, and .77 at 45–64. These ratios are work-injury ratios and are derived by dividing the percentage of all work injuries experienced by an age group by the percentage of all workers represented by that age group. For example, persons age 65 and over represent 2.2% of all workers but account for only .9% of all injuries, or $.9\% \div 2.2\% = 0.41$. Home accidents, however, occur more often to people over 65 (falls, burns, fires that result in injury, ingesting food poorly, poisoning by liquids, or asphyxiation by gas). The older age group also experiences more accidents while in hospitals and nursing homes, when, because of weakness or lack of experience, they fall getting in or out of wheelchairs and when using the bathroom. Snow, ice, and areas with rough or rocky ground also cause problems, as do dropping of cigarettes, neglect of cooking devices, and misuse of drugs or medicines.

Sterns, H. L.; Barrett, G. V.; and Alexander, R. A. "Accidents and the Aging Individual," in Birren, J. E., and Schaie, K. W., *Handbook of the Psychology of Aging* (2nd ed.). New York: Van Nostrand Reinhold, 1985.

acculturation The process of the rapid cultural change that occurs when two different cultures are brought into contact is known as acculturation. Studies confirm that cultural variables are important in inducing biological changes that contribute to HYPERTENSION and coronary heart disease.

Three acculturation indices were used in a study of Japanese-Americans: (1) culture of upbringing; (2) culture assimilation (the degree to which new customs, language and diets were accepted); and (3) social assimilation (the degree to which contacts were made outside the Japanese community). Those who were most acculturated to Western cul-

1

ture had three to five times higher prevalence of coronary heart disease.

In the tribes of the Solomon Islands, those who were most Westernized had higher blood pressure, higher cholesterol levels, and higher stress levels than those tribes maintaining the traditional tribal lifestyle.

Researchers conclude that repeated stressful situations, as can be found in adapting to a new culture, have a negative effect on the aging process. They emphasize the importance of a stable society whose members can enjoy support in a closely knit environment as the best protection against the various forms of social stress.

Marmot, M. G., and Syme, S. L. "Acculturation and Coronary Heart Disease in Americans." *Amer. J. of Epidermology* 104: 225–247 (1976).
Page, L. B. *et al*. "Antecedents of Cardiovascular Disease in Six Solomon Islands Societies." *Circulation* 49: 1132–1146 (1974).

acculturation rank   Acculturation ranks are used to single out cultural variables that may affect the rate of aging. A study that was conducted on the Solomon Islands identified different acculturation factors:

1. Evidence of demographic change
2. Increases in adult height
3. Length and intensity of contact with Western culture
4. Religious change
5. Education
6. Availability of medical care
7. Extent of entry into cash economy
8. Adoption of European-style diets

It was found that the members of the Solomon Island community who were the most Westernized had higher blood pressure, higher cholesterol levels, and higher stress levels. These individuals appeared older than the individuals who were less Westernized.

Page, L. B., *et al*. "Antecedents of Cardiovascular Disease in Six Solomon Islands Societies." *Circulation* 49: 1132–1146 (1974).

ACE (Active Corps of Executives)   See SCORE.

achievements at an advanced age
Many well-known people made major accomplishments in old age. The following is a list of such examples.

1. At 100, Grandma Moses was painting.
2. At 94, Bertrand Russell was active in international peace drives.
3. At 93, George Bernard Shaw wrote the play *Farfetched Fables*.
4. At 91, Eamon de Valera served as president of Ireland.
5. At 91, Adolph Zukon was chairman of Paramount Pictures.
6. At 90, Pablo Picasso was producing drawings and engravings.
7. At 89, Mary Baker Eddy was directing the Christian Science Church.
8. At 89, Arthur Rubinstein gave one of his greatest recitals in New York's Carnegie Hall.
9. At 89, Albert Schweitzer headed a hospital in Africa.
10. At 88, Pablo Casals was giving cello concerts.
11. At 88, Michaelangelo did architectural plans for the church of Santa Maria degli Angeli.
12. At 88, Konrad Adenauer was chancellor of Germany.
13. At 85, Coco Chanel was the head of a fashion design firm.
14. At 84, Somerset Maugham wrote *Points of View*.
15. At 83, Aleksandr Kerensky wrote *Russia and History's Turning Point*.
16. At 82, Winston Churchill wrote a *History of English Speaking People*.
17. At 82, Leo Tolstoy wrote *I Cannot Be Silent*.
18. At 81, Benjamin Franklin effected the compromise that led to the adoption of the U.S. Constitution.
19. At 81, Johann Wolfgang von Goethe finished *Faust*.

20. At 80, George Burns won an Academy
    Award for his performance in *The Sun-
    shine Boys.*
    See also LATE GREAT ACHIEVERS.

Avery, A. C., *et al. Successful Aging.* New York:
Ballantine Books, 1987.

ACTION ACTION was created by Congress in 1971 as the umbrella agency for
federal volunteer programs. The emphasis
of all ACTION programs is to enable communities to address local needs through volunteer service.

ACTION programs include FOSTER
GRANDPARENT PROGRAM (FGP), RETIRED SE-
NIOR VOLUNTEER PROGRAM (RSVP), SENIOR
COMPANION PROGRAM (SCP), Volunteers in
Service To America (VISTA), National Cen-
ter for Service Learning (NCSL), and Young
Volunteers in ACTION (YVA).

The Office of Volunteer Liaison (OVL)
provides links at national, state, and local
levels among public and private organizations.

There are 10 regional offices throughout
the country as well as state offices and numerous local offices, which coordinate, fund
and administer all programs within their given
areas, including those specifically for
the elderly. For more information write:
ACTION,
806 Connecticut Avenue, N.W.,
Washington, DC 20525

Active Corps of Executives See SCORE.

activity theory The common-sense idea
behind many programs and services for older
adults rests on the proposition that activities
in and of themselves have important benefits
and that they contribute to increased life
satisfaction for everyone. No one had tested
this notion scientifically until the early 1970s
when Dr. Vern Bengtson of the Andrus
Gerontology Center, University of Southern
California, and others developed a formal
activity theory that could be used as the
foundation for systematic research on the
effect of activities on the well-being of older
people.

Activity theory holds that people construct
ideas about themselves from two major
sources: the things that they do and the roles
that they fill in life. According to activity
theory people give up many roles as they
age—they retire from work, become widows
or widowers, drop out of professional and
other organizations, leave clubs and unions,
and so on. These changes challenge the ideas
that people hold about themselves; they may
create a reduced sense of identity; and they
sap the strength of one's inner "self." For
this reason people need to, and most actually
do, engage in activities that develop substitute roles for those that have been abandoned. Hence, activities in late life are essential to restore one's "self" and boost
one's sense of well-being.

Research developed to test activity theory
has shown that most people do indeed benefit
from a high level of activity in age. For
instance, the General Social Survey (an annual sampling of the American population
designed by professors Jim Davis of Harvard
University and Tom Smith of the University
of Chicago, and conducted by the National
Opinion Research Center at the University
of Chicago) shows a much higher level of
happiness among those who are most active
at all stages of life. But, investigators have
also discovered other things—that new activities are not necessarily substitutes for
previous activities and that the quality of an
activity is also important. Activity carried
on merely for the sake of being "active"
may even have negative effects.

To be worthwhile, activities must have
meaning to the participant: They can be
solitary (hoeing a garden, knitting, reading,
solo visits to museums); informal (chatting
with friends on the telephone, greeting fel-
low shoppers at the supermarket); or formal
(joining an AARP club, SCORE, or RSVP). A
few individuals may actually prefer and benefit most from *inactivity,* but most find that

hobbies, crafts, volunteer work, housework and home repairs, caring for pets, sharing life with family and friends, and generally getting out and about, have the greatest value for a positive sense of well-being.

Possuth, P. M., and Bengtson, V. "Sociological Theories of Aging: Current Perspectives and Future Directions," in Birren, J. E., and Bengtson, V. L., eds., *Emergent Theories of Aging.* New York: Springer Publishing Company, 1988.

acute respiratory disease (ARD; upper respiratory infection, URI) Acute respiratory disease (ARD) is a term used to characterize mild to severe inflammation of the pharynx, nasopharynx, sinuses, eustachian tube–middle ear apparatus, larynx, epiglottis, and trachea. The most frequent cause of ARD is a viral organism, but secondary bacterial infections also cause a variety of complications.

Acute respiratory disease is seen frequently in the elderly. Several factors may contribute to the increased susceptibility to respiratory disease in the elderly. These include age-related physiological alteration in the lung, a decrease in mucociliary clearance, probable decline in the immune function, and the frequent presence of other pulmonary diseases.

One of the most common viruses, the INFLUENZA virus, is responsible for widespread, often epidemic, diseases with devastating complications. The elderly are especially vulnerable. Severe malaise, fever, nausea, headaches, and diffuse pains result. BRONCHITIS and secondary bacterial PNEUMONIA are common complications. The single most effective preventive measure is an annual influenza vaccination. All high-risk people should obtain one each year.

Treatment of uncomplicated ARD and influenza is symptomatic. Antibiotics are of no value in uncomplicated cases. Treatment usually consists of rest, plenty of fluids, and aspirin or aspirin substitutes for pain and fever.

It is important to treat promptly any respiratory infection because of the likelihood of progression to bronchitis or pneumonia in the elderly.

See also SINUSITIS.

Ballenger, J. J. *Diseases of the Nose, Throat, Ear, Head and Neck,* 13th ed. Philadelphia: Lea & Febiger, 1985.

adenocarcinoma, renal See CANCER, KIDNEY.

adult children, relationships with As individuals grow older there is a tendency for their children to take on the authority role. Unless older people are mentally incapable, they should be allowed to handle their own affairs. Older people should make it perfectly clear that, although there may be some things that they need help with, they can still make their own decisions. Older people living with their children will welcome responsibilities that give them a sense of belonging to the family. The elderly cherish their independence and are sensitive about being a burden to their children.

On the other hand, many older individuals forget that their children are grown responsible adults. There is a tendency for the parent to correct or criticize the child much as he or she did when the child was dependent. The child should not tolerate this.

Many children feel they owe a parent a place in their home. There is no automatic obligation. If a parent and child did not get along well early in life they frequently will not get along in later years. If personality conflicts still exist the older parent should not live with the child.

On occasion, an adult child may move back in with the parent because of divorce or financial strain. These situations work out better if a length of stay is prearranged, if privacy can be maintained for both the offspring and the parent, if responsibilities can be shared so that no one feels like a guest, and if the offspring contributes financially.

If the offspring is unable to contribute, the parents should enforce the notion that they are taking care of the child.

Deedy, J. *Your Aging Parents.* Chicago: The Thomas More Press, 1984.

Lester, A. D., and Lester, J. L. *Understanding Aging Parents.* Philadelphia: The Westminster Press, 1980.

African Masai   See MASAI.

African pygmy

For a long time, environmental physiologists have studied the biological adaptation of humans to the extremes of heat, cold, and altitude and its role in the aging process.

None of the studies of tropical populations show evidence of accelerated aging. Two African pygmy populations—the Mbuti of northeastern Zaire and the Babinga of the Central African Republic—did not age at a different rate than people who live in more moderate climates. They were well adjusted to the hard conditions of the rain forest, and their endurance was remarkable despite exposure to a broad spectrum of parasites.

The increase in systolic and diastolic blood pressure between 20 and 60 years of age was small in both tribes. The serum cholesterol levels of the Mbuti were consistently low and did not increase with age, though the levels were somewhat higher in the Babingas. No MYOCARDIAL INFARCTION was found in either tribe.

Thus, the conclusions from the studies contradict widely held beliefs that natives of the tropics are in poorer health and age more quickly than people in temperate climates.

See also CLIMATES, EXTREME.

Mann, G. V., *et al.* "Cardiovascular Disease in African Pygmies." *J. of Chronic Diseases* 15: 341–371 (1961).

age

One of the most useful and yet misleading of all folk sayings in America relates to age: People often declare "You're as old as you feel!" Psychologists have found this saying to be true in the respect that inwardly people remain "themselves" throughout life. They experience inner continuity as they age irrespective of the way that they change physically and socially. Gray hair, wrinkles, and a bulging waistline may come upon one, others may think of one as "old," and one may even qualify for certain government benefit programs for the elderly and fit into elderly social categories (Social Security or the label "Grandpa" or "Grandma"), but these events do not mean that one has become another person when he or she enters advanced stages of maturity. Inwardly people still feel that they are the same "selves" as they were when they were children, teenagers, young adults, or at any other point on the journey of life.

Yet, this commonplace piece of folk wisdom can be misleading because it may grow out of an attempt to deny to oneself and to everyone else that one has become "old." People do not like to think of themselves as "old," they do not like to be called "old," and many conceal their age throughout their maturity. When people assert that "You're as old as you feel," they often fling the words out aggressively as if to say, "You'd better not say or think that I'm old" no matter how old they may appear to others.

Gerontologists agree with the statement to the extent that they know the way one feels about oneself does not necessarily coincide with one's chronological age (age in years), nor even with one's biological or social age. As a result they use several different terms when they speak of age. One of these is *cognitive age,* which has been defined as the age that one thinks of oneself as being; often one feels that one is younger than other people who are the same chronological age.

Chronological age is also recognized as a way of classifying people socially; one tends to think of someone under 10 as a child, someone 15 or 16 as a teenager, a person in their forties as middle-aged, and 70- and 80-year-olds as old, and so forth. Chronological age is also used as the official standard for qualifying for certain social services—children must be age 6 to qualify for admission to school in some states, and older people must reach 65 before they qualify for full Social Security benefits.

The tendency to classify people into age categories has also led to the idea of *social age*. It has been observed that people in different countries, centuries and circumstances have thought about age differently. In Africa, for instance, people have used a system known as *functional age* as a way of assigning age classifications. Functional age refers to an individual's ability to walk distances and carry out tasks without need to rest.

Different times and societies have looked on the status of being old more or less favorably. Americans tend to view the idea of being old with aversion, but some social groups consider age the greatest period of life. The old hold a high status and are esteemed for their WISDOM because they understand the traditions of their social group, and they stand nearest the ancestors who can help the group in day-to-day life. In some nations with such beliefs the old must be supported by their children, a practice that some gerontologists describe as a kind of social security system.

Yet another concept used in speaking about age scientifically appears in the term *age cohort*. This applies to people born in a particular year, or set of years, who share in common the experiences of their historical period. While each individual may have experienced his or her times in a unique way, people over 85 in 1991, for example, were born about the time that the Republican Party was ascendant under Teddy Roosevelt, lived through World War I, the Jazz Age, the depression, World War II, the television and computer ages, Vietnam era, etc. The BABY BOOM GENERATION did not experience the depression and the two world wars but came to maturity during the explosion of youth culture and tribulations of the 1960s, lived through the difficulties of the 1970s and

early 1980s, and then was able to join in riding on the wave of prosperity of succeeding years.

Because of their times each generation shares unique characteristics. For example, the old are more religious than the young today and have different attitudes about divorce and sex because they grew up in more religious times. New arrivals at age 65 are also less likely to experience poverty than were people who reached 65, and died before the improvements in Social Security benefits adopted in the early 1970s.

Many people in America today think that the old in this country had greater social status and enjoyed better treatment in times gone by, or that the old in nations like Japan are much better off than they are in America. The reality is that the status of older people has changed little in America since at least 1790 and, further, that every country that has become modernized assigns older people a lesser status than they hold in countries that have not yet achieved modernization. The simple fact is that the great majority of Americans long ago did not live long enough to enjoy an old age (the average life expectancy remained less than 50 years until after 1900), and the old did not, as many people think, receive extensive support from nor live with their children.

It was through the introduction of science and technology that the trend toward modernization wiped out the special status for the old. In past times the older population possessed knowledge and skills in crafts and farming that could be learned only slowly over a life time. Today science, technology, and the educational revolution have transferred the highest levels of skills and knowledge to the younger generation. Tied to the superior knowledge and skill of the old was the fact that most people before 1800 were farmers, and the old held the economic power and dominated daily life because they owned the farms. Wherever it has occurred, modernization has destroyed the historic foundations of status for the older generation.

This worldwide trend has been rooted in our history, and has made our attitude toward age what it is today.

Yet, whatever changes have occurred in the status of the old since times long ago, old people in America today are better off than they were in the past. As David Wolfe, founder of the National Association of Senior Living Industries, has said, America's old people today are the healthiest, wealthiest, and longest-lived older generation in our history. America may not yet have reached the pinnacle of perfection in attitudes, services, and status for the old, but this nation has reached a level where each person as an individual can convert the last years of a long life (a life that has increased more than one-third—over 25 years—in length since the turn of this century) into their best years.

Achenbaum, W. A. *Old Age in a New Land: The American Experience Since 1790*. Baltimore: The Johns Hopkins University Press, 1978.

Birren, J. E., and Cunningham, W. R. "Research on the Psychology of Aging: Principles, Concepts, and Theory" in Birren, J. E., and Schaie, K. W., eds., *Handbook of the Psychology of Aging*, 2nd ed. New York: Van Nostrand Reinhold Company, 1985.

Simmons, L. *The Role of the Aged in Primitive Society*. New Haven: Yale University Press, 1945.

age bias in employment   Age bias has been and remains a problem in the United States, as indicated by a Louis Harris and Associates public opinion poll that showed that eight out of 10 Americans think that employers discriminate against the elderly. Partly due to the passage some years ago of the Age Discrimination in Employment Act, and to the growing public awareness of rights of older people under this law, the number of age discrimination complaints has increased from about 11,000 per year in 1980 to approximately 27,000 per year at the present time. The provisions of this act are administered nationally by the Equal Employment Opportunities Commission, which

has had to take to court some 700 cases per year that could not be settled by local hearings.

By far the most common age-discrimination complaint concerns improper discharge from a job for reasons of age rather than of poor performance. In a recent year over 100,000 such cases were filed across the nation, and age accounted for about 15 percent of all such cases, ranking only behind race and sex as the reason for such complaints. Other major causes for age-discrimination complaints included unreasonable terms and conditions of employment, discrimination in hiring, improper layoffs, unfair treatment in promotions, and wage discrimination.

Some of the reasons for employment discrimination include favoring people with youthful appearances when appearance is not a reasonable criterion for job performance; higher rates for insurance benefit packages; and inadequate opportunity for training older employees for modern technology. Observers also note that older people may be denied loans or access to apartments for reasons of age.

Equal Employment Opportunities Commission, *20th Annual Report*. Washington, D.C.: The Commission, 1988.

House of Representatives Hearing, "Age Discrimination in Employment," January 28, 1988. Committee Publication No. 100–656. Washington, D.C.: U.S. Government Printing Office, 1988.

ageist language   *Ageist language* is the term for words and phrases commonly used to refer disparagingly to older people. While there are some terms that are intended to honor the old (e.g., senior citizen, golden ager, old-timer, mature citizen), others are derogatory. They include some that apply to older women—*bag, hag, harridan, crone, biddy,* and even *witch*. For men the terms are fewer and perhaps not quite as unpleasant—*codger, coot, geezer, mossback*, etc.

Other terms attribute disagreeable habits and personality traits to older individuals: *crank, fogy, fossil, fuddy-duddy, grump, miser, reprobate, DOM (dirty old man)*, and *cantankerous*. Yet others single out the physical weaknesses of the older generation—*doddering, tottering, rickety, decrepit, frail, shriveled, long-in-the-tooth, moribund*. Older people are sometimes characterized as mentally incompetent, as when a well-intended younger person will comment that an older person is "still sharp as a tack," as if to suggest that the old in general are mentally dull. Terms that disparage the mental state of the old include *rambling, doty, driveling, gaga, second childhood*.

Even the names of nursing homes and retirement communities may inadvertently contribute to the ageist lexicon by calling facilities by such soppy titles as Tender Care, Crystal Pines, Leisure World, Forest Villa, Happy Time Rest Home, instead of employing more straightforward language.

Two publications designed to prevent ageist portrayal of older people now exist: *Truth About Aging: Guideline for Accurate Communication* and *Media Guidelines for Sexuality and Aging*. Continual vigilance will be necessary if ageism is to be reduced significantly, if not eradicated from our language and literature. One positive step has already begun in this regard. The newly established national intergeneration organization, Understanding Aging, Incorporated, has recently established an award for authors who portray the elderly in a realistic and nonstereotype fashion.

Nuessel, F. "Old Age Needs a New Name," in *Aging*, Goldstein, E. C., ed. Vol. 2, Art. 70. Boca Raton, Fl.: Social Issues Resource Series, Inc., 1981.

Spencer, M. E. "Truth About Aging: Guidelines for Accurate Communications." Washington, DC: AARP, 1984.

Wisnieski, C. J. "Media Guideline for Sexuality and Aging," in *Television and the Aging Audience*. San Diego: University of Southern California Press, 1980.

aging, biological theory of   Researchers are testing two major sets of theories to explain the biological causes of human aging. One set of theories rests on the idea of "wear-and-tear" of the body, and envisions a situation in which the body accumulates a series of "environmental insults" over time. According to this view, the body can normally repair itself during youth, but its capacity to do so eventually becomes worn down under the steady bombardment of environmental attack.

The "somatic mutation" theory represents one branch of this thinking, and it holds the background radiation from various sources in the environment—not necessarily manmade—produces mutations and genetic damage in our cells, which, in turn, cause our cells to fail to properly reproduce themselves. Research, however, has shown that human, animal, and even insect patterns of aging are much too varied and rapid to be explained by externally caused cell mutation.

Another variant of the wear-and-tear theory is that faulty protein molecules in human genes may sometimes contain errors that build up over time and eventually cause an "error catastrophe" that results in death. Although research has shown that faulty proteins do build up in cells and tissues, there is no evidence yet that such proteins result from genetic errors or end in an "error catastrophe."

A second set of theories perceives aging as a continuous process and a normal development that may be programmed in human genes before birth. One branch of this theory suggests that the endocrine organs, which produce hormones and control nerve impulses, decline in function as people grow older. A particularly popular and successfully researched version of this theory is that the hypothalamus (a specialized cluster of cells in the central part of the brain that joins with other glands to regulate growth, sexual development, the menstrual cycle, the onset of menopause, etc.) and the pituitary glands function as master timekeepers of the body. Over time neuroendocrine tissues in human bodies lose the capacity to respond to signals from the control mechanisms, and the result is that people age.

Another line of thinking in this branch of theory is that the genetic consitution, which faithfully regulates the reproduction of genes within cells, undergoes internally caused changes (mutations) that produce errors. Although the cells manage to repair these errors throughout life, their capacity to do so begins to fail as the years go on. Again, the result is aging.

Yet a third approach arising out of the concept of normal aging relates to the working of the immune system. About 20 years ago researchers determined conclusively that the effectiveness of the immune system declines with the years. The consequence is that people become increasingly vulnerable to disease, whether it be from acute infections like pneumonia or from slower-working malignancies like cancer. Specialists on the immune system also observe that this system loses the power to distinguish between hostile invaders of the body and the body itself. While still providing some protection against outside invaders, the immune system becomes an attacker of the body, a process known as "autoimmunity," or immunity against oneself. Some researchers, however, question the validity of the autoimmune theory on the ground that organisms with immune systems far less complex than those of humans also experience aging.

Many people may be familiar with the term *collagen,* which introduces another of the ideas about why people age. According to this approach, there are molecules in the body that form stable links with other molecules, and these in turn eventually change the molecules that create them. The result is

a loss of elasticity in body tissues. Because the changes in process especially affect the skin, it is the cross-links that carry the main blame for the wrinkles that normally mark people during aging. Loss of elasticity in blood vessels may also contribute to high blood pressure.

Finally, there is a theory that holds that "free radicals" (a free radical is a small molecule with an unpaired electron) escape during the normal cellular process of burning food (metabolism), and that these free radicals cause damage that builds up as life goes on. Although human bodies produce enzymes that usually destroy free radicals, these unwanted products slowly accumulate rather like a buildup of rust or carbon in an automobile engine. Ultimately they cause human bodies to break down.

One of the interesting byproducts of this last theory is the finding that restriction of calorie intake can increase the life span of several species of laboratory animals by as much as 50 percent. Were humans to experience such an increase it would be equivalent to raising the possible biological length of their lives to over 180 years. The well-known researcher Dr. Roy Walford of the University of California is carrying on a unique test of this theory by experimenting on himself. He is consuming a carefully controlled low-calorie diet that may provide striking confirmation of the theory if Walford lives to the extended human life span of 120 years.

Although research is still far from determining the whole truth about the causes of aging, there are a few clearly established findings. One is that certain specific environmental factors under human control do influence the process of biological aging. For example, it is well documented that exposure to the sun speeds up the aging of the skin, and also that the sun worship so widely practiced by Americans contributes to cancer of the skin. It has also been well documented that a high-cholesterol diet may contribute to high blood pressure by building up fatty deposits in the arteries and veins. Environmental factors under human control, therefore, contribute to ill health, and it is increasingly recognized that ill health, rather than the passage of years, underlies the physical changes that people most often refer to when they speak of aging.

Research also suggests that sensescence, the process of growing old, may be built into human cells. Some years ago Dr. Leonard Hayflick performed a simple but elegant experiment where he maintained human cells alive in a laboratory culture medium. He found that the cells continued to reproduce themselves and to proliferate, but that eventually this process slowed down and stopped, resulting in the death of the cells. Accordingly, it appears that human cells, and consequently our entire bodies, have a limited lifetime.

People may never be able to find the key to the biology of human aging, and even if they do, they may never be able to prevent, halt, or reverse the aging process completely. Research findings, however, clearly show that individuals who maintain intelligent and healthful lifestyles have a greater chance of living longer and achieving a better quality of life. They actually modify the seemingly unalterable course of human mortality simply by their own choice to live with moderation.

Cristofalo, V. J. *Atherogenesis*. Frankfurt, New York, London, Tokyo: Springer-Verlag, 1986.
Weindruch, R., and Walford, R. L. *Retardation of Aging by Dietary Restriction*. New York: Raven, 1987.

alcohol abuse   Alcohol abuse occurs when there is a deep-seated, compulsive craving for alcohol. It is not as common a problem in the elderly as it is in younger age groups; however, about one-fourth of older alcoholics began their excessive drinking after age 60, usually because of the various stresses associated with aging.

Like alcoholics of all ages the elderly rarely admit to themselves or to their physician that they have a drinking problem. Yet their consumption may be significant. Alcoholism is a common problem among the aged admitted to hospitals as mentally ill. The majority of these patients have been alcoholics for many years.

Alcohol abuse may occur in response to loneliness, grief over the loss of a spouse or friend, a recent social decline, tension between the elderly and their children or perhaps a forced change in residence. It can also be the product of a life-long habit.

Within a few minutes of ingestion, alcohol reaches the brain where it first depresses those functions that have to do with inhibition and judgment. The drinker may feel friendlier and more gregarious. But with increased consumption, some drinkers suffer radical mood changes, from euphoria to self-pity, for example. Some may have personality changes and become aggressive or cruel. Motor ability, muscle function, reaction time, eyesight, depth perception, and night vision are affected next. A combination of headache, stomach upset, and dehydration is also a common side-effect.

Alcohol permeates easily into every cell and organ of the body. Thus, its effects are wide-ranging and complicated. The primary damage is to the liver, the organ that breaks down alcohol in the body. The central nervous system, gastrointestinal system, and the heart suffer severe damage as well. Other effects of alcohol abuse include sluggish circulation, malnutrition, water retention, weakening of both bones and muscles, skin disorders including permanent dilation of the blood vessels near the skin's surface, and decreased resistance to infection. These functions, already impaired by the natural aging process, are further complicated by alcoholism. Alcoholics who continue to drink decrease their life expectancy by 10 to 15 years.

Treatment for alcohol abuse varies depending on the type of abuser. Some may need hospitalization or care in a rehabilitation facility. Others may abstain with outpatient counseling and psychotherapy. The underlying cause, when known, should be addressed. Alcoholics Anonymous continues to be the primary source for information and support for family members as well as for the alcoholic.

See also DRUG ABUSE.

O'Brien, R., and Chafetz, M. *The Encyclopedia of Alcoholism*. New York: Facts On File, 1991.
Steinberg, F. U. *Care of the Geriatric Patient*, 6th ed. St. Louis: C. V. Mosby Co, 1983.

Alzheimer's disease   The term *Alzheimer's disease* in everyday language has come to designate nearly every variety of mental problem experienced by older people. The disease itself, however, with its typically associated deterioration of the organic structure of the brain, can at present be diagnosed with certainty only following an autopsy after death. Among the organic features of the brain in Alzheimer's disease (often referred to medically as ''AD'') are: senile plaques, rather like clots of nerve cells in the brain, neurofibrillary tangles, and granulovacuolar degeneration of the neurons in the cerebral cortex (the surface of the brain).

Alzheimer's disease is the most common cause of organic brain syndrome (OBS), but it is not the exclusive cause, nor is senility a normal consequence of aging. It is estimated that 15 percent of the older population may have mental health problems but that only from 4 to 6 percent of the population over 65 suffers from OBS. Of this proportion, 10 to 20 percent of the cases can be treated and reversed. Mental problems often attributed to Alzheimer's disease may be due to misuse of medications, alcohol abuse, and functional psychological disorders that can be treated by psychiatric interventions. The speed of mental response does seem to slow with age, and the proportion of persons with OBS does reach over 20 percent after age 85, but senility is not the norm even in late

life—close to 80 percent do not experience mental problems.

The cause of Alzheimer's disease today is unknown in spite of several promising avenues of research currently underway. Some researchers have discovered a ''slow virus'' infection whose clinical picture mimics Alzheimer's disease. Once this virus is isolated it is felt that a vaccine can be developed. The autoimmune theory speculates that, due to the progressive aging of brain neurons, a pseudo-foreign body response is triggered in the immune system. The incidence of Alzheimer's disease is somewhat increased in families that have a history of a familial occurence. Researchers have found diminished levels of the neurotransmitter acetylcholine and increased levels of aluminum in the brains of people with Alzheimer's disease, which supports a chemical imbalance theory. Presently, however, there is no vaccine or cure for Alzheimer's disease.

Some of the symptoms of Alzheimer's disease are deterioration of social skills, progressive memory loss, decline in the ability to perform routine tasks, impaired judgment, confusion, disorientation, personality change, speech and communication defects, difficulty in learning and retaining information, belligerence, and incontinence. In many cases, the disease will progress to the point that its victims are totally incapable of caring for themselves.

Even though the person's thought process is impaired, his or her senses are still functioning well. Brightly colored objects may be visually stimulating, music may have a calming effect, and foods and fragrances that have been the person's favorites will still be enjoyed. Touch and eye contact give the person a sense of well-being.

There is at present no treatment for Alzheimer's disease comparable to antibiotics used against bacterial infections. A major step forward in the treatment of the disease, however, occurred when it was recognized that mental decline is not a normal consequence of aging; that it can be treated; and that interventions by means of care are as important as medical cures. Current treatments for AD and other mental disorders stress behavioral approaches. They include such alternatives as close supervision most often provided by placing the affected individual in a nursing home, giving respite help to relieve stress on family members caring for the AD victim, and training of AD patients to deal with the impaired state of their memory. While no one can predict how rapidly researchers will succeed in finding the causes, treatment, and a cure for AD, it is notable that the National Institute on Aging has targeted the disease for a major research effort, and that progress so far has caused much enthusiasm and hope. People who need to know more about AD and other mental disorders can contact such organizations as that named below, as well as relying on physicians and other professional resources.

For more information, write or call:
Alzheimers Society National Headquarters
70 E. Lake Street
Chicago, IL, 60601
(312) 853–3060

Kelly, W. E. *Alzheimer's Disease and Related Disorders.* Springfield, Ill: Charles C. Thomas Co., 1984.
Reisberg, B., ed. *Alzheimer's Disease: The Standard Reference.* New York: The Free Press, 1983.

Alzheimer's disease, treatment   The progressive deterioration of brain cells is inevitably fatal in Alzheimer's disease. There are treatments that ease the burden on the person and family. These treatments for Alzheimer's disease include reality orientation, tactile contact, maintaining and maximizing current functional abilities with physical exercise and social activity, and tranquilizers. Tranquilizers can lessen agitation, anxiety, and unpredictable behavior, improve sleep patterns, and help create a calm and pleasant environment.

Current functional abilities with physical exercise and social activity should be continued as much as possible.

It is important to keep the environment safe around people with Alzheimer's. Medicines, cleaning supplies, sharp knives, and tools should be kept out of reach. Rugs need to be secured to prevent sliding and tripping and handrails should be installed.

AD victims can remain independent longer when living in familiar surroundings. Furniture and cupboards, for instance, should be consistent. Keeping doors locked will prevent the person from wandering outside alone and getting lost.

The transition from a totally independent person to one of dependence can be a trying time. Unusual situations should be handled in a quiet calm manner so that the person with Alzheimer's keeps his or her respect and as much independence as possible.

Powell, L. S., and Courtice, K. *Alzheimer's Disease.* Reading, Mass: Addison-Wesley Publishing Company, 1983.

amaurosis fugax (transient loss of vision)   The term *amaurosis fugax* describes repeated transient episodes of visual loss in one eye. These may be caused by GIANT CELL ARTERITIS or migraine headaches. However, most are due to carotid artery insufficiency as a result of atherosclerotic lesions in the neck. In the majority, the immediate cause is temporary closure of an artery of the retina by a blood or cholesterol embolus. Rarely, it is caused from a reduction in blood pressure and flow in the major artery of the eye from severe narrowing or total closure of the internal carotid artery.

Symptoms of amaurosis fugax include a transient loss of vision in one eye that may be recurrent. Some people with amaurosis fugax suffer permanent loss of sight.

Treatment for amaurosis fugax involves determining the cause of the vascular insufficiency. Generally, once the blood flow is restored, either through medications or surgery, the amaurosis fugax is resolved. Full

medical assessment is necessary to evalute
the need for an endarterectomy (opening the
artery). Aspirin may reduce the frequency
of attacks of amaurosis fugax, presumably
by inhibiting the accumulation of platelets.
Systemic steroids are immediately used if
there is any evidence of giant cell arteritis.

Amaurosis fugax may be a warning signal
preceding a STROKE or heart attack. If amaurosis fugax occurs frequently, a prompt
physical checkup is indicated.

See also TRANSIENT ISCHEMIC ATTACK.

Newell, F. W. *Ophthalmology Principles and
Concepts,* 6th ed. St. Louis, C. V. Mosby
Co., 1986.
Slatt, B. J., and Stein, H. A. *The Ophthalmic
Assistant Fundamentals and Clinical Practice,*
4th ed. St. Louis: C. V. Mosby Co., 1983.

American Association of Retired Persons (AARP)

The American Association
of Retired Persons was formed in 1958 by
the National Retired Teachers Association
to extend its membership beyond the ranks
of retired teachers. Originally, it was located
in Washington, D.C., but has now grown to
include local chapters in all 50 states with a
membership of over 28 million. It is the
largest organization for the elderly with
membership recently increasing over 20 percent a year. Membership (dues are $5 per
year) is open to any person aged 50 or more.

Services to members include the Pharmacy Service, with emphasis on low-cost
generic products; Group Health Insurance
Program (GHIP), the nation's largest; Automobile and Homeowners Insurance Program; Motoring Plan; Travel Service; and
the AARP Investment program, rising at a
rate of $50 million per week. The monthly
magazine *Modern Maturity* continues to increase in circulation and is one of the top-
ranked magazines in the country. At the end
of 1986, 28 AARP books were in publication.

The Legislation, Research, and Public
Policy Division is active at the federal and
government levels, and plays a significant
and active role in legislative and regulatory
programs affecting health and retirement income, tax reforms, Social Security benefits,
mandatory retirement, and other programs.

For more information, write or call:
AARP
1909 K Street, N.W.
Washington, DC 20049
(202) 872–4700

anemia Anemia is a decrease in the blood
hemoglobin concentration or erythrocyte
mass, which occurs in 5 to 20 percent of the
elderly population. It may be caused by
inadequate diet, loss of blood, chronic diseases, or industrial poisons. Hemoglobin
transports oxygen from the lungs to the tissues of the body and is, along with cardiac
output, a key determinant of how much
oxygen can be transported, delivered, and
consumed. Due to decreased hemoglobin,
anemia causes a decrease in oxygen delivery
to the body tissues. This causes an increase
in cardiac output, which can lead to CONGES-
TIVE HEART FAILURE, fatigue, and ANGINA.
Symptoms of anemia develop slowly and
frequently go unnoticed because they are
common to other aging problems.

Symptoms of anemia include fatigue,
VERTIGO, congestive heart failure, pedal
edema, angina, dyspnea, headaches, confusion, urinary incontinence, increased sensitivity to cold, irritability, pale skin, arrhythmia, spoon-shaped nails, and a red, sore
tongue.

See also ANEMIA, CHRONIC DISEASE; ANE-
MIA, IRON DEFICIENCY; ANEMIA, MEGALOB-
LASTIC; FOLIC ACID DEFICIENCY; VITAMIN
B$_{12}$ DEFICIENCY.

Ham, R. J. *Geriatric Medicine Annual—1987.*
Oradell, N.J.: Medical Economics Books, 1987.
Reichel, W. *Clinical Aspects of Aging.* Balti-
more: Williams & Wilkins Co., 1979.

anemia, chronic disease Chronic disease anemia refers to anemia that is associated with chronic inflammatory states such
as RHEUMATOID ARTHRITIS, chronic infec-

tions, and malignancies. It is caused by a blockage in the release of iron from the reticuloendothelial cells. It differs from IRON DEFICIENCY ANEMIA in that this anemia is generally mild with a relatively stable course after about one month. Treatment of chronic disease anemia involves establishing the underlying disease and treating that disorder.

Ham, R. J. *Geriatric Medicine Annual—1987.* Oradell, N.J.: Medical Economics Books, 1987.
Reichel, W. *Clinical Aspects of Aging.* Baltimore: Williams & Wilkins Co., 1979.

anemia, iron deficiency   Iron deficiency anemia occurs because of improper dietary intake, poor gastrointestinal absorption, or blood loss.

The quality and quantity of food a person eats may change as a person ages due to several factors. The expense of a balanced diet with iron-rich foods may become prohibitive for a person who lives on a fixed income. Lack of transportation may limit a person's purchasing power of fresh foods. Physical disabilities may impair a person's willingness or ability to prepare foods properly. Loss of teeth may result in avoidance of certain foods. Depression may lead to self-neglect and poor nutrition.

Symptoms of iron deficiency anemia include fatigue, VERTIGO, CONGESTIVE HEART FAILURE, pedal edema, angina, dyspnea, headaches, confusion, urinary incontinence, increased sensitivity to cold, irritability, pale skin, arrhythmia, spoon-shaped nails, and red sore tongue.

Iron supplements are frequently prescribed to replace deficits. Generally, supplements are oral medications, but iron injections may also be necessary, particularly when malabsorption, iron intolerance, excessive iron needs, or noncompliance preclude the oral treatment. Blood transfusions are rarely necessary and are reserved only for severe cases.

Oral iron therapy can cause gastrointestinal intolerance and severe constipation. This may be particularly bothersome for the el-derly since constipation is frequently a problem anyway. Laxatives may be necessary while the person is on iron therapy. Since iron supplements are absorbed in the duodenum, the use of antacids hinders this absorption and should be avoided.

Nutritional consultation is frequently necessary to educate the patient on the types of foods that should be eaten. These foods include beef, clams, peaches, beans, soybean flour, and liver.

If the anemia is due to blood loss, the patient may be suffering from a gastrointestinal disorder such as a PEPTIC ULCER, DIVERTICULOSIS, HEMORRHOIDS, chronic GASTRITIS, COLON CANCER or HIATAL HERNIA. Diagnosis of these disorders may require further testing, such as barium studies, stool cultures, or colonoscopies, to determine the source of bleeding.

Ham, R. J. *Geriatric Medicine Annual—1987.* Oradell, N.J.: Medical Economics Books, 1987.
Reichel, W. *Clinical Aspects of Aging.* Baltimore: Williams & Wilkins Co., 1979.

anemia, megaloblastic   Most megaloblastic anemias are due to vitamin B_{12} or folic acid deficiencies. Symptoms of megaloblastic anemia include neurologic changes, smooth tongue, confusion, and dizziness. Treatment for megaloblastic anemia involves properly identifying the deficiency and replacing it. Replacement can be accomplished by a proper diet and supplemental oral folic acid or vitamin B_{12}.

See also FOLIC ACID DEFICIENCY; VITAMIN B_{12} DEFICIENCY.

Ham, R. J. *Geriatric Medicine Annual—1987.* Oradell, N.J.: Medical Economics Books, 1987.
Phipps, W. J., *et al. Medical Surgical Nursing.* St. Louis: C. V. Mosby Co., 1983.
Reichel, W. *Clinical Aspects of Aging.* Baltimore: Williams & Wilkins Co., 1979.

anemia, pernicious   See VITAMIN B_{12} DEFICIENCY.

aneurysm   An aneurysm is a localized or diffuse enlargement of an artery at some point along its course. Aneurysms occur when the vessel wall becomes weakened from trauma, infection, and atherosclerosis. Most aneurysms occur in people over 60 years of age and are predominantly seen in males. Once an aneurysm develops there is a tendency for it to progress.

Symptoms of an aneurysm include acute pain in the chest or abdomen, abdominal mass, and shock. Symptoms usually do not occur until the aneurysm becomes quite large or begins to leak.

If the aneurysm is small and nonprogressive, conservative treatment can be used. Antihypertensive medications, pain medications, and negative inotropic agents, such as Inderal, are usually the treatments of choice. Negative inotropic agents decrease the force of cardiac or vascular wall muscular contraction. If the aneurysm enlarges or ruptures, surgical intervention is required. The aneurysm is removed and is replaced with a Teflon or Dacron prosthesis.

See also ANEURYSM, ABDOMINAL.

Anderson, H. C. *Newton's Geriatric Nursing,* 5th ed. St. Louis: C. V. Mosby Co., 1971.
Ham, R. J. *Geriatric Medicine Annual—1986.* Oradell, N.J.: Medical Economics Books, 1986.
Phipps, W. J., *et al. Medical Surgical Nursing.* St. Louis: C. V. Mosby Co., 1983.

aneurysm, abdominal   An abdominal aneurysm is a sac formed by the dilation of the wall of the aorta as it traverses the stomach cavity. The abdominal aneurysm is the most common aneurysm, particularly in the elderly. If it ruptures, it can be life-threatening. An untreated ruptured aneurysm is 100 percent fatal. For patients with a ruptured aneurysm who live long enough to reach the operating room the mortality rate is 50 percent.

A key factor in considering aneurysm treatment in an elderly person is to weigh the risk of a ruptured aneurysm against the risk of the operative procedure. Generally, aneurysms less than five centimeters (two inches) in diameter and calcified can be observed and no surgery is necessary. Aneurysms that are greater than five centimeters, those that begin to enlarge, or those that become symptomatic should be repaired immediately. Ultrasound is extremely useful in measuring the size and other characteristics of the aneurysm.

Symptoms of an abdominal aneurysm include abdominal pain and a pulsating mass in the abdomen. Many times the aneurysm is found unexpectedly on a routine X-ray. Few symptoms occur until the aneurysm becomes quite large or begins to leak. Symptoms of a ruptured abdominal aneurysm include acute abdominal pain, profound shock, and an abdominal mass. This constitutes a medical emergency and treatment should be sought immediately. Treatment consists of a surgical replacement of the aneurysm with a Teflon or Dacron prosthesis.

Anderson, H. C. *Newton's Geriatric Nursing,* 5th ed. St. Louis: C. V. Mosby Co., 1971.
Ham, R. J. *Geriatric Medicine Annual—1986.* Oradell, N.J.: Medical Economics Books, 1986.
Phipps, W. J., *et al. Medical Surgical Nursing.* St. Louis: C. V. Mosby Co., 1983.

anger   Anger is considered a crucial element in DEPRESSION. There are many manifestations of anger, which include violence, hostility, sarcasm, defiance, tantalizing, teasing, sneering, passive obstructiveness, gossip, withdrawal, and self-destructive behavior to the point of SUICIDE. Anger can be a cover for deeper problems that may be centered around the need for intimacy and a profound sense of deprivation.

One of the emotional manifestations of old age is a sense of rage at the seemingly uncontrollable forces that confront older people as well as the indignities and neglect of the society that once valued their productive capacities. Some older people rage against the inevitable nature of aging and death.

Some older people use anger to control others. They may see it as strategy for maintaining some sense of power over their own lives because as long as they remain angry or resistant people will notice them. Some older people express resistance to any suggestions or new ideas. This resistance is a way of maintaining a sense of personal identity, which may be threatened by change.

Sometimes simple things, such as the inability to thread a needle, remember a name, or do a physical task, can be the cause of anger. A person should not wrestle with anger, but handle it by controlling the cause. The older person should identify the source of the anger and attempt to correct it. A tranquilizer might also help to control anger, but after the effects of the medication wear off, the problem will remain.

Although some anger is therapeutic in relieving stress, anger caused by failure is pointless.

Deedy, J. *Your Aging Parents.* Chicago: The Thomas More Press, 1984.
Lester, A. D., and Lester, J. L. *Understanding Aging Parents.* Philadelphia: The Westminster Press, 1980.

angina See ANGINA PECTORIS.

angina pectoris (angina) Common in people over the age of 60 years, angina pectoris occurs when myocardial oxygen demand exceeds myocardial oxygen supply. Although it is usually caused by ATHEROSCLEROSIS of the coronary vessels, the incidence of angina pectoris is high in people with hypertension, DIABETES MELLITUS, THROMBOANGIITIS OBLITERANS, POLYCYTHEMIA VERA, PERIARTERITIS NODOSA, and AORTIC REGURGITATION.

Classically, angina is characterized by recurrent deep chest pain, often radiating down the inner aspect of the left arm. The angina is frequently precipitated by exertion, anger, emotional stress, cold, or eating.

The main symptom of angina is chest pain in the sternal area, but dyspnea, pallor, sweating, and faintness can also occur. The pain is described as a burning pressure, much like indigestion—a squeezing, a choking feeling in the upper chest or throat or a tightening in the chest that may radiate to the shoulder, left arm, jaw, neck, or teeth. The duration of the pain is usually less than five minutes. Frequently, rest and sometimes belching alone will alleviate the pain.

Medical therapy is aimed at reducing myocardial oxygen demand. The precipitating factors that bring on the angina—such as hypertension, obesity, and smoking—should be identified and avoided if possible. Frequently, an exercise program is prescribed. The purpose in the exercise program is to reduce the rise in blood pressure and pulse rate upon exertion. The result is a decrease in myocardial oxygen demand and an increase in the amount of exercise an individual can do without experiencing angina.

When people who have angina pectoris must be exposed to the cold they should dress warmly and avoid heavy exertion. It is unwise, for instance, to sleep in a cold bedroom or to walk against a cold wind. The person with angina may be advised to eat small meals rather than large ones to reduce cardiac output. Excessive emotional strain may cause vasoconstriction by releasing epinephrine into the circulation. People with angina need to accept situations as they find them and avoid emotional outbursts and stress whenever possible. As optimistic outlook helps to relieve the work of the heart and therefore reduces angina.

Treatment for angina is primarily with the use of nitroglycerin. This may be used when the pain starts by placing a tablet under the tongue. If the pain is not relieved within 15 minutes (one tablet taken every five minutes) a physician should be contacted. Nitrol ointment or Nitro patch (long-acting forms of nitrates) is being used more commonly to diminish attacks and increase exercise capacity. Nitroglycerin loses its potency after six months so individuals should be instructed to keep this medication in a dark brown bottle and to check the expiration date regularly. If the nitroglycerin is fresh it should cause a burning sensation on the tongue, flushing, and sometimes a headache. These side effects diminish as the individual develops a tolerance to the drug. The person should also be cautioned not to stand or sit up abruptly after taking nitroglycerin because it decreases the systolic blood pressure and may cause dizziness or faintness. Nitroglycerin therapy is successful in the great majority of angina cases. However, when medical therapy does not control the angina, artery expansion or coronary bypass surgery may be considered.

Frequent evaluations of angina should be obtained, since the chest discomfort is similar to that of a heart attack, hernia, gall bladder disease, and esophagitis and can cause these diseases to go unnoticed.

It is important not to ignore angina. Angina pain is a warning that the myocardium is not receiving enough blood and something needs to be done. With use of medication, resting, or altering daily habits, most people continue to live active, productive lives despite attacks of angina pectoris.

See also MYOCARDIAL INFARCTION.

Phipps, W. J., et al. Medical Surgical Nursing. St. Louis: C. V. Mosby Co., 1983.
Scherer, J. C. Introductory Medical-Surgical Nursing. Philadelphia: J. B. Lippincott Co., 1982.

anosmia (loss of smell) Anosmia is a total loss of the sense of smell. The causes can be varied but most commonly there is an interference with the intranasal diffusion of the odorous particles. This is mostly due to obstruction from swelling due to allergies, the common cold, or nasal polyps.

In the elderly, senile atrophy of the nasal mucous membranes is a prime contributing factor in anosmia. Intracranial lesions from tumors, vascular lesions, head injury, or infections may also be found. In a patient with severe atrophy or crusting of the nasal mucosa, both trigeminal and olfactory (nose) nerve endings may be destroyed.

In testing for anosmia, two odors are used: One is a strong trigeminal stimulant (ammonia) and the other a pure olfactory stimulus (freshly ground coffee). Normally, a person can easily detect both ammonia and coffee. In organic anosmia, the patient cannot detect coffee but does note a tingling or slight burning with ammonia.

There is no specific treatment for anosmia, but control of the underlying intranasal disease processes often result in recovery of the sense of smell.

See also SINUSITIS.

Ballenger, J. J. Diseases of the Nose, Throat, Ear, Head and Neck, 13th ed. Philadelphia: Lea & Febiger, 1985.

anti-aging diet Scientists have repeatedly demonstrated that undernutrition (as distinguished from malnutrition) extends the lives of laboratory animals. Researchers Dr. Roy Walford and Richard Weindruch of the University of California at Los Angeles School of Medicine recently achieved a 30 percent increase in the maximum life span of animals whose diets were restricted in adulthood. They gradually reduced the intake of their animals, down to about 60 percent of their normal diet. Experimental underfeeding did not merely delay death, it delayed aging. The lack of extra calories forestalled the development and hence the decay of the immune system. In other underfeeding experiments, the cancer rate dropped markedly.

Because undernutrition can easily lead to malnutrition, a doctor's supervision is necessary before undertaking such a program. An optimal human diet is being developed.

At Temple University Medical School in Philadelphia, Dr. Arthur Schwartz is working with an adrenal-gland product called dehydroepiandrosterone, or DHEA. He suggests that use of DHEA may duplicate the anti-aging and anti-cancer effects of caloric restriction.

See also AGING, BIOLOGICAL THEORY OF.

Conniff, R. *"Living Longer,"* in *Aging,* Goldstein, E. C., ed. Vol. 2, Art. 8. Boca Raton, Fl.: Social Issues Resource Series, Inc., 1981.

Walford, R. *The 120-Year Diet: How to Double Your Vital Years.* New York: Simon and Schuster, 1987.

antioxidants   With normal metabolism, free radicals (a free radical is a small molecule with an impaired electron) are a normal byproduct. Antioxidants prevent or neutralize free radicals.

Antioxidants are a diverse group of chemicals that include vitamins A and C, selenium, cysteine, and the food preservative BHT.

The Life Extension Foundation in Florida advocates high doses of antioxidants as one of the regimens for prolonging life. However, detractors, including the House Select Committee on Aging, believe such views are false and misleading with no evidence to support retarding, much less reversing, the aging process. Many of the food-related ingredient antioxidants are dangerous in very large quantities, although they are quite safe in the much smaller amounts found in a normal diet. The known risks of the antioxidants include headaches, intestinal disorders, and kidney damage. Megadoses of vitamin C actually shortened the lives of guinea pigs in laboratory experiments. Long-term consumption of two grams a day of vitamin B_6 has been shown to produce disabling sensory neuropathy in humans. Selenium is an essential nutrient and may play an antioxidant role in the body, but in excessive amounts is toxic.

There may be additional risks that have not yet been identified.

See also AGING, BIOLOGICAL THEORY OF; FREE RADICAL THEORY OF AGING.

Lardner, J. "The People Who Want to Live Much, Much Longer," in *Aging,* Goldstein, E. C., ed. Vol. 2, Art. 48. Boca Raton, Fl.: Social Issues Resource Series, Inc., 1981.

Meister, K. "The 80's Search For The Fountain of Youth Comes Up Very Dry," in *Aging,* Goldstein, E. C., ed. Vol. 2, Art. 76, Boca Raton, Fl.: Social Issues Resource Series, Inc., 1981.

anxiety (stress)   Anxiety is a feeling of uneasiness, apprehension, or dread that all people experience at various times in their lives. When normal fear or nervousness becomes irrational or is not related to a specific cause then it becomes neurotic and needs to be treated medically.

Anxiety is common in the elderly with quite varying symptoms. Some people have nonspecific complaints such as apprehension, "nerves," or a feeling of going to pieces. Others have complaints related to cardiac function, bowel function, or genitourinary symptoms. Still others complain of sweating, tremor, dry mouth, and blurring of vision.

Anxiety can be a major symptom of physical illness in the elderly but frequently is a reaction to conditions of everyday existence such as personal loss, fear of dying, dependence on others, or perhaps the need to make a change in residence. Often it is a prominent part of depressive illness or organic brain disease.

Symptoms include INSOMNIA, loss of appetite or obsessive eating, fear, panic, helplessness, tearfulness, tension, rapid heartbeat, shortness of breath, loss of the ability to concentrate, confusion, hypchondria, and poor compliance with established medical therapies.

In approaching the anxious elderly, both physician and family should establish an atmosphere of warmth and concern. A pat and a gentle hug convey a sense of caring. In assessing these people, it is important to remember the many losses to which they are vulnerable at this time in life. The anxiety may be a response to the loss of a friend or spouse, to reduced income, impaired health, and to a decline in coping capacity.

Anxiety in response to such losses can usually be managed by psychotherapeutic means alone. The opportunity to discuss the situation and explore possible solutions are often sufficient for the older patient to gain better control of his or her anxiety, although this may take place only after several sessions. Reassurance, understanding, and a recognition of the physical symptoms involved by family and physician are encouraging to the anxious person.

Treatment should include making an effort to identify and alleviate the cause of anxiety. The person should be told when psychological stress appears to be related to the symptoms of his or her illness.

Environmental intervention should be used to create calmer, quieter surroundings. Sometimes use of deep muscle relaxation techniques, regular exercise programs, and mild analgesics or a small amount of alcohol before bed are helpful.

Occasionally mild tranquilizers are helpful but should not be used for indefinite periods of time. At times, anxiety may coexist with DEPRESSION. In this instance, tranquilizers are definitely contraindicated.

See also DEPRESSION; PARANOIA.

Steinberg, F. U. *Care of the Geriatric Patient,* 6th ed. St. Louis: C. V. Mosby Co., 1983.

ARD See ACUTE RESPIRATORY DISEASE.

arrhythmias, cardiac Cardiac arrhythmia refers to the presence of a heart rate and rhythm other than normal sinus rhythm. There are numerous types of arrhythmias, including sinus bradycardia, atrial fibrillation, sinus tachycardia and premature ventricular contractions.

The incidence of cardiac arrhythmias rise with age and all types may be encountered. The causes also vary and include digitalis intoxication, increase of heart fibrous tissue, hypertension, and underlying heart disease. Symptoms include fatigue, fainting, confusion, light-headedness, heart flutter, and

anxiety. Many arrhythmias, however, may be asymptomatic and found unexpectedly in a routine exam.

Treatment for arrhythmias involves determining the exact cause. This is generally done through a workup that may include laboratory tests, X-rays, EKG, and Holter monitors. (A Holter monitor is a constant EKG recorder that is worn for 24 to 48 hours, to detect nonconstant problems.)

A variety of antiarrhythmic drugs are available and may be prescribed to control the arrhythmias. If the arrhythmia involves a complete heart block the treatment of choice is to implant surgically an artificial pacemaker.

Arrhythmias, particularly atrial fibrillation, are frequent early manifestations of CONGESTIVE HEART FAILURE or other heart disease. Because of this, people with arrhythmias should be checked frequently for other heart disease.

See also ATRIAL FIBRILLATION; BRADY-CARDIA, SINUS; TACHYCARDIA, SINUS; VEN-TRICULAR CONTRACTIONS; VENTRICULAR FI-BRILLATION.

Phipps, W. J., et al. *Medical Surgical Nursing.* St. Louis: C. V. Mosby Co., 1983.
Scherer, J. C. *Introductory Medical-Surgical Nursing.* Philadelphia: J. B. Lippincott Co., 1982.

arteries, hardening of See ARTERIO-SCLEROSIS.

arteriosclerosis Arteriosclerosis is the thickening and loss of the elasticity of the arteries. Mineral and fatty deposits collect on the inner lining of arteries (plaque). This plaque encroaches on the passageway and gradually obstructs the flow of blood.

The exact cause of arteriosclerosis is not known. However, several factors contribute to the age of onset and the severity of the disease. These factors include heredity, alterations in the sex hormones, diabetes, hypertension, gout, obesity, smoking, and a diet high in cholesterol and fats. Arteriosclerosis is frequently the cause of other diseases, including ANEURYSM, ANGINA, MYOCARDIAL INFARCTION, THROMBOSIS, cerebrovascular disease, and decreased hearing and vision.

Symptoms of generalized arteriosclerosis include coldness or numbness of the feet, dizziness, shortness of breath, headache, fatigue, leg cramps, and loss of memory. Recent reports indicate that certain drugs combined with a low-fat diet and exercise can lower blood cholesterol levels and help prevent the artery clogging plaque. Some individuals so treated demonstrate a shrinkage of the artery-choking deposit.

Chronic reduction of circulation may be ameliorated by vascular surgery and replacement of the diseased arterial segment. In severe arteriosclerosis the affected extremity may develop gangrene. In these cases amputation may be necessary.

Vasodilator medications may be prescribed, although these are of help only for increased skin circulation.

Most treatment concentrates on preventing the condition from becoming worse. The person with arteriosclerosis should stop or greatly curtail smoking, control weight, and treat and control any disease, such as diabetes, high blood pressure, or gout, that accentuates arteriosclerotic changes. The person should follow a diet low in cholesterol and fats and should participate in a regular exercise program, such as walking or bicycling. Stress reduction through relaxation therapy or other means may also be helpful.

See also ANEURYSM; GANGRENE.

Ross, R. "The Pathogenesis of Atherosclerosis." *New Engl. J. Med.* 314: 488, 1986.
Schaefer, E. J., and Levy, R. I. "Pathogenesis and Management of Lipoprotein Disorders." *New Engl. J. Med.* 312: 1300, 1985.
Steinberg, F. U.: *Care of the Geriatric Patient,* 6th ed. St. Louis: C. V. Mosby Co., 1983.

arteritis, giant cell (temporal arteritis)

Giant cell arteritis, or temporal arteritis, is a condition characterized by proliferative granulomatous inflammation (many focal lesions) of the aorta and its major arteries. The cervical segments of the internal and external carotid arteries and the temporal, ophthalmic and occipital arteries are particularly affected. Those portions of the carotid and vertebral arteries that have a high elastic tissue content are most prone to be involved.

The cause of giant cell arteritis is unknown, and it is rarely seen before age 50. Women are affected more often than men. The most common symptoms are pain and tenderness in one or both frontal-temporal areas and diminished or absent pulsation over the temporal arteries. Headaches may be localized or radiate to the face, jaw, and neck. Tenderness of the scalp may cause sleeplessness from the head touching the pillow. Combing or brushing the hair may be intolerable. Intermittent claudication in the tongue is a common finding causing slurred speech.

Visual complications occur frequently as a result of severe ischemic optic atrophy (narrowing of the artery) or of occlusion of the central retinal artery. When diplopia (double vision) is present it is frequently indicative of potential visual loss.

Fever, weight loss, and depression may precede local symptoms by several weeks. Joint pain may occur even earlier.

A markedly high erythrocyte sedimentation rate (degree of rapidity with which the red cells sink in a mass of drawn blood) is the characteristic finding. Corticosteroid therapy should begin immediately. With adequate dosage, symptoms should subside within 48 hours. Treatment with maintenance doses is continued for 18 months but is often needed for much longer.

Brocklehurst, J. C. *Textbook of Geriatric Medicine and Gerontology,* 3rd ed. New York: Churchill Livingstone, 1985.

arteritis, temporal See ARTERITIS, GIANT CELL.

arthritis See OSTEOARTHRITIS.

arthritis, infectious (septic) Infectious arthritis has always been common among children and adolescents. However, in the last two decades an increasing number of cases have been found in the elderly.

The usual symptoms of infectious arthritis are fever, pain, redness, swelling and effusion in the involved joint. In the elderly, however, the symptoms are less acute and may occur in the same joints previously involved in rheumatoid arthritis or osteoarthritis. The hip or knee is the most common site affected. Leucocytosis (excessive white blood cells), anemia, and an elevated erthrocyte sedimentaiton rate (rapidity with which red cells sink in drawn blood) are the most frequent abnormalities found in laboratory tests. The diagnosis is made by joint aspiration, which usually reveals purulent fluid.

Once the diagnosis is made treatment is begun on the basis of either a Gram stain or culture results. The most frequent causative organism of infectious arthritis in the elderly is *Staphylococcus aureus*, although various streptococci, *Mycobacterium tuberculosis,* and gram negative bacilli may occasionally be the causative agent.

If treatment is initiated before the cartilage is destroyed, full return of function may be expected. Because of limited blood supply, late therapy of septic arthritis of the hip may result in avascular necrosis (death of tissue). Degenerative arthritis and decreased range of motion may complicate a poor result. In the elderly it is not uncommon for limitation of motion to persist even though the joint may not be severely damaged.

Covington, T., and Walker, J. *Current Geriatric Therapy*. Philadelphia: W. B. Saunders, 1984.

arthritis, rheumatoid Rheumatoid arthritis is a chronic progressive disease with marked inflammatory changes and atrophy of the tissue to the joints. The disease may begin at any age but is more predominant between the ages of 20 and 60, peaking at ages 35 to 45. Women are affected two to three times more often than men, and there is often a family history of the disease.

Onset of the disease is usually insidious with stiffness and aching joints followed by gradual swelling, warmth, redness, and tenderness with limitation of motion. In most patients, the small joints of the hands and feet are commonly involved. Other affected joints are the wrists, knees, elbows, ankles, shoulders, hips, and, rarely, the cervical spine. The muscles of affected extremities may become severely weakened and atrophied to a greater degree than would be expected to result from disuse alone.

Symptoms include fatigue, malaise, low-grade fever, TACHYCARDIA, weakness, weight loss, ANEMIA, and joint deformities. Subcutaneous nodules may appear over pressure joints, especially the elbow. People with rheumatoid arthritis appear to be more susceptible to peptic ulcers, and this tendency is increased when the patient takes drugs such as aspirin, ibuprofen, indomethacin (Indocin), phenylbutazone, (Butazolidin) and corticosteroids (Prednisone).

The basic treatment for rheumatoid arthritis consists of rest, physical therapy, and anti-inflammatory drugs. Surgery is only necessary in a small number of people. A proper balance of rest and exercise should be part of the person's daily program. Heat, particularly moist heat, is helpful as a muscle relaxant. Therapeutic exercise is best done after the application of heat when the person is comfortable and muscle spasm is reduced.

The person must be encouraged and motivated to make the most of his or her capabilities. The elderly are especially prone to depression and passivity and benefit from a trusting, caring relationship with their physician and family. Local chapters of the Arthritis Foundation can provide assistance in directing people to self-help devices and rehabilitative facilities.

For additional information write or call:
National Arthritis Foundation
1314 Spring Street, N.W. #103
Atlanta, GA 30309
1-800-282-7023

Reichel, W. M. *Clinical Aspects of Aging.* Baltimore: The Williams & Wilkins Co., 1979.

aspiration   Part of the aging process produces depressed cough and gag reflexes. Patients with arteriosclerotic vascular disease may have cranial nerve dysfunction, further diminishing these reflexes. Thus, pulmonary aspiration, or intake into the airways of food particles, fluids, or foreign bodies, can be a significant problem in the elderly, even a cause of death.

Sudden aspiration of a large piece of food can lead to death by asphyxiation. The suddenness of this event has frequently led to an incorrect diagnosis of acute myocardial infarction. When smaller food particles are aspirated, an extensive hemorrhagic pneumonia may be seen in about six hours. With repeated food aspirations, X-ray findings may show small objects that look like miliary tuberculosis (small discrete multiple lesions).

Patients with varying states of consciousness should not be fed orally. They should be placed in bed in such a position as to ease the drainage of upper airway secretions and gastric contents. A patient should never be placed flat in bed. Tube-fed patients should be observed for delayed gastric emptying. Positioning nearer a sitting position after feeding may prevent regurgitation.

See also PNEUMONIA.

Covington, T., and Walker, J. *Current Geriatric Therapy.* Philadelphia: W. B. Saunders, 1984.

asthma   Asthma is an airway disorder characterized by intermittent episodes of smooth-muscle spasm, mucosal edema, and retained thick secretions. It is marked by recurrent attacks of wheezing and dyspnea. These attacks are chronic and may be associated with emphysema. The degree of airflow obstruction is directly related to the severity of the above mechanisms.

There are two types of asthma, immunologic and nonimmunologic. Immunologic or allergic asthma usually occurs in childhood. Nonimmunologic asthma usually develops in adults over 35 years of age. These attacks are precipitated by an infection in the sinuses and bronchial tree. Asthma can also be classified as mixed asthma, where attacks are initiated by viral or bacterial infections and allergens. Hypoxemia (lack of O_2), hypercapnia (excess CO_2), and the use of bronchodilators may lead to an acute asthmatic attack.

A careful history by the physician can be helpful in determining causative factors. These attacks often occur at night. The person experiences choking, dyspnea, and the characteristic wheezing sound. The person may become cyanotic and diaphorectic. Most attacks subside in 30 minutes to one hour.

Treatment is aimed at symptomatic relief and control of specific causative factors. In people whose asthma is caused by contact with the allergen, an attempt may be made to desensitize this individual. However, this is rarely used with adult-onset asthmatics. Oxygen is usually not necessary unless the patient develops cyanosis. Oxygen may be given by nasal prong, mask, or intermittent positive pressure breathing.

Bronchodilators are divided into two groups: the adrenergic drugs, epinephrine and isoproterenal; and the xanthine derivatives, aminophylline and theophylline. These drugs reduce bronchospasm by causing relaxation of the smooth muscle lining of the bronchi and bronchioles. They are very effective when given by nebulizer. The effectiveness of bronchodilators is dependent on the dose and delivery of the drug into the lung. Overuse of these drugs can lead to loss of effectiveness and should be used cautiously in patients with arteriosclerotic heart disease.

Humidification of inspired air is important therapy. Dehydration of the respiratory mucous membrane can lead to bronchial asthma attacks. Humidification causes liquification of the secretions, which promotes more effective clearing of the airways. Increased fluid intake will help replace fluids lost by perspiration during an acute attack. The patient should avoid antihistamines. Sedatives and tranquilizers can be used to control anxiety. Care must be taken to avoid suppression of respirations and the cough reflex. Narcotics are avoided because of their respiratory depressant effects.

If the acute asthmatic state is complicated by an infection, it is treated with antibiotics. The environment should be as free as possible of factors that contribute to respiratory infections. The patient should be protected from exposure to allergens that may set off attacks.

See also EMPHYSEMA.

Phipps, W. J., et al. Medical Surgical Nursing Concepts and Clinical Practice. St. Louis: C. V. Mosby Co., 1983.

Scherer, J. C. Introductory Medical Surgical Nursing. Philadelphia: J. B. Lippincott Co., 1982.

astigmatism   Astigmatism is the condition in which rays of light in the eye are not refracted equally in all directions, so that a point focus on the retina is not attained. In most instances astigmatism occurs because the radius of curvature of the cornea is not equal in all directions; this is called corneal astigmatism. Astigmatism can also occur as a result of tight suturing following an intraocular surgery, such as cataract surgery. Since over one million cataract surgeries are performed each year in the United States on the elderly, the incidence of astigmatism is greater in this age group than in others.

While the hyperopic person can normally see efficiently at a distance and the myopic person sees well close up, the person with astigmatism most often complains of an inability to see well either at a distance or near without glasses.

Treatment of astigmatism usually involves wearing glasses with a corrective lens. A surgical procedure is available to help correct astigmatism.

See also HYPEROPIA; MYOPIA; AND PRESBYOPIA.

Newell, F. W. Ophthalmology Principles and Concepts, 6th ed. St. Louis: C. V. Mosby Co., 1986.

Slatt, B. J., and Stein, H. A. The Ophthalmic Assistant: Fundamentals and Clinical Practice, 4th ed. St. Louis: C. V. Mosby Co., 1983.

atrial fibrillation   Atrial fibrillation is a totally disorganized series of rapid unsystematic contractions of the upper heart chambers (atria). The atria beats chaotically at rates of 350 to 600 beats per minute. The ventricles respond to the atrial stimulus with an irregular rhythm. Some of the ventricular beats are so weak that they are ineffective in opening the aortic valve and propelling the blood. In the presence of mitral stenosis, thrombi may form affecting the lungs or periphery of the body. Atrial fibrillation may be transient or it may be chronic.

Chronic atrial fibrillation is commonly associated with underlying heart disease such as coronary atherosclerotic heart disease, hypertension, pericarditis, and thyrotoxicosis. Other diseases that can be associated with atrial fibrillation include pulmonary embolism and chronic lung disease.

Symptoms of atrial fibrillation include heart flutter, anxiety, weakness, and dizziness. The treatment goal of atrial fibrillation is to attain a resting heart rate of 60 to 80 beats per minute or to restore sinus rhythm.

Atrial fibrillation is usually treated medically with drugs such as digitalis, quinidine, beta-adrenergic blockers, or calcium-channel blockers. Sometimes anticoagulants are prescribed to prevent blood clots. Cardioversion, which is a method of electrical countershock, may be necessary in people who have persistent atrial fibrillation or recurrent embolization.

See also ARRHYTHMIAS, CARDIAC.

Phipps, W. J., et al. Medical Surgical Nursing. St. Louis: C. V. Mosby Co., 1983.

Steinberg, F. U. Care of the Geriatric Patient, 6th ed. St. Louis: C. V. Mosby Co., 1983.

autogenic training   Autogenic training, developed in 1905 by Johannes Schultz, was a combination of relaxation techniques that evolved earlier in Germany. The treatment consists of carefully selected and significant phrases. The patient repeats these phrases to himself, allowing the mind and body to relax and go into a state in which the mind can discharge disturbing material. The seemingly innocuous phrase, "My right arm is heavy," has been sufficient to enable the one elderly participant with hypertension to drop her blood pressure. This type of therapy is useful in older patients to control certain body functions such as high blood pressure.

See also BIOFEEDBACK TRAINING; GESTALT DREAM ANALYSIS; HATHA YOGA; POSITIVE ATTITUDE; SELF-IMAGE EXERCISE; TAI CHI CHUAN.

Fields, S. "Sage Can Be a Spice in Life," in Aging, Goldstein, E. C., ed. Vol. 1, Art. 26. Boca Raton, Fl.: Social Issues Resource Series, Inc., 1981.

B

Baby Boom generation, aging of   The Baby Boom generation born between 1946 and 1964 makes up nearly one-third of the nation's population—76 million strong. Because this generation is rapidly reaching the threshold of age, and by 2030 will boost the total elderly population to its highest point in U.S. history, it is important to review the role it has played in American life.

It was this generation that touched off the "age of Aquarius" in the 1960s and that was responsible for the Woodstock concert, the spread of a hippie lifestyle, and the dominance of youth fashions in clothing and hairstyles. It was the Baby Boom generation primarily that fought the Vietnam war and played the major part in the protests against that futile episode.

By the 1970s most of the Baby Boomers had reached working age, their numbers swelling the U.S. labor force by 24 percent. Although there were pockets of unemployment among younger people (most notably among minorities and teenagers) during the 1970s and 1980s, the growth of jobs kept pace with the growth of the labor force, and Baby Boomers have experienced a period of relative prosperity. Along with the expanding young population entering the labor force, women of the Baby Boom have joined the labor market in unprecedented numbers, so that today about half of the U.S. work force is made up of women.

The Baby Boom generation has attained the highest level of education ever achieved in U.S. history, with close to 85 percent having graduated from high school and more than 45 percent having attended or graduated from college. This compares with about 25 percent high school graduates and less than 20 percent college attendees and graduates in the over age 65 population. These high levels of education were achieved as a result of the efforts of generations of Americans who reached old age before the Baby Boom. The older generation expanded the public education system, created community colleges and technical schools, and expanded state colleges, universities, and private higher education so that the oncoming wave of the Baby Boom would acquire the know-how to function and provide leadership during this present technical age. As a result more members of the Baby Boom workforce will occupy higher prestige jobs than any previous generation, and many will be in the $50,000 and up income bracket.

As the Baby Boom generation has reached maturity America experienced its highest divorce rate ever, with an increase from 2.2 divorces per 1,000 population in 1960 to a peak of 5.3 divorces per 1,000 in 1981, the year when divorce began a slow but steady decline. The rate of childbearing slowed, perhaps influenced by the high costs of family formation (rent, purchase of residence, furnishing a home, etc.) as much as by the new workforce commitment of both partners to marriages and the changing styles in family planning. Child bearing has now begun to rise again.

With this already notable history, the next phase of life for the Baby Boom generation—its imminent entry into the ranks of the aging—may well be its most interesting time ever. Already those born at the start of the boom, 1946, have entered middle age and will soon reach 50, with their younger fellows waiting in the wings to join them. During the next century the Baby Boom generation will boost the proportion of the population over age 65 to more than 21 percent of the total, and to over 67 million persons (compared to the 30–34 million of recent years)—the highest level in American history.

What circumstances and values will the baby boom generation carry with it into age? In view of its unique history as a generation, together with new lifestyles, higher levels of income, and more education, it can be predicted that this group of future elderly will have a prosperous and well-filled old age. No one can forecast the future with certainty, but there are reasons to believe that the aging Baby Boom population and its successors will live their advanced maturity with an unprecedented quality of life. Advances in biological research and medical science have already reduced premature death, and it can be expected that increasing numbers of individuals in the future will reach

more and more closely to the biological limit of the human life span—120 years.

In the financial sphere, social planning is providing a foundation for retirement income through the Social Security program. At the same time private business pension coverage of employees has grown from only 12 percent of all workers and 4 million persons in the late 1930s to half of all workers and over 40 million persons in the 1980s. With over 90 percent of government employees, representing approximately another 15 million workers, also covered by public pension plans, it is evident that the majority of the work force in the future ought to have a sufficiently high level of income to experience a financially comfortable old age.

In recent years the United States has begun to develop new patterns for retirement living that ensure an increasing level of enjoyment of leisure for the future older population. Retirement communities, retirement housing centers, and lifecare centers (see RESIDENCES) now number well over 2,500 across the land. Facilities like these provide recreation, relieve their older residents of the burdens of home maintenance and care of surroundings, and offer maximum opportunity for social relationships and support from peers. While such patterns of living are still new and only involve about 10 percent of the elderly population, their rapid growth suggests a trend that may well become the pattern for future residential living by the elderly population.

The higher levels of education of the Baby Boom generation give it an unprecedented opportunity to plan life with wisdom. Insight, good judgment, and thoughtful planning all rest on the fund of knowledge that people possess, and if what Thomas Jefferson said—''knowledge is power, knowledge is safety, knowledge is happiness''—is true, then the Baby Boomers should have attained these qualities in greater abundance than any generation in history. Given such foundations, the work of the AARP (American Association of Retired Persons) and organizations like Ken Dychtwald's Age Wave of Emeryville, California, and Edith Tucker's *United Retirement Bulletin* published by United Business Services of Boston, Massachusetts, should achieve outstanding success in supplying the elderly with solid information on mature living.

American business is recognizing the older population as a consumer market and is beginning to develop products and marketing systems directed to it. Advertisers increasingly portray older people in their photographs and displays, featuring mature models in upbeat advertisements for cosmetics, automobiles, and fashions. Manufacturers have developed specially designed clothing and lightweight golf clubs, and the leisure industry has designed travel tour packages—to mention only a few such adaptions—for the mature market.

Ultimately, developments during the present, and in the probable future of the baby boom generation, suggest that American attitudes about age will become more positive than they have been traditionally. Instead of shunning or looking on age with aversion, future generations of Americans may look forward with pleasure to the advanced years of life. Social customs and social attitudes may even change enough so that the last years become the best years.

Keeney, C. "Baby Boomer," in *Aging*, Goldstein, E. C., ed. Vol. 2, Art. 80. Boca Raton, Fl.: Social Issues Resource Series, Inc., 1981.
U.S. Bureau of the Census, *Statistical Abstract of the United States: 1989*, 109th ed. Washington, D.C.: U.S. Government Printing Office, 1989.

backache   Back pain afflicts as many as four out of five adults at least once during their lives. It is one of the leading causes of hospitalization and lost work days to industry. The majority of back pain results from stress, physical exertion, and muscle strain.

Pain is a symptom of injury. Tense muscles do not have the flexibility to function properly and may pull or tear, causing in-flammation and pain. Ligaments, the tough elastic tissues that connect bone to bone, are subjected to the same strains that muscles are and can suffer similar injuries.

Though muscle strain is the most common cause of backaches, disk disease is another common disorder, particularly in the elderly. The disks are the back's shock absorbers and are sandwiched between the vertebrae to provide cushioning and flexibility. In the middle of the disk is a jellylike material that is held in place by tough, fibrous bands that surround the disk. As people age, these bands lose some of their strength and elasticity. They may become brittle and prone to injury. Rest is the primary course of treatment though surgery may be necessary to repair a ruptured disk.

The most important consideration for a healthy back is prevention of injury. Proper exercise, weight control, diet, good posture, and adequate rest all contribute to a healthy back.

See also BACK PAIN AND BACK INJURY, PREVENTION OF.

Gutman, R. *The Healthy Back Book*. Chicago: Blue Cross/Blue Shield, 1986.

back pain and back injury, prevention of   The most common cause of back pain is muscle strain. Because of the pace of modern life, people's muscles remain tense and may not have the flexibility to function properly. Such simple acts as reaching for the phone or bending over can trigger pain.

Regular physical exercise is the best way to relieve stress and build strong muscles. The lumbar region of the spine—the lower back—is especially dependent on strong muscles for support.

Aerobic exercise is the most effective type of exercise.

Any exercise that raises the pulse rate and maintains it at an appropriate level for 20 or 30 minutes is considered aerobic. This can include brisk walking, bicycling, swimming, jogging, cross-country skiing, jumping rope, or aerobic dancing. Each exercise session should begin with a period of stretching and warm-up exercise to increase flexibility and prevent injury. To be effective, aerobic exercise should be undertaken three or more times each week. It is important to work up gradually to the prescribed level. A doctor should be consulted before beginning a vigorous exercise program, especially if there is a history of chronic back pain. In these cases, activities that involve pounding movements in the legs or sudden twisting should be avoided. Brisk walking may be best.

A daily program of specific exercises for the back can help build strength, flexibility, and range of motion. These can include sit-ups done with knees bent, curl-ups, and pelvic tilts. The exercises must be done smoothly while breathing normally. Exercises that cause pain should be avoided.

There are a number of ways to reduce back strain during daily routines. The following should be kept in mind:

1. Always bend at the knees—not the waist.
2. Prop one leg up to reduce stress when standing.
3. Lean on the sink when shaving or brushing teeth.
4. Distribute weight evenly when carrying packages or luggage.
5. Support your lower back when sitting, using a small pillow if necessary.
6. When lifting, bend at the knees, keeping the body straight, and holding what is being lifted close to the body.
7. Push heavy objects rather than lifting or pulling.

Gutman, R. *The Healthy Back Book*. Chicago, Blue Cross/Blue Shield. 1986.

badminton   See TENNIS.

baldness   See HAIR TRANSPLANTS.

Basedow's disease   See HYPERTHYROID-ISM.

bathing (skin care)   Body odors are a major problem for physically and mentally disabled older people, due to loss of bladder and bowel control and a faster rate of dying cells. Because of this, frequent bathing is necessary.

Although daily bathing is not advisable—aging skin has less oil and too-frequent baths may exacerbate this condition—daily local bathing is necessary. The face, groin, underarm and other body creases should be cleansed daily.

People who are physically handicapped may find it necessary to place a chair in the shower or attach a bathtub rail to assure safety. Substituting a handheld shower head with an extra long hose may also be useful. Putting a few drops of bath or baby oil on a washcloth and rubbing over the body helps to prevent itching from dry skin.

Gillies, J. *A Guide to Caring for and Coping with Aging Parents*. Nashville: Thomas Nelson Publishers, 1981.

bedsores   See DECUBITI.

Belgian elderly   Belgium has recently seen a decline of the ratio between working members of the population and welfare recipients, including pensioners. In 1950 there were 4.2 people holding jobs to every one on welfare. This ratio has dropped in recent years to 1.7 to one. Statistics from 1984 show that 13.7 percent of the Belgian population is 65 years of age or older.

The health and hospital services committees in Belgium are the responsibility of public assistance committees in each town. The committees pay for relief patients in private hospitals, administer public hospitals, and organize nursing services and clinics.

Social Security applies to all workers subject to employment contracts. The Central National Social Security Office collects Social Security and distributes the money to respective committees.

Twigg, H. D. "Enter the Age of Age," in *Aging*, Goldstein, E. C., ed. Vol. 2, Art. 17. Boca Raton, Fl.: Social Issues Resource Series, Inc., 1981.

bereavement As a term, *bereavement* normally applies only on the occasion of loss of a very close family member, most commonly a spouse, through death. The psychological consequences of bereavement—grief—can, however, accompany a number of other life events, such as the death of a child, sibling, close friend, business partner, or even divorce, abandonment, loss of a pet, destruction of a residence by fire, and sometimes financial loss. While bereavement involving loss of a spouse may occur at any adult stage of life, it is most likely to take place in advanced maturity. According to the *Handbook of the Psychology of Aging*, for example, after age 65, 51 percent of women and 13.6 percent of men have experienced widowhood at least once.

When men and women are taken together the General Social Survey shows that the highest rate of death of family members does not necessarily occur in the most advanced years of life, that is, beyond age 85. This source shows that the peak years for experiencing the death of a relative in the past 5 years (in many cases a spouse) are from age 55–84. The percentages of people reporting such a loss range from 54 percent at age 55–64, down to 52 percent at 75–84. By comparison only about 50 percent of those over 85 report a loss within the past five years.

Differences occur between the sexes. The highest years for loss for women come between ages 55 and 64, when more than 55 percent report the death of a relative in the past five years—most commonly their husband. For men the peak years occur after age 85, when 65 percent report a loss, many of which involve their wives. These differences between the sexes undoubtedly exist because the average man marries a woman who is younger than himself, and he dies at a younger age than his wife. Men who do live beyond 85 may quite likely lose their spouse because the average life expectancy of women is about 78 years.

The death of a child preceding the death of a parent becomes increasingly common as the years pass. Exact statistics on the frequency of this type of loss are not available, but one can surmise that child deaths become quite frequent after 85 if we observe, first, that the average age of beginning parenthood comes in the early 20s and then note that the frequency of death is about 1,300 per 100,000 at age 55–64, or over a quarter of a million deaths, when more than 3 1/4 million persons over age 85 remain alive. Some of these death inevitably occur to people whose parents are over 85; in fact, people over 85 may well have lost all their relatives and be the only surviving members of their families.

No one should underestimate the severe psychological impact of bereavement. A number of studies have documented increased depression, illness, and death among widows and widowers. If there can be good news in the face of so grave a personal loss as the death of a spouse, it is that long-term studies of widows and widowers show lower rates of clinical depression (depression that is measurably severe) than might be expected—33 percent in a month following death and 13 percent after a year. Authors La Rue Asenath, Connie Dessonville and Lissy Jarvik comment in the *Handbook of the Psychology of Aging* that, "Relatively few older people appear to develop protracted and disabling depressive illness following age-appropriate loss of loved ones."

Asenath, L. R.; Dessonville, C.; and Jarvik, L. F. "Aging and Mental Disorders," in Birren, J. E., and Schaie, K. W., eds., *Handbook of the Psychology of Aging*, 2nd. ed. New York: Van Nostrand Reinhold Company, 1985.
Kastenbaum, R. "Dying and Death: A Life-Span Approach," in Birren, J. E., and Schaie, K. W., eds., *Handbook of the Psychology of Aging*, 2nd. ed. New York: Van Nostrand Reinhold Company, 1985.

Russell, C. M., and Megaard, I. *The General Social Survey, 1972–1986: The State of the American People.* New York: Springer-Verlag, 1988.

biliary colic   See GALL BLADDER DISEASE.

biofeedback training   Biofeedback instruments monitor physiological changes through sensors placed on the body. The signals from the sensors are usually amplified as an auditory or visual display. Elderly people can learn relaxation techniques through biofeedback, and many medical complaints of older people have been eliminated through this instrumental teaching of relaxation.

See also AUTOGENIC TRAINING; GESTALT DREAM ANALYSIS; HATHA YOGA; POSITIVE ATTITUDE; SELF-IMAGE EXERCISE; TAI CHI CHUAN.

Fields, S. "Sage Can Be a Spice in Life," in *Aging,* Goldstein, E. C., ed. Vol. 1, Art. 26. Boca Raton, Fl.: Social Issues Resource Series, Inc., 1981.

bladder cancer   See CANCER, BLADDER.

blepharochalasis (excessive upper lid skin)   Blepharochalasis is a common elderly abnormality in which there is eyelid atrophy and loss of skin elasticity and turgor. Usually a fold of tissue from the upper eyelid hangs over the upper eyelid margin. Up to 60 percent of elderly may exhibit some degree of blepharochalasis.

Symptoms of this condition include a decrease in the visual field and ocular irritation from the lashes being pushed onto the cornea.

Treatment is not usually necessary. If the fold of skin interferes with the person's visual field, causes excessive ocular irritation, or is cosmetically unacceptable, the excess skin may be surgically excised.

Newell, F. W. *Ophthalmology Principles and Concepts,* 6th ed. St. Louis: C. V. Mosby Co., 1986.

blepharoplasty   See COSMETIC SURGERY.

blepharoptosis   See PTOSIS.

blood clot   See THROMBOPHLEBITIS.

blood pressure, high   See HYPERTENSION.

blood pressure, low   See HYPOTENSION, ORTHOSTATIC.

body temperature reduction   Reduction in body temperature in animals slows the aging process. In studies done on cold-blooded animals, a tenfold increase in longevity has been achieved by lowering body temperature. This cooling method has also been experimented with on warm-blooded mammals. The results are the same, slower aging process, but not as drastic. It has been predicted that lowering the body temperature by three degrees Farenheit could add 30 years to a human life. There is currently no practical long-term way to lower body temperature in humans.

See also AGING, BIOLOGICAL THEORY OF.

Rosenfield, A. "The Longevity Seekers," in *Aging,* Goldstein, E. C., ed. Vol. 2, Art. 1. Boca Raton, Fl.: Social Issues Resource Series, Inc., 1981.

bones, brittle   See OSTEOPOROSIS.

bowel obstruction (volvulus, strangulated hernia)   The most common cause of intestinal obstruction is cancer, occurring more frequently in older people. The tumor gradually grows until it completely obstructs the bowel. If the obstruction is partial, changes in bowel habits may be noted. These changes include alternating constipation and diarrhea. Prompt diagnosis and treatment may avert complete obstruction.

Volvulus, a twisting or kinking of a portion of the intestines, and strangulated hernia are other causes of acute intestinal obstruction.

With an obstruction symptoms may arise suddenly. The portion nearest to the obstruction becomes distended with intestinal contents, and the portion furthest away from the obstruction is empty. If the obstruction is complete, no gas or feces are expelled rectally. Peristalsis (movement of the intestine) becomes very forceful in the proximal portion as the body attempts to propel the material beyond the point of the obstruction. This can cause severe cramps, which tend to occur intermittently.

When the obstruction occurs high in the intestinal tract, vomiting usually results. If the obstruction is low in the colon vomiting usually does not occur.

The patient becomes dehydrated due to an inability to take oral fluids and from losing water and electrolytes through vomiting. The failure of the mucosa to reabsorb the secretions contributes to the water and electrolyte imbalance.

The increased pressure on the bowel due to severe distention (expansion and swelling) and edema (swelling due to an accumulation of fluid) may impair circulation and lead to gangrene of a portion of the bowel. Perforation of the gangrenous bowel causes the intestinal contents to seep into the peritoneal (abdominal) cavity, resulting in peritonitis. Intestinal obstruction may prove fatal if prompt treatment is not given.

Diagnosis is based on patient history and physical examination. X-ray of the intestinal tract is usually necessary.

Mechanical obstruction is usually treated surgically. The obstruction is relieved by a minor surgical procedure, such as a temporary colostomy (surgical opening between colon and surface of body) or cecostomy (surgical opening into the cecum). When the patient's condition has improved as a result of relief of the obstruction and supportive therapy, more extensive surgery may be undertaken. A permanent colostomy may be necessary depending on the location and extent of the malignant process.

Intestinal decompression, intravenous fluids, and antibiotics help stabilize the person's condition prior to surgery.

See also CANCER, COLON; AND RECTAL HERNIA.

Scherer, J. C. *Introductory Medical-Surgical Nursing*, 3rd ed. Philadelphia: J. B. Lippincott Co., 1982.

Steinberg, F. U. *Care of the Geriatric Patient*, 6th ed. St. Louis: C. V. Mosby Co., 1983.

braces of teeth   See ORTHODONTIA.

bradycardia, sinus (cardiac arrhythmia)   Sinus bradycardia is a cardiac arrhythmia characterized by atrial and ventricular rates of less than 60 beats per minute and a regular rhythm.

Sinus bradycardia is normal in athletes and laborers who have enlarged hearts from regular strenuous exercise. Bradycardia is sometimes seen in people with increased intracranial pressure, hypothyroidism, digitalis toxicity, carotid sinus or eyeball pressure, with the Valsalva maneuver, and during anesthesia.

Generally, sinus bradycardia is a benign rhythm. If, however, the heart rate is not adequate to maintain proper cardiac output, congestive heart failure or syncope may occur.

Treatment for sinus bradycardia may involve the use of cholinergic blocking agents (atropine). If the bradycardia is chronic and not controlled well with medication a cardiac pacemaker may be surgically implanted. The purpose of the pacemaker is to generate a pulse and maintain effective cardiac output. The person with a cardiac pacemaker should check his or her pulse once or twice daily. If any change is noted the physician should be seen since battery failure and displacement of wire electrodes is possible. Some physicians outfit their pacemaker patients with special equipment that transmits the electrocardiagram (ECG) over the telephone. See also ARRYTHMIAS, CARDIAC.

Phipps, W. J., et al. *Medical Surgical Nursing*. St. Louis: C. V. Mosby Co., 1983.

Scherer, J. C. *Introductory Medical-Surgical Nursing*. Philadelphia: J. B. Lippincott Co., 1982.

breast cancer See CANCER, BREAST.

British elderly Currently, in Britain, retirement benefits are paid to men at age 65 and to women at age 60. The government provides services for the handicapped. Ninety-eight percent of Britain's practicing general physicians are part of the National Health Service. The service provides full, and in most cases, free service to all residents. A patient is free to choose his or her own doctor and pays only part of the costs for such things as prescriptions, eyeglasses, and dentures. The program is financed through taxation. Each resident contributes about $30 per year in taxes.

Twigg, H. D. "Enter the Age of Age," in *Aging*, Goldstein, E. C., ed. Vol. 2, Art. 17. Boca Raton, Fl.: Social Issues Resource Series, Inc., 1981.

bronchitis, chronic Chronic bronchitis is characterized by the presence of a productive cough resulting from an excessive production of mucus. The mucosal surface of the tracheobronchial tree is lined by cilia. Their function is, specifically, to propel excess secretions to the trachea where a cough will remove the material. Air pollutants decrease ciliary activity, with retention of secretions. These secretions form plugs within the bronchi where infection readily ensues.

Diagnosis is made by evaluating the patient's symptoms, performing a careful history, physical examination, X-ray of the chest, fluoroscopy, and pulmonary function tests. A sputum culture may be obtained. Keeping a record of the volume expectorated

per day may be helpful in assessing the disease.

Treatment of chronic bronchitis requires long-term planning. It is usually palliative in nature, directed at preventing infections and relieving symptoms.

Maintaining optimal health and preventing respiratory infections are important in maintaining the patient's resistance. A diet containing adequate protein, vitamins, and other nutrients is important. Maintaining an increased humidity in the home assists in the liquification of secretions and prevention of mucus plugs. Sufficient rest and avoiding emotional stress is helpful with the overall disease.

Rogers, S. C., and McCue, J. D. *Managing Chronic Disease*. Oradell, N.J.: Medical Economics Co., 1987.

Scherer, J. C. *Introductory Medical-Surgical Nursing*. Philadelphia: J. B. Lippincott Co., 1982.

bruises (senile purpura) Senile purpura is a common condition of easy bruisability seen most commonly on forearms and legs of older individuals. It is usually caused by the loss of subcutaneous (under the skin) fat and is occasionally caused by the excessive use of aspirin or other blood thinners. Thrombocytopenia (lack of platelets), steroids, diabetes mellitus, vasculitis (blood vessel inflammation), scurvy, and connective tissue diseases may also be contributing factors.

Symptoms of senile purpura include purple bruises with small red patches on the skin, which fade to a permanent brown pigmented area over a span of a few weeks.

There is no treatment for senile purpura, unless it is caused by certain drugs. If so, the medications may be altered to reduce the senile purpura. Otherwise, the therapy of full explanation and reassurance may be the best treatment for senile purpura. If senile purpura does not seem to be in exposed areas, the capillary fragility test may be useful in distinguishing whether ecchymoses (the escape of blood into the tissue from leaking blood vessels) are due to a bleeding disorder or to trauma. Other tests for suspected clinical entities might be necessary, such as blood sugars, skin biopsy, blood cultures, or platelet vitamin C levels.

Rossman, I. *Clinical Geriatrics,* 3rd ed. Philadelphia: J. B. Lippincott Co., 1986.
Steinberg, F. U. *Care of the Geriatric Patient,* 6th ed. St. Louis: C. V. Mosby, 1983.

bunions   A bunion is the swelling of the bursa, fluid-filled sacs in the tissue, below the base of the big toe. Bunions are usually caused by shoes that fit improperly, flat feet, arthritic contractures and deterioration of the fat pad of the feet. Sometimes bunions are hereditary. Twenty-five percent of the people with bunions are 65 years of age or older. In the elderly, atrophy (wasting away) of muscles, ligaments, and tendons and arthritis increase the likelihood of developing bunions.

Symptoms include pain, swelling, and limping. Foot soaks and emollients to lubricate the skin can temporarily relieve swelling and pain. Over-the-counter pads and toe separators can help. Molded shoes, which eliminate pressure on friction areas, may also help relieve pain. Occasionally steroid, whirlpool, and ultrasound treatment may be necessary for relief of inflammation. Analgesics or other pain medication may also be required. Surgery is sometimes necessary. Surgical treatment of bunions in the older person is indicated if pain and shoe-fitting difficulties persist after nonoperative treatment.

See also CORNS.

Shea, T. P., and Smith, J. K. *The Over Easy Foot Care Book.* Glenview, Ill.: Scott, Foresman and Co., 1984.

burial   See FUNERAL.

bursitis (tendonitis, "tennis elbow")
Bursitis is the inflammation of the bursa, a fluid-filled sac in the tissue, which usually prevents friction. The bursa facilitates the gliding of muscles and tendons over bony surfaces.

The most common joint affected by bursitis is the shoulder, although the elbow, foot, knee, and hand can be affected. Bursitis is the most common cause of shoulder pain in older people. With recurring inflammation of the area, calcium deposits and fluid may remain, which may lead to a chronic condition. Often, inflammation of the underlying tendon of the rotator cuff is the primary cause of shoulder pain in adults. Any abnormality of the rotator cuff results in a frozen shoulder where the range of motion is restricted with extreme discomfort when movement exceeds a few degrees in any direction.

Symptoms of bursitis include localized pain, limitation of motion, swelling, and redness. Pain may be so severe that the person will immobilize the affected area, which rapidly leads to stiffening of that joint.

Treatment of bursitis includes anti-inflammatory agents, analgesics, and in severe cases injection of steroids into the affected area. Physical therapy and range of motion exercises may be beneficial. In severe cases, it may be necessary to remove calcium deposits or repair bursa tears surgically. A shoulder rotation done under anesthesia loosens adhesions in a frozen shoulder that does not respond to more conservative treatment.

Tennis elbow is seen in older individuals and is more common in men than in women. Any activity that involves forceful turning of the hand or forceful extension of the wrist can produce tennis elbow. Pain may radiate upward from the elbow toward the shoulder and down into the hand or may be localized in the elbow.

This condition is treated by resting the affected area, avoiding activities that cause pain, and wearing an elbow guard. It is important to avoid activities that put stress on the wrist and finger extensors until pain has been absent for several weeks.

Steinberg, F. U. *Care of the Geriatric Patient,* 6th ed. St. Louis: C. V. Mosby Co., 1983.

bushmen of the Kalahari desert   The study of other cultures and lifestyles helps give insight into disease processes and aging. Study of the bushmen of the Kalahari desert helps with blood pressure studies.

The bushmen of the Kalahari desert age much in the same ways as tropical forest populations. Mean blood pressure did not rise between the ages of 20 and 83. No cases of hypertension or coronary heart disease were found in the population. The serum cholesterol levels were found to be very low. The low cholesterol levels are probably due to the bushmen's diets. Their major sources of food are mongongo nuts and game. The meat they eat has a much lower fat content than that of farm animals.

This population, especially the elderly, living on low-calorie diets that are particularly low in saturated animal fats, enjoy the definite advantage of low blood pressure and low lipid values.

This supports the well-documented view that changes in blood pressure is a function of lifestyle rather an inevitable part of the human aging process.

See also MASAI; NEW GUINEAN HIGH-LANDERS; POLYNESIANS; SOLOMON ISLAND TRIBES; SOMALI CAMEL HERDSMEN; TARA-HUMARA INDIANS; YANOMANO INDIANS.

Brocklehurst, J. C. *Textbook of Geriatric Medicine and Gerontology.* New York: Churchhill Livingstone, 1985.

C

calcium   See VITAMINS.

cancer   Cancer is an aberration of normal cells in which the cells grow in a wild, undisciplined manner. It is the second greatest cause of death in the elderly, led only by cardiovascular disease. The most frequent age for the occurrence of cancer is between 60 to 65 years. Increasing age and accompanying physiologic changes make the older person more susceptible to carcinogens.

The three most common cancers and causes of cancer-related deaths are lung cancer, breast cancer, and colorectal cancer. This is true for the elderly as well as younger people. In men over 75 years of age, prostate cancer is the leading cause of cancer-related deaths. In women breast cancer is the most common type at all ages. Skin cancer is possibly the most prevalent cancer, though it is not usually life-threatening.

For each site of origin of cancer, there are "low stage" cancers, which are localized and generally cured by surgery, and "high stage" cancers, which are more extensive, less often curable, and usually treated with radiotherapy or chemotherapy. The staging of cancer reveals the extent of the tumor and allows for the best approach in treatment. Once cancer has been diagnosed and staged, a treatment program can be designed using surgery, radiation therapy, or chemotherapy as needed.

Early detection is extremely important in the future management of cancer, for many cancers can be cured if found early. Some warning signs to be aware of are: a sore that does not heal; change in wart or mole; hoarseness or cough; difficulty in swallowing; a lump or thickening in breast or elsewhere; a change in bowel or bladder habits; unusual bleeding or discharge.

Of course, prevention is most important. Certain changes in lifestyle can be practiced by the older person to reduce the possibility of cancer. For example, avoidance of sun exposure can decrease the incidence of skin cancer and elimination of the use of tobacco products will lessen the number of cases of lung, mouth, and throat cancers.

During the treatment and rehabilitation of the cancer patient, every effort should be made to consider the patient and family as a unit, to focus therapeutic efforts on supportive care, and to make a special effort to manage the patient in a loving, caring surrounding. This is especially important in the terminal phases of a fatal illness. Total care of the cancer patient is of primary importance whether or not treatment is successful and whether life expectancy can be measured in years or days.

For additional information write or call: American Cancer Society, National Office
4 West 35th Street
New York, NY 10001
(212) 736-3030

See also cancer, bladder; cancer, breast; cancer, colon and rectal; cancer, lung; cancer, ovarian; cancer, prostate; cancer, uterine.

Steinberg, F. U. *Care of the Geriatric Patient*, 6th ed. St. Louis: C. V. Mosby Co., 1983.

cancer, bladder   The earliest symptom of a malignancy of the bladder is painless hematuria (blood in the urine). Diagnosis is made by cystocopic examination (looking with an instrument into the bladder) and biopsy. If the muscle wall of the bladder is not penetrated by the tumor, metastases have usually not occurred.

Small tumors may be removed by transurethral resection or fulguration. In larger tumors, segmental resection (partial removal of bladder) or cystectomy (total removal) may be performed. In elderly patients who are poor operative risks, some success can be achieved with radiation or chemotherapy.

Following cystectomy, the patient is usually quite ill. He or she is prone to surgical shock, thrombosis, cardiac decompensation, and other circulatory disturbances. Management is similar to that of the patient with major abdominal surgery.

Cancer of the bladder is currently considered incurable and is usually fatal within five years. Surgery and treatment with anticancer drugs can prolong and improve the quality of life. Pain and other symptoms can be relieved or controlled. The medical literature cites a few instances of unexplained recovery.

Scherer, J. C. *Introductory Medical-Surgical Nursing,* 3rd ed. Philadelphia: J. B. Lippincott Co., 1982.
Steinberg, F. U. *Care of the Geriatric Patient,* 6th ed. St. Louis: C. V. Mosby Co., 1983.

cancer, breast   In American women, the breast is the most common site of cancer. The disease can occur at any age, but it is most common during and after menopause. The longer a women lives the greater her chance of developing breast cancer. However, if it is discovered and treated early, the five-year level of cure for small lesions is about 80 percent.

In order to discover carcinoma of the breast early, it is necessary that a woman examine her breasts on a regular, monthly basis, reporting any unusual signs or lumps immediately to her physician. A lump may be a cyst, a benign tumor, or a malignancy. Characteristically, malignant lumps are painless in their early stages. Other symptoms of breast cancer are nipple discharge, pain, and a change in the appearance of the breast.

A mammogram, a soft tissue X-ray examination, is an excellent diagnostic tool. On these films, it is possible for the radiologist and the surgeon to distinguish with considerable accuracy a benign lump from a malignant one and to discover lesions too small to feel. Each woman over the age of 40 should have a mammogram annually.

When a malignancy is suspected a biopsy is usually taken to confirm the diagnosis. If the results are positive, a lumpectomy or some type of mastectomy is performed. There is continuing medical debate and controversy about which surgical procedure offers the most favorable prognosis. The various procedures are: lumpectomy—removal of the tumor only; partial mastectomy—the tumor and small amount of breast tissue are removed; simple mastectomy—the breast is removed; subcutaneous mastectomy—all breast tissue is removed but the skin and nipple are left intact; modified radical mastectomy—the breast and axillary lymph nodes are removed; and radical mastectomy—the breast, axillary lymph nodes, and pectoral muscles are removed. Frequently, surgery will be followed by radiation therapy or chemotherapy.

Exercises are an important part of a patient's postoperative care, enabling her to again become independent and self-sufficient. When the wound is sufficiently healed a prosthesis may be fitted. Reconstruction is also a possibility depending upon the extent of the cancer and preference of the patient.

Unfortunately, metastases of breast cancer occurs in many patients. Lymph nodes are most commonly affected followed by bone and pulmonary involvement, though many organs can be affected. The methods of treatment for metastatic cancer include hormonal therapy, radiation therapy, and chemotherapy. All forms of treatment carry the possibility of unpleasant side effects and complications. At present, metastatic carcinoma of the breast is incurable. The goal of treatment is to prolong the patient's life and make her more comfortable.

Breast amputation is a devastating experience, irrevocably altering a woman's body and her self-image. The emotional comfort of the postmastectomy patient is as great a necessity as her physical comfort. Often she feels isolated with no one to help her face her worries about social acceptance and her concerns about death. The patient needs a great deal of support from members of her health-care team as well as her family and friends. Volunteer agencies can be contacted through the American Cancer Society to help patients, spouses, and other family members through this traumatic experience.

Rossman, I. *Clinical Geriatrics*, 3rd ed. Philadelphia: J. B. Lippincott Co., 1986.

Scherer, J. C. *Introductory Medical-Surgical Nursing*, 3rd ed. Philadelphia: J. B. Lippincott Co., 1982.

cancer, colon and rectal   Cancer of the colon and rectum are among the most commonly occurring malignancies in the United States. More than 40,000 cases of colon and rectum cancer occur in people over the age of 65 yearly. The incidence of bowel cancer is higher in developed countries. Two thirds of the malignancies occur in the sigmoid colon and rectum.

Diet plays a significant role in the incidence of bowel cancer. Eating foods high in dietary fibers and low in animal protein, fats, and refined carbohydrates may offer protection against bowel cancer. Early diagnosis and treatment offer the best chance for a cure. A change in bowel patterns such as constipation or diarrhea, a change in the shape of the stool, or passing of blood should be investigated.

Polyps growing in the lumen of the colon may develop into colon cancer. Partial or total obstruction may result in the lower colon from the formed stool unable to pass through the narrowed lumen. Bleeding may result from ulceration of the lesions.

Colon cancer may spread by direct extension or through the lymphatic or circulatory systems. The liver is the major organ of metastasis.

Diagnosis of cancer of the colon is made by physical examination, sigmoidoscopy, colonoscopy, and barium enema examination. Cancer of the rectum is diagnosed by biopsy of a lesion during a proctoscopic examination. The stool is examined for occult blood.

Cancer of the colon is always treated surgically, with the tumor, colon, and lymph nodes being resected. If the growth cannot be treated surgically or has caused an obstruction with inflammation, an opening may be made into the cecum or transverse colon as a palliative measure for fecal contents to escape. When the edema and inflammation around the tumor subside the growth is resected, the bowel sections are rejoined (anastomesed), and the cecostomy or colostomy is closed.

See also CANCER, STOMACH.

Phipps, W. J. *Essentials of Medical-Surgical Nursing.* St. Louis: C. V. Mosby Co., 1985.
Steinberg, F. U. *Care of the Geriatric Patient,* 6th ed. St. Louis: C. V. Mosby Co., 1983.

cancer, esophageal   Carcinoma is the most common cause of obstruction of the esophagus in the elderly. Symptoms develop very slowly. By the time difficulty in swallowing (dysphagia) is noticeable the cancer may have invaded surrounding tissues and lymphatics. Prognosis is generally poor.

In the beginning, symptoms may be mild with only vague feelings of discomfort and difficulty in swallowing. As the disease progresses, solid foods become almost impossible to swallow and the patient resorts to a liquid diet. Weight loss occurs with progressive dysphagia.

Treatment of cancer of the esophagus depends on the extent of the lesion and evidence of metastasis. Radiation is used for inoperable lesions but, if possible, surgical resection of the esophagus is performed. If the patient is too ill to withstand surgery, a gastrostomy may be performed, permitting food to be introduced directly into the stomach through an opening in the abdomen. Sometimes this will be a temporary measure used until the patient's nutritional status has improved enough to permit surgery. Gastrostomy is a relatively minor procedure and can be performed even if the patient is very weak.

Scherer, J. C. *Introductory Medical-Surgical Nursing,* 3rd ed. Philadelphia: J. B. Lippincott Co., 1982.
Steinberg, F. U. *Care of the Geriatric Patient,* 6th ed. St. Louis: C. V. Mosby Co., 1983.

cancer, kidney (malignant hypernephroma, renal adenocarcinoma)

Cancer of the kidney is seen in adults over the age of 40; however, the risk increases in adults over 60 years of age. Both sexes can be affected, but cancer of the kidney is twice as common in men as women.

Cancer of the kidney is known as malignant hypernephroma or renal adenocarcinoma. Since these tumors are deeply seated in the body, they can become quite large before they cause symptoms. They are dangerous because they usually metastasize early but do not present distressing symptoms until late in the disease.

Symptoms of a malignant tumor may include weight loss, unexplained fever, malaise, and blood in the urine. Sometimes symptoms do not appear until the disease has metastasized.

Removal of the primary cancer is the preferred treatment if the tumor is localized or if there is severe pain, bleeding, or infection. Nephrectomy (removal of the kidney) has been done for metastatic disease but is discouraged because the mortality of the operation is greater than the likelihood of improvement. Radical nephrectomy is a hazardous procedure in the geriatric patient. When these tumors invade blood vessels and then metastasize to lung and bone, systemic therapy is of little benefit. Regression from radiation or chemotherapy only lasts several months.

An important part of treating patients with these tumors is managing a variety of syndromes. In addition, the patient should be kept as comfortable as possible with the use of analgesics and pain medication.

Scherer, J. C. *Introductory Medical-Surgical Nursing,* 3rd ed. Philadelphia: J. B. Lippincott Co., 1982.
Steinberg, F. U. *Care of the Geriatric Patient,* 6th ed. St. Louis: C. V. Mosby Co., 1983.

cancer, lip   Lip cancer is the most common cancer of the head and neck, accounting for approximately 30 percent of these cancers. Lip cancer is predominatedly seen in cigarette smokers in the sixth or seventh decades, and in blond, light-complexioned males who have occupations with sun exposure. Women are at less risk and it is thought that lipstick affords some protection. Since melanin blocks ultraviolet absorption, the incidence is lower in dark-skinned people.

About 95 percent of lip cancers are squamous cell carcinomas involving the lower lip. The early lesion may be a persistent "cold sore" with crusting, peeling, or mild ulceration that is painless. The lesions are usually present six to 24 months before treatment is initiated. These lesions grow slowly and rarely metastasize. The tendency is to spread laterally rather than deeply. Prognosis is excellent regardless of treatment. Both surgical procedures and radiation therapy are usually successful.

However, with cancer of the upper lip, the prognosis is poor. It arises spontaneously, metastasizes early and spreads more quickly. Recurrence rates are also higher.

Following treatment, patients will frequently need rehabilitative training, including speech therapy. They also need to be counseled on proper oral habits, nutrition, and the need for elimination or reduction of tobacco and alcohol products. Postoperative management is necessary to closely watch for any recurrence.

Ballenger, J. J. Diseases of the Nose, Throat, Ear, Head and Neck, 13th ed. Philadelphia: Lea & Febiger, 1985.
Steinberg, F. U. Care of the Geriatric Patient, 6th ed. St. Louis: C. V. Mosby Co., 1983.

cancer, liver The liver is commonly involved with malignancy, either from metastatic spread or as the primary site. Primary tumors are classified as hepatomas and are rare. They are most often found in males between 50 and 70 years of age. The most common malignant tumor of the liver is a metastatic lesion from the breast, lung, or gastrointestinal tract. At autopsy, 30 percent to 50 percent of all cancer patients have secondary spread to the liver.

Symptoms of a hepatoma may be vague and can be confused with cirrhosis. Once the tumor is large enough, the patient may complain of pain in the right upper quadrant of the abdomen and a sudden onset of abdominal distention. Metastatic lesions lead to changes in liver function with the liver being markedly enlarged, hard and tender.

Metastatic tumors are inoperable because they are scattered throughout the liver. Chemotherapy and radiation therapy may be attempted but are rarely successful. If a hepatoma is confined to a single lobe of the liver surgery may be attempted. The prognosis is very grim with the five years survival rate at almost zero. Radiation therapy and chemotherapy are also ineffective.

Following surgery, the patient's postoperative care is similar to that for abdominal or chest surgery. Complications may include hemorrhage, hepatic failure, metabolic abnormalities, hypoglycemia, and respiratory problems.

Rossman, I. Clinical Geriatrics, 3rd ed. Philadelphia: J. B. Lippincott, Co., 1986.
Scherer, J. C. Introductory Medical-Surgical Nursing, 3rd ed. Philadelphia: J. B. Lippincott Co., 1982.

cancer, lung Lung cancer has shown a significant increase during the last several decades. This is in part due to more accurate diagnosis, a growing number of older people in the population, an increase of cigarette smoking, and an increase in air pollution. Exposure to asbestos, radioactive dust and gases have also been implicated in lung cancer.

This is the most common fatal malignancy in males and may soon replace breast cancer as the most common malignancy in females. High-risk patients should have periodic screening with yearly chest X-rays and sputum cytology. Early detection will reduce mortality.

Cancer of the lung may be primary or metastatic. Bronchogenic carcinoma is the most common type of primary lung cancer.

The tumor initially produces no symptoms. As the tumor enlarges, the patient may experience a productive cough of mucopurulent or blood-streaked sputum. The cough may be slight at first and attributed to smoking. As the disease advances the patient may experience fatigue, weight loss, and anorexia. Dyspnea (shortness of breath) and chest pain occur in the later stages of the disease. Hemoptysis (spitting up blood) is not uncommon.

Metastasis to the lung may be found before the primary lesion is known. The mortality of persons with lung cancer is dependent on the specific type of cancer and size of tumor. Squamous cell carcinoma is the most common. Adenocarcinoma and undifferentiated small cell cancer are the least common.

Early diagnosis is difficult because symptoms do not appear until the disease is well established. X-ray and other diagnostic tests such as bronchoscopy, biopsy, examination of the sputum, and surgical exploration are used for definitive diagnosis.

Surgical removal is the treatment of choice. It is usually successful in the early stages of the disease. Depending on the size and location of the tumor, removal of lung lobe (lobectomy) or excision of entire lung (pneumonectomy) may be performed. Radiation therapy is used as an adjunct to surgery and for palliation. Chemotherapy is used to slow the course of the disease and alleviate symptoms.

Phipps, W. J., *et al. Medical Surgical Nursing.* St. Louis: C. V. Mosby Co., 1983.

Rossman, I. *Clinical Geriatrics,* 3rd ed. Philadelphia: J. B. Lippincott Co., 1986.

Scherer, J. C. *Introductory Medical-Surgical Nursing,* Philadelphia: J. B. Lippincott Co., 1982.

cancer, mouth, throat, and larynx

The most significant etiologic (cause-related) factor associated with cancer of the mouth and throat is the use of tobacco products. Cancer risk increases dramatically when five cigars or pipe bowls of tobacco are used daily or more than a pack of cigarettes is smoked daily. Chewing tobacco and the use of snuff are also factors in mouth cancer. Other high-risk factors include vitamin deficiency (especially vitamin A), malnutrition, and poor oral hygiene. Almost 60 percent of these tumors are advanced at the time of diagnosis. Survival rate is only 50 percent.

Symptoms of cancer of the mouth, throat and larynx include hoarseness, lumps in the neck, difficulty swallowing, coughing, loosening of teeth, weight loss, and swelling, pain, and ulceration. Squamous-cell carcinoma is found in almost 95 percent of cancers of the nose, mouth, and throat. The usual treatment is surgery, radiation therapy, or a combination of surgery and radiation therapy. Chemotherapy is used less frequently.

Complications in treatment are more common in patients over 70 years of age. Postoperative wound breakdown is more frequent in patients who have diabetes mellitus, cardiovascular disease and chronic obstructive pulmonary disease (COPD). Also at risk are patients who suffer a preoperative weight loss of 20 pounds or more, have a hemoglobin count of less than 10, and have a total protein count of less than 3.5. Alcoholics may have gastrointestinal bleeding. Dietary intake and negative nitrogen balance should be corrected prior to surgery.

Patients undergoing neck irradiation and/or surgery are susceptible to hypothyroidism and should have levels of thyroid hormones checked preoperatively. Hypercalcemia is also a postoperative complication. Calcium levels should be monitored preoperatively.

Following treatment, patients will frequently need rehabilitative training, including speech therapy. They also need to be counseled on proper oral habits, nutrition, and the need for elimination or reduction of tobacco and alcohol products. Postoperative management is necessary to closely watch for any recurrence.

Ballenger, J. J. *Diseases of the Nose, Throat, Ear, Head and Neck*, 13th ed. Philadelphia: Lea & Febiger, 1985.

Steinberg, F. U. *Care of the Geriatric Patient*, 6th ed. St. Louis: C. V. Mosby Co., 1983.

cancer, nose   Cancer of the nose is seen most commonly in adults over 60 years of age, probably due to a lifetime of excessive exposure to sunlight. Overexposure to X-rays and chronic skin ulcers may also increase the risk of cancer of the nose.

Squamous cell carcinoma is the most common malignant tumor of the nose and paranasal sinuses. Clinical manifestations of these tumors are not consistent. There may be pain or no pain. Nasal discharge may be serous (watery) or purulent (pussy). If pain is present, it is apt to be worse at night. Symptoms may involve the upper teeth or an upper denture may become ill-fitting. Swelling may occur on the affected side of the face, the side of the nose, or at the inner corner of the affected eye. Orbital manifestations are often found such as proptosis (bulging of eyeball in the orbit) or enophthalmos (eyeball back in the orbit).

Surgery is the usual form of treatment. Often, radiation therapy is conducted pre-operatively to shrink the size of the lesion and block the regional lymphatics. Surgery is then performed six weeks after completion of the radiation. At this time there has been maximum regression of the tumor, the radiation reaction in normal tissue is subsiding and secondary changes in the normal tissue that interfere with healing have not occurred.

Postoperative management is necessary to closely watch for any recurrence. Prosthesis may be constructed to minimize the cosmetic defect.

Ballenger, J. J. *Diseases of the Nose, Throat, Ear, Head and Neck*, 13th ed. Philadelphia: Lea & Febiger, 1985.

Steinberg, F. U. *Care of the Geriatric Patient*, 6th ed. St. Louis: C. V. Mosby Co., 1983.

cancer, ovarian   Malignant tumors of the ovary are frequently far advanced when they are first detected and are thus inoperable. It is believed many of these tumors arise from ovarian cysts. The greatest number of patients appear between the ages 50 to 80 years of age, but the peak incidence is about age 77.

Usually there are not symptoms with ovarian cancer but some women complain of vague abdominal symptoms for a long time before the diagnosis is made. Pressure on the bladder may occur, leading to frequent urination. It is, therefore, important to rule out ovarian cancer in any woman over 40 years of age, especially if she has a history of multiple spontaneous abortions, involuntary sterility, enlarged abdomen, abnormal vaginal bleeding, or a family history of ovarian cancer.

The ovary is unique in that not only does it give rise to a great number of tumors, but it is the recipient of tumor metastases from other organs. Two of the most common cancers that metastasize to the ovaries are breast and colon cancers.

Treatment for carcinoma of the ovary is surgical removal of the uterus, fallopian tubes, ovaries, and appendix. This is commonly followed by chemotherapy rather than radiation therapy. Since many of these patients are elderly, it is important to evaluate the renal function and electrocardiogram before certain drugs are used.

Management of the patient following surgery is similar to that following general abdominal surgery. Since this surgery is usually so invasive, recovery is usually less than 25 percent after five years.

See also CANCER, UTERINE.

Rossman, I. *Clinical Geriatrics*, 3rd ed. Philadelphia: J. B. Lippincott Co., 1986.

cancer, pancreatic   The incidence of cancer of the pancreas is, inexplicably, steadily rising. The disease in males over the age of 75 is eight to 10 times that in the general population. Early diagnosis is often difficult because symptoms may not be apparent until the disease is far advanced.

Abdominal pain is the predominant symptom and manifests as a dull ache or boring pain. Weight loss occurs in almost all patients and can be rapid and progressive despite maintaining a good appetite and adequate food intake. Jaundice is also typical. Bowel symptoms such as constipation, diarrhea, bloating, and flatulence are also common.

Radiation therapy or chemotherapy are used on inoperable tumors but do not offer a cure. The most that can be hoped for is to enable the patient to be more comfortable. In some cases, surgery may be performed but the mortality rate is very high.

The course of pancreatic cancer is rapidly progressive and metastatic spread occurs early. Survival from the time of diagnosis to death is usually less than six months.

Rossman, I. *Clinical Geriatrics,* 3rd ed. Philadelphia: J. B. Lippincott Co., 1986.
Scherer, J. C. *Introductory Medical-Surgical Nursing,* 3rd ed. Philadelphia: J. B. Lippincott Co., 1982.

cancer, prostate   Cancer of the prostate is a major health problem in the geriatric male. It is the second most common cause of cancer deaths in men. As life expectancy increases, more and more men live to an age when the incidence of this disease is highest.

Initially, there are no symptoms. However, when the tumor grows large enough, it will obstruct urinary flow. Thus, when a patient complains of urinary symptoms, such as retention, painful urination, or blood in the urine, the disease is already in a more advanced stage.

Radiation therapy is the usual method of treatment and is at least as effective as surgical removal in controlling the disease. The advantage of this method of treatment is a lower incidence of incontinence and impotence. However, if urinary obstruction occurs, surgical treatment may be necessary. The disadvantages of this treatment are that it virtually guarantees impotence and may result in serious urinary control problems.

If the cancer spreads, it is by way of the blood stream and lymphatics to the pelvic lymph glands and bones, particularly the lumbar vertebrae, pelvis, and hips. The first symptoms may be back pain or sciatica due to metastases to the nerve sheaths. Systemic hormonal therapy is the method of treatment when metastases develop.

After surgery, some dietary control may be indicated if the patient experiences bladder or bowel incontinence. Perineal exercises to improve muscle tone may also be helpful.

See also PROSTATE HYPERTROPHY, BENIGN.

Scherer, J. C. *Introductory Medical-Surgical Nursing,* 3rd ed. Philadelphia: J. B. Lippincott Co., 1982.
Steinberg, F. U. *Care of the Geriatric Patient,* 6th ed. St. Louis: C. V. Mosby Co., 1983.

cancer, skin   The skin is the most frequent site of carcinoma. Fortunately, skin cancer is not usually life-threatening since the lesions can be detected when they are still small and more readily curable. The incidence of skin cancer increases with age, partly due to the cumulative effects of a lifetime exposure to the sun and the elements, such as winds. Chronically exposed areas such as the forehead, hands, and nose are commonly affected.

Symptoms of skin cancer include sores or ulcers that do not heal, and sudden changes in color, size, and texture of moles, warts, or birthmarks.

Basal-cell carcinoma is the most common form of skin cancer. This is a slow growing carcinoma, locally invasive, with little tendency to metastasize. The most common type of basal cell carcinoma begins as a small, smooth, rounded, pearly or waxy-looking papule with telangiectatic (dilated, tortous) vessels on the surface.

These tumors may be treated by curettage and electrodesiccation, surgical excision, irradiation, or topical chemotherapy. In the vast number of patients the cure rate is 95 percent or better.

Squamous-cell carcinomas of the skin are found less frequently than basal cell carcinomas but are more likely to metastasize. This type of cancer is found on chronically sun-damaged skin of the backs of the hands, arms, ears, neck, and face. Surgical excision is the most common form of treatment.

Those with skin cancers should be cautioned to avoid, as much as possible, further sun exposure. Sunscreens, long-sleeved shirts, and wide-brimmed hats are encouraged when the person is outdoors.

Steinberg, F. U. *Care of the Geriatric Patient,* 6th ed. St. Louis: C. V. Mosby Co., 1983.

cancer, stomach   Ninety-five percent of malignant stomach neoplasms are adenocarcinomas. Thus, the term gastric cancer generally refers to adenocarcinoma of the stomach. Adenocanthoma, squamous-cell carcinoma, and carcinoid tumors also occur in the stomach.

Stomach cancer occurs more frequently in men than women, and occurs most often between the ages of 50 and 70. It usually occurs in the distal third and extends directly through the stomach wall into adjacent tissues, lymphatics, and other abdominal organs. It may metastasize through the bloodstream to the lungs or bones.

Heredity and chronic inflammation of the stomach appear to be causative factors. Early symptoms of gastric cancer are often vague. As the tumor enlarges it begins to obstruct either the pyloric or cardiac openings. The patient then may notice a prolonged feeling of fullness after eating, anorexia, weight loss, and weakness from anemia. The stool usually contains concealed (occult) blood. Pain is a late symptom.

Diagnosis is made by fluoroscopy (dynamic x-ray exam), gastroscopy (looking with a scope), and a barium swallow gastroscopy. Gastric analysis may show the absence of free hydrochloric acid. The treatment of cancer of the stomach is partial (subtotal) or total gastrectomy. The type of surgery depends on the location of the tumor and whether metastasis has occurred. Following a total gastrectomy, the jejunum is anastomased to the esophagus. A subtotal gastrectomy may be possible depending on the location and the size of the tumor. Retaining part of the stomach preserves a more normal function.

Patients with a total gastrectomy must eat frequent small meals because they are unable to tolerate large meals. They should eat easily digested foods. Injections of vitamin B_{12} are usually necessary for the rest of the patient's life, once the stomach is removed to prevent pernicous anemia. The intrinsic factor from the stomach necessary for absorption of vitamin B_{12} is no longer produced.

Scherer, J. C. *Introductory Medical-Surgical Nursing,* 3rd ed. Philadelphia: J. B. Lippincott Co., 1982.
Steinberg, F. U. *Care of the Geriatric Patient,* 6th ed. St. Louis: C. V. Mosby Co., 1983.

cancer, uterine   Cancer of the uterus is most likely in postmenopausal women. High-risk patients suffer from obesity, hypertension, diabetes mellitus, or a family history of uterine cancer.

Bleeding is the earliest and most common symptom of uterine cancer. At first there may be spotting, especially after intercourse. If untreated, the discharge continues, growing bloody and malodorous. There may be pain and symptoms of pressure on the bladder or bowel.

All vaginal bleeding after menopause should be considered to be cancer and must be investigated. An examination and PAP smear are conducted first and if cancer is suspected, the patient may require a diagnostic dilatation and curettage under anesthesia.

Treatment of cancer of the uterus may include a hysterectomy (surgical removal of the uterus), chemotherapy, radiotherapy, hormonal therapy, or a combination of any of these.

Women who have been treated for uterine cancer should have regular gynecologic exams because of the possibility of recurrence or metastases. Possible complications include the fatal spread of cancer to the bladder, rectum, and distant organs. Regular PAP smears can detect early uterine cancer. With early diagnosis and treatment, 90 percent of women with this cancer survive at least five years.

See also CANCER, OVARIAN.

Scherer, J. C. *Introductory Medical-Surgical Nursing,* 3rd ed. Philadelphia: J. B. Lippincott Co., 1982.
Steinberg, F. U. *Care of the Geriatric Patient,* 6th ed. St. Louis: C. V. Mosby Co., 1983.

cardiac decompensation   See CONGESTIVE HEART FAILURE.

cardiac incompetence   See CONGESTIVE HEART FAILURE.

cardiac insufficiency   See CONGESTIVE HEART FAILURE.

caregiver   One who provides care and assistance to an aged and infirm loved one is known as a caregiver. Because of the great improvements in modern medicine and public health, people are living longer. Many of these elderly suffer chronic ailments and the usual infirmities that go with increasing age. Thus, as the population ages, the need for long-term care and caregivers will increase.

With the increasingly high costs of long-term care facilities, more families are assuming the role of caregiver. In the vast number of cases, it is a female who is the primary caregiver—a daughter, daughter-in-law, sister, or niece.

When men do assume the caregiver role they tend to devote far less time to it than women do, and they frequently employ assistance, according to an article that appeared in *Modern Maturity,* the magazine of the American Association of Retired Persons (AARP). In many instances men assume an indirect and secondary role in caregiving, such as managing finances or doing home repairs because they learn (or are "socialized" in the language of the social sciences) to hold jobs and provide financial support—the primary adult male roles.

Women have usually assumed household duties and personal care of elderly family members because these have been the major feminine roles that begin even in childhood with dressing, feeding, and playing with dolls. Because of their roles women are thought to develop more sympathetic reactions to pain and suffering. For this reason they may become more prone to the "compassion trap"—undertaking labors of love that may cause hardship and offer little else than emotional compensation.

Sometimes middle-aged women who have completed childrearing responsibilities, and were about to become free to relax and enjoy life, are compelled to care for a disabled parent—a mother who has fallen and broken her hip or a father diagnosed to have disabling hypertensive disease. The empty nest becomes refilled, and the newly freed woman finds herself once again providing daily care to others: feeding, bathing, cooking, helping, visiting doctor's offices for appointments, providing transportation, giving medicines, watching diets, and always being available.

According to research carried out at Princeton University, the proportion of women engaged in caregiving to older parents and relatives has probably increased in recent years. Sixty-five percent of 50-year-old women in the United States had living mothers in 1980, whereas in 1940 the figure was 37 percent. Further, the average age of caregivers today is 57, with one-third of them over 65 and nearly one-quarter in only fair health themselves.

While some women find the care of their parent(s) personally fulfilling—an opportunity to pay back their childhood nurturing—guilt is considered to be the primary reason that many caregivers push themselves to fulfill unrealistic expectations. The dual mistake many make is to assume that they must take care of their parents just as their parents cared for them as children, and that their parents want and expect them to provide round-the-clock care.

Caring for an older person is not the same as caring for a child. A child progresses in development, even if incapacitated in some way. An older person, in most cases, will probably decline. Not all older people are sweet and loveable, and caregivers occasionally fight resentment in caring for their unloving or unloved parents.

There is a misconception that parents want and expect their children to take them into their homes. When given a choice, most of the elderly prefer to maintain a home separate from their children. They do not want to lose control of their lives and need to remain independent. But most important, they do not want to be a burden. Parents want their children to care about them—not for them.

Whatever the future development of gender roles in providing support to elderly parents, programs to help caregivers have developed rapidly in the 1980s (note, for instance, the Alzheimer's Society National Headquarters in Chicago, Ill. mentioned in Appendix II), and there is growing attention to financing these through public funds and company benefit programs. Research shows that both those who receive as well as those who give the care may benefit from the following types of assistance: educational training to increase adaptive coping; respite from care activities provided by day-care services or short nursing home stays for the elderly dependent person; and psychotherapy for the caregiver designed to manage feelings of anxiety, guilt, frustration, and depression. Growing public awareness of the burden of responsibility for older family members promises increasing help for caregivers in the future.

A Guide for Long Distance Caregivers. AARP booklet, 1986.
Wood, J. "Caregiver," in *Modern Maturity,* August–September, 1987.

caregiving, long-distance Society today is highly mobile. Many families relocate, sometimes frequently, for employment reasons. Likewise, older people move more often than in the past. During the 1970s, for instance, the number of retirement-age people who moved from state to state increased by 58 percent.

In consequence, families with ailing older relatives who live far away may face difficult problems in caring for them. Travel to provide help is costly in itself, but the greatest problems arise in finding and accessing services needed by the elderly relative.

State units on aging offer a good starting point for needed guidance. By law these are required to offer information and referral services at no cost. States are divided into smaller areas, each with a designated Area Agency on Aging to spearhead local services for the elderly. These, too, can be contacted for information about community resources for elder care.

People who need assistance can refer to the government section of the telephone book under state, city, and county headings; these list home care services, human services, mayors' or governors' agents for aging, and the Social Security Administration. The current local "Silver Pages Directory" may identify local area agencies on aging.

Others that may provide help are the United Way, Catholic Charities, Jewish Family Services, Protestant Welfare Agencies, and Family Services of America. Neighbors and friends who have used elder services may be able to offer advice on getting started, and direct referrals to service agencies for the elderly are often provided by physicians, nurses, social workers, and clergy.

A Guide for Long Distance Caregivers. AARP booklet, 1986.

caries, senile (cavities of teeth)   One of the chief disorders affecting the teeth of the older person is known as senile caries. This is decalcification or decay of the tooth at the cervical area—the junction of the crown of the tooth and the gingival epithelium (the gum area). As the soft tissue and bone recedes, the cementum of the root surface is exposed and these areas may decay.

The chief etiologic factors in cervical caries in the aged are changes in the quality and quantity of saliva production. This is complicated by the soft, easy to chew diet, high in refined carbohydrates, to which many elderly people must resort. Also, older individuals frequently lack the manual dexterity necessary for good oral hygiene due to arthritic changes, the effects of a stroke, or other physical disabilities.

Symptoms of dental caries include a visible defect in the tooth, with air or cold sensitivity and pain.

Proper brushing and flossing remain basic to preventive dentistry. A battery-operated tooth brush or Water Pik may be useful to the person with physical limitations. Artificial saliva and fluoride gel are available over the counter and help alleviate the symptoms of senile caries. Treatment for dental caries involves removal of the decayed portion and replacing it with a simple filling, inlay, or crown.

When decay has reached the pulp of a tooth, it may be necessary to extract the tooth or have root canal therapy. It is, therefore, crucial that the elderly patient attend to his or her dental health thoroughly and routinely.

Steinberg, F. U. *Care of the Geriatric Patient,* 6th ed. St. Louis: C. V. Mosby Co., 1983.

carotid obstruction   See TRANSIENT ISCHEMIC ATTACK.

cataract   A cataract is a clouding of the lens of the eye, which blurs normal vision.

Cataracts can be the result of heredity, trauma, inflammation, diabetes mellitus, a birth defect, or the use of drugs such as steroids. The cause of the vast majority of cataracts is unknown and presumed to be a part of the aging process. This type of cataract is referred to as a senile cataract and is the type seen in approximately 90 percent of all cataract patients.

Symptoms of cataracts include a gradual decrease of vision, double vision, and a decrease in color perception.

Treatment for cataracts involves surgical removal of the opaque lens. There are no medicines, drops, or treatments that will dissolve a cataract. Protection from ultraviolet light may help prevent cataracts.

When the lens of the eye is removed it is necessary to replace it in order to see well. There are three ways of replacing the lens: cataract eyeglasses, a contact lens (lens that is worn on the outside of eye), and an intraocular lens (lens that is implanted inside the eye at the time of surgery).

Cataract glasses are the simplest optical correction, although they make objects appear 25 percent larger, and severely restrict peripheral vision. Many people adjust to cataract glasses fairly well, but special care should be taken during the adjustment period. These people may at first have difficulty driving, going up and down stairs, pouring liquids, and walking.

Contact lenses can also be used for an optical correction after cataract surgery. Contacts only magnify objects by 8 percent and allow full peripheral vision, therefore reducing the visual distortion. Contact lenses are not suitable for everyone, however. Frequently older people, especially those with arthritis, find they lack the manual dexterity to handle contact lenses. Extended-wear contacts can be fitted in some cases. These are contacts that can be left in the eye for several weeks at a time. When necessary, these lenses are removed, cleansed, and replaced at the doctor's office. This may be a suitable alternative for people who have difficulty handling their lenses.

The third method for optical correction is the intraocular lens. This is an artificial plastic lens that is implanted inside the eye immediately following the cataract removal. The intraocular lens allows full side vision and objects appear their normal size. There is a slight increase of risk at the time of surgery with intraocular lens implantation; however, approximately 95 percent of cataract surgeries with lens implants are successful.

Most of the time the intraocular lens is the most effective way to replace the opaque lens in an older person. Most cataract patients have an intraocular lens implant after lens removal.

Newell, F. W. *Ophthalmology Principles and Concepts*, 6th ed. St. Louis: C. V. Mosby Co., 1986.

Slatt, B. J., and Stein, H. A. *The Ophthalmic Assistant Fundamentals and Clinical Practice*, 4th ed. St. Louis: C. V. Mosby Co., 1983.

cavities, teeth   See CARIES, SENILE.

centenarians   The 1980 census reported 25,000 United States citizens over 100 years of age, and the Bureau of the Census estimated that this figure would grow to 45,000 by 1985 and to 100,000 by the year 2000. Because of the increasing effectiveness of strategies for prolonging life, projections are that the number of centenarians in America may reach 19 million by 2080.

Thompson, L. "After Age 30, Survival Is Infinite," in *Aging*, Goldstein, E. C., ed. Vol. 3, Art. 17. Boca Raton, Fl.: Social Issues Resource Series, Inc., 1981.

Twigg, H. D. "Aging Inches Across America," in *Aging*, Goldstein, E. C., ed. Vol. 2, Art. 69. Boca Raton, Fl.: Social Issues Resource Series, Inc., 1981.

U.S. Bureau of the Census. *Statistical Abstract of the United States: 1989*, 109th ed. Washington, D.C.: U.S. Government Printing Office.

centrophenoxine   Centrophenoxine is a drug that reduces the accumulation of "age pigments," called lipofuscin, in the body tissues of some laboratory animals. Whether or not the pigments affect longevity is not known at present. Centrophenoxine treatment has increased life expectancies and lifespans in mice and fruit flies. In humans, the therapy has improved blood glucose levels and maximum oxygen consumption. The animals and humans in these experiments lost weight, leading the scientists to conclude that the drug's possible life-extending effects could be related to weight loss.

See AGING, BIOLOGICAL THEORY OF.

Kurz, M. A. "Theories of Aging and Popular Claims for Extending Life," in *Aging*, Goldstein, E. C., ed. Vol. 2, Art. 88. Boca Raton, Fl.: Social Issues Resource Series, Inc., 1981.

cerebral vascular accident (CVA, stroke)   A stroke is a sudden onset of neurologic deficit due to disruption of vascular function. This may be caused by partial or total blockage of blood vessels to the brain by a hemorrhage, or blood clot, of the brain.

In the United States 50 percent of the people suffering their first stroke are 70 or older. Stroke is more prominent in males than females.

There are three groups who are at a high risk for stroke. People with transient or mild neurologic events, those with a cardiac disease that predisposes to embolism, and asymptomatic people with a carotid bruit (indicating a blockage) comprise this group. Those who have experienced TIAs (transient ischemic attacks) also have a high risk for stroke. TIAs are indications of cerebrovascular disease and are a warning that a CVA could occur at any time.

Stroke caused by an embolism occurs suddenly. When a stroke is caused by a cerebral embolism, there is usually not a loss in consciousness although there is an alteration in the state of consciousness. Some neurologic symptoms such as hemiplegia (paralysis of one side of body), aphasia (inability to speak), or hemianopia (loss of side vision of both eyes) may also be noted.

Stroke caused by hemorrhage may occur suddenly or may be slowly progressive. It is generally caused by an aneurysm that bursts or a congenital malformation of the vessel. Nausea, vomiting, headaches, and stiff neck are symptoms of this type of hemorrhagic stroke.

Symptoms of a stroke depend upon the cause of the stroke as well as the part of brain affected. Generally the symptoms include a decrease in the level of consciousness, sensory loss on one side, paralysis, visual field loss, speech defects, mental confusion, hypertension, headache, nausea, vomiting, and difficulty breathing.

Hypertension is the single most important risk factor for stroke. Other factors include heart disease, diabetes, smoking, and hyperlipemia (elevated blood cholesterol).

Once a stroke has occurred, there is nothing that can be done to restore the dead brain tissue. Treatment includes preventing the recurrence of stroke with anticoagulation medication and medical control of the hypertension. Agents are available to control cerebral edema. Some forms of aneurysms and hemorrhages can be treated surgically. Rehabilitation is important to maximize the degree of functional adaptation and self-care. Physiotherapists and speech therapists may also help with the person's rehabilitation.

CVAs can cause permanent damage to the brain. Because of the seriousness of strokes, high-risk patients should be well informed about the possible warning signals and symptoms of a cerebral vascular accident.

See also ANEURYSM; ARTERIOSCLEROSIS; TRANSIENT ISCHEMIC ATTACK.

Scherer, J. C. *Introductory Medical-Surgical Nursing,* 3rd ed. Philadelphia: J. B. Lippincott Co., 1982.

Steinberg, F. U. *Care of the Geriatric Patient,* 6th ed. St. Louis: C. V. Mosby Co., 1983.

"change of life"   See MENOPAUSE.

CHF   See CONGESTIVE HEART FAILURE.

Chinese elderly   China will have a population of 80 million people over age 65 by the year 2000 and more than 178 million people by 2025—the largest elderly population in the entire world. In 1983 the China National Committee on Aging, made up of physicians, social scientists, and health and welfare officials, was set up to plan for an improved life and social role for Chinese elderly, and this group is addressing the problem of providing for the world's greatest number of older people. The Committee advises the government on programs for the elderly, including social insurance, relief, and medical services.

Unlike the practice in many Western nations where the government is expected to take a major role in assistance to the elderly, the family in China is explicitly held responsible for helping and supporting parents. The constitution of the nation contains clauses designating the family as the responsible agent. Consistent with this provision, maltreatment of the elderly is prohibited by law.

In China, men in government offices retire at 60 and women at 55, a provision designed to ensure that there are enough jobs to provide employment for young people in the vast 600 million–person Chinese workforce (the U.S. workforce is approximately 130 million persons). In factories and offices retirement age is 55 for men and 50 for women. Seventy-five percent of the Chinese workforce is employed in agriculture, however, and it is uncertain just what a compulsory retirement age means for this segment of the population. Retired workers receive a pension of 75 percent of their wages if they have worked 20 years or longer.

Most retired Chinese live in the countryside and do light work to support themselves. Some prefer to live with their children and others to live independently. Childless people without incomes in the cities and countryside are guaranteed their livelihood from the collective, which is either a small community that functions as an economic unit (e.g., a farm town), or the equivalent of a city government. There are 23,000 retirement homes in the countryside. In many cities neighborhood committees have organized volunteer groups to care for old people who are experiencing problems, and in some cases these groups take on the entire support of individuals.

Chinese policy toward the elderly has aimed to maintain older people in active roles consistent with their knowledge, interest, and ability levels. Old workers and technicians come back to their factories to help train young workers. Forty percent of veteran workers and cadres work as advisors and consultants in local associations, government offices, and enterprises. Many take up hobbies they never had time for before; they visit relatives and friends.

Over 70 senior citizen schools have been established. They have been turned into activity centers for the elderly. Over 10 million retired people do physical exercises each day. Many places have clubs and recreational centers for them.

Hen Chong Wei, *et al.* "Addresses to the Sino-American Workshop on Gerontology." Beijing National University, Tuesday, September 18, 1986. Unpublished.
Zheng. S. "New Problems, New Prospects," in *Aging,* Goldstein, E. C., ed. Vol. 3, Art. 16. Boca Raton, Fl.: Social Issues Resource Series, Inc., 1981.

cholecystectomy See GALL BLADDER DISEASE.

cholelithiasis See GALL BLADDER DISEASE.

chromium Chromium is a substance researchers believe slows the aging process. It is useful in preventing and lowering high blood pressure. It also helps reduce cholesterol levels and hardening of the arteries. Therefore, it may be helpful in fighting the mental changes that accompany senility.

Foods that are rich in chromium are liver, beef, whole grain bread, brewer's yeast, and fresh vegetables, especially beets. Though it is not proven that chromium will add years to life, chances are good that it will help to keep individuals functioning better.

See also AGING, BIOLOGICAL THEORY OF.

Martin, P. "Good News About Growing Older," in *Aging,* Goldstein, E. C., ed. Vol. 2, Art. 41. Boca Raton, Fl.: Social Issues Resource Series, Inc., 1981.

chronic and acute conditions Because one or more chronic health conditions (such as arthritis, high blood pressure, heart trouble, diabetes, poor hearing, and eyesight) affect nearly 90 percent of the older population, it is common to think that illness is normal for the old. Chronic illness, however, needs to be distinguished from specific episodes of acute illness (such as a heart attack, a bout with pneumonia, or a bone fracture). Individuals who have chronic conditions can usually manage things by themselves by modifying their diets and lifestyles, taking medications, or using devices such as hearing aids. Acute conditions, however, are usually much more serious, often requiring hospitalization and attention from physicians, nurses, physical therapists, or other trained health personnel.

Contrary to what one might expect, incidents of acute illness are three times more frequent among children under age 6 than for people over 45 because of the common childhood diseases. The figures on acute health problems for various age groups are reported by the U.S. Bureau of the Census as follows:

Acute Disease Rate per 100 Population

Age	Infective and Parasitic	Respiratory		Digestive System	Injuries
		Upper	Other		
>5	55.5	96.6	81.3	8.2	23.4
5–17	39.9	51.2	88.2	8.3	34.5
18–24	19.6	37.8	60.7	7.2	32.9
25–44	19.5	27.0	59.8	5.1	27.9
45–64	9.5	20.4	46.3	4.5	20.4
65+	8.8	19.6	28.6	7.3	21.3

SOURCE: National Center for Health Statistics.

Two significant points with respect to chronic disease among the elderly relate, first, to the individual's feelings about his or her health, and, second, to restricted activity caused by chronic disease. As long as people continue to feel satisfied with their health, chronic illness does not interfere with their quality of life, and as long as they do not need assistance with activities of daily living (cooking, bathing, toileting, etc.) they do not require support from others nor do they incur personal or public expenses for assistance.

An indication of the importance of the first point can be seen from data elicited in the General Social Survey. This shows that only about 52 percent of the population over 65 describes their health as "good" to "excellent," but that over 75 percent rate themselves as fairly satisfied or a great deal satisfied with their health. (The National Health Interview Survey carried out by the National Center for Health Statistics, incidentally, reports a more positive picture of self-assessed health than the GSS—it shows that over 70 percent of the population over 65 rates its health as good to excellent).

In regard to the problem of disability due to chronic conditions, the National Long-Term Care Survey showed that over 60 percent of the population over 65 had no disability, and that less than 20 percent had any limitation in a major activity of daily living (i.e., that they were unable to carry on one or more activities of daily living, such as

Age and Chronic Health Problems

Chronic Conditions	Number of Conditions per 1,000 Population	
	Under 45 Years	65 and Over
Arthritis	30.2	480.4
High Blood Pressure	42.1	394.4
Hearing Impairment	39.6	295.6
Heart Disease	32.5	276.6
Orthopedic Impairment	93.8	172.7
Chronic Sinusitis	130.2	169.4
Diabetes	6.3	98.3
Visual Impairment	22.3	95.0

dressing and eating). Statistics on chronic conditions show the greater frequency among people over 65 when compared with people aged 18–44. These figures also suggest that most activity limitation is due to heart conditions, high blood pressure, and arthritis.

Physician visits for chronic conditions are also more frequent among the elderly than among younger age groups. The annual rate of such visits per person is 4.7 at age 25–44, and these then rise to 6.6 at 45–64, 8.1 at 65–74, and to 10.6 after age 75. The very young (under age 5) also have a fairly high rate of physician visits for chronic conditions—6.3 visits per person per year.

Problems of chronic illness are often controlled and even overcome by individuals acting by their own initiative and without help from others. Physical fitness and exercise—activities that should be maintained throughout life—are especially beneficial in late life when an affirmative effort is needed to keep healthy, and when individuals have more time for them than during working and childrearing years. People who have chronic health problems should not undertake physical activity and exercise without consulting a physician; nor does exercise need to be strenuous—walking, swimming, bicycling on a stationary bicycle, etc. will promote good health and also maintain muscle and joint conditioning even when done with moderation.

Other measures to control chronic illness include good nutrition to reduce blood pressure and cholesterol levels. Avoiding drugs (except when prescribed by a physician) and alcohol, controlling stress, and discontinuing smoking can all reduce sickness, ameliorate chronic poor health, and promote a long life of high quality. The major obstacle to adopting a sound health regimen often does not lie in the condition of one's health itself, but rather in developing the willpower and determination needed for self-control and for engaging in pursuit of fitness activities. When motivation is a problem, joining with others who are participating in activity programs, reading inspirational books, and seeking out training programs to overcome bad habits and promote good ones will frequently supply the willpower to begin an exercise regimen.

National Center for Health Statistics, Dawson, D. A., and P. F. Adams. Current Estimates from the National Health Interview Survey; United States, 1986. *Vital and Health Statistics.* DHHS Pub. No. (PHS) 87–1592. Series 10, No. 164. Public Health Service. Washington, D.C.: U.S. Government Printing Office, 1987.

Russell, C. H., and I. Megaard. *The General Social Survey, 1972–1976: The State of the American People.* New York: Springer-Verlag, 1988.

U.S. Bureau of the Census. *Statistical Abstract of the United States: 1989,* 109th ed. Washington, D.C., 1989.

climacteric   See MENOPAUSE.

climates, extreme   The biological adaptation of humans to extreme climates was one of the earliest subjects to interest gerontological researchers. The pygmy population in hot, humid rain forests has been studied extensively, and no evidence of accelerated aging has been found. The Eskimos, who are exposed to extreme cold, do not appear to age any more rapidly than people who live under more moderate climatic conditions. High altitudes (above 10,000 feet) do not speed up the aging process, and, in fact, the incidence of high blood pressure and ischemic (lack of blood) heart disease is consistently lower among people living at high altitudes than those living at sea level. These findings suggest that aging is not caused by external environmental influences but may be programmed into the human and animal genetic structure.

See also AFRICAN PYGMY; ESKIMOS.

Brocklehurst, J. C. *Textbook of Geriatric Medicine and Gerontology.* New York: Churchhill Livingstone, 1985.

clothing   Common standards on old age in the past did not generally consider older people in terms of fashion. To satisfy prevailing tastes, older men were expected to wear formal suits while women had to wear pale, muted, or dull colors. The effect of clothing on the self-image of the old went unnoticed. Fortunately, the dull, drab tradition of elder-wear was swept aside in the clothing style revolution of the 1960s, though perhaps not to the same degree as among the youth. On the whole, however, older people today have greater latitude to indulge personal tastes, express their freedom, and chose clothing for style or comfort as they will.

For people who need to assist dependent older family members with the choice of clothing, it is important to keep in mind certain principles that should govern the selection of clothing throughout life. Clothing helps to give one a measure of personal identity, a high (or low, unfortunately) self-image, and a sense of comfort and security. For individuals who have restricted body movement due to arthritis, an injury, or an operation, a sense of competence can be maintained by use of apparel that's easy to put on—clothing with Velcro fasteners, large-sized buttons and button holes, zippers, pre-tied neck ties, and simple buckles, for example.

Practical clothing choices also make sense. Long robes and slip-on slippers, while seemingly comfortable and casual, need to be avoided because they can cause the wearer to trip. Shoes with laces and low broad heels can prevent tripping.

Because circulation slows with age, garters and girdles don't make sense for older women, nor do rolling down or twisting of stocking tops below the knee. Older men need to shun the calf strangling elastic top socks that have become standard in most department stores. Likewise, underclothes should not constrain nor restrict the crotch or armpits. Because incontinence, due to weakening of muscles used to control elimination, can sometimes be a problem, it may be necessary for some persons to wear underclothing that is absorbent and easy to launder. Warm clothing, made of smooth fabric that does not irritate the skin, with full-length sleeves, also makes sense.

To overcome visual disabilities that may interfere with dressing, it is sensible to provide bright lights in dressing areas, arrange clothing in drawers and closets according to color schemes, and hang blouses and matching slacks and jackets on the same hanger. If a member of the family must move to a nursing home, it is useful to remember that nursing homes and summer camps share something in common—laundry gets mixed up—so the wise relative will see to it that the nursing home resident's clothing is labeled with indelible ink.

Gillies, J. *A Guide to Caring for and Coping with Aging Parents.* Nashville: Thomas Nelson Publishers, 1981.

coenzyme Q   See CoQ.

colon cancer   See CANCER, COLON AND RECTAL.

communicating with the elderly   Nearly all individuals experience some degree of sensory loss as they age, whether it be in taste, touch, sight, hearing, or sensitivity to pain (pain threshold). Of these diminished senses, the loss of hearing is very common in later life. It stands next to arthritis as a chronic condition (90 percent of the U.S. population experiences some degree of joint degeneration by the age of 40). About 30 percent of the population over age 65 has a hearing impairment, with males, at about 34 percent, leading females, at about 25 percent.

While hearing aids and training can do much to alleviate hearing difficulties, they do not always eliminate them. Nor do aids overcome other problems that can affect communication—problems of poor eyesight; the speed of speech that an older person can comprehend; difficulty in distinguishing tones; weakened power to transmit messages by speech; and physical weakness following illness.

Awareness that the older person may experience a variety of communication problems can do much to improve family and personal relationships. Simple measures often help, as by turning down the radio or TV during conversation, standing before the person or leaning close when talking, slowing down one's rate of speech, and enunciating carefully and clearly.

Raising one's voice can help also, but this practice requires good judgment because older people who may be quite deaf to high tones can often hear deep tones perfectly clearly. Under such circumstances loud shouting should be replaced with a deeper voice pitch, which will avoid a sharp reprimand from the older person—"Stop shouting at me! I'm not deaf!" Some individuals shout at old people because the old tend to respond slowly. This impulse should be curbed because the slow response may not be due to deafness but to the slower rate at which the elderly process and respond to information mentally.

Planning conversational topics before visits can help, especially so if an older person is disoriented or senile. It is also well to focus conversation on routine subjects—the time of day, the day of the week, the weather, and doings and visits of friends and family members. Nor is there any need to feel discomfort over gaps or even long conversational silences; sometimes just sitting quietly by or gently touching an older person are the best forms of communication.

See also CORRESPONDENCE; REALITY ORIENTATION; VISITING, TO HOMEBOUND AND INSTITUTIONALIZED ELDERLY.

Gillies, J. *A Guide to Caring for and Coping with Aging Parents.* Nashville: Thomas Nelson Publishers, 1981.

confusional state, acute   See DELIRIUM.

congestive heart failure (heart failure, cardiac decompensation, cardiac insufficiency, cardiac incompetence, CHF)   Congestive heart failure (CHF) develops when the heart is unable to pump an adequate supply of blood to meet the demands of the body. This condition affects three to four million Americans. Seventy-five percent of affected people are older than 60. There are about 45 cases of congestive heart failure per 1,000 after the age of 65.

Congestive heart failure can be caused by a variety of things, including arteriosclerosis, myocardial infarction, myocarditis, ventricular aneurysm, mitral or aortic regurgitation, atrial or ventricular septal defects,

hypertension, pericarditis, constrictive cardiomyopathies, and hyperthyroidism. Frequently, in the elderly, congestive heart failure is caused by a combination of factors.

Symptoms may develop acutely and include syncope (fainting), shock, acute pulmonary edema, cardiac arrest, or sudden death. Acute congestive heart failure may be seen following a myocardial infarction. Chronic congestive heart failure symptoms develop gradually and include pitting edema of the feet and ankles (which disappears during the night), fatigue, confusion, weight gain, persistent cough, abnormal respirations, difficulty breathing while lying flat, and dyspnea (shortness of breath) on exertion.

The primary goals of treatment for congestive heart failure are to restore a balance between the supply and demand for blood by the body and to remove excessive fluid.

In the acute phase of congestive heart failure the person may require bed rest, supplemental oxygen, diuretics, and digitalis.

Treatment of congestive heart failure should involve identifying the underlying condition and correcting it, if possible. If the underlying condition cannot be controlled, congestive heart failure may become a chronic problem. Therapy for chronic congestive heart failure includes a salt restricted diet, diuretics, heart stimulants, and sometimes a change in lifestyle. Generally the person can continue his or her activities with moderation. Diuretics combined with a salt-restricted diet remain the mainstay of therapy in older people. Potassium supplements will probably be necessary to counteract the potassium loss caused by diuretics. Digitalis may be prescribed to help the heart to be more effective in pumping blood. Treatment is not curative and recurrences are frequent, especially when the person deviates from his or her medication and diet.

People with congestive heart failure are particularly vulnerable to infection, especially pneumonia and influenza. An infection often aggravates the underlying heart disease and leads to rapid, frequent recurrences of the congestive heart failure.

If possible, the older person with congestive heart failure should weigh daily. If a sudden weight gain is detected, prompt consultation with a physician may prevent an acute attack of congestive heart failure.

See also PULMONARY EDEMA, ACUTE.

Phipps, W. J., *et al. Medical Surgical Nursing*. St. Louis: C. V. Mosby Co., 1983.
Rogers, C. S., and McCue, J. D. *Managing Chronic Disease*. Oradell, N.J.: Medical Economics Books, 1987.
Scherer, J. C. *Introductory Medical-Surgical Nursing*, Philadelphia: J. B. Lippincott Co., 1982.

constipation (see Tables 9, 19, 20) Constipation is decreased motility of the colon or retention of feces in the lower colon or rectum. The longer feces remains in the colon, the greater the reabsorption of water and the dryer the stool becomes. This makes it more difficult to expel.

Bowel habits vary greatly from person to person. Some people have daily bowel movements, whereas others only have two or three BMs a week. A major factor leading to constipation in the elderly is lack of mobility due to stroke, senility, or other chronic diseases. Lack of appetite, poor dentition, inability to pay for meals, and psychological unwillingness to prepare and eat a meal alone are underlying reasons for constipation in the aged.

Many prescription drugs can cause constipation. For example, codeine, antidepressants, aspirin, and antacids can cause constipation. Fecal impaction can occur as a complication of constipation. Fecal impaction occurs when the stool remains in the colon and becomes hard.

Symptoms of constipation include abdominal pain, decreased appetite, headache, and fatigue. With a fecal impaction the symptoms may include watery diarrhea-like stools with intermittent constipation.

Emphasis is placed in teaching the person habits that promote normal elimination. Avoiding laxatives allows the bowels to function normally. Eating raw fruits, vegetables, whole grain bread and cereal, increasing fluid intake, and regular rest and exercise are important. When initial attempts at retraining the bowel are unsuccessful, the patient needs to be encouraged to continue efforts, as it may take time to change this condition.

See also FECAL IMPACTIONS.

Phipps, W. J., *et al. Medical Surgical Nursing*. St. Louis, C. V. Mosby Co., 1983.
Steinberg, F. U. *Care of the Geriatric Patient*, 6th ed. St. Louis: C. V. Mosby Co., 1983.

COPD See LUNG DISEASE, CHRONIC OBSTRUCTIVE.

CoQ (coenzyme Q) CoQ is a drug that is sold in Japan to treat heart disease and other disorders that affect much of the elderly population. This drug is currently being investigated because of a theory that proposes that immune system declines are caused partly by a deficiency of quinone compounds. When administered to mice, the drug protected them from tumors, a cause of premature death in elderly people. This drug is being further investigated because it may have damaging effects, especially on tissues that lack adequate blood supply.

See also AGING, BIOLOGICAL THEORY OF.

Kurz, M. A. "Theories of Aging and Popular Claims for Extending Life," in *Aging*, Goldstein, E. C., ed. Vol. 2, Art. 88. Boca Raton, Fl.: Social Issues Resource Series, Inc., 1981.

corns A corn is a circular mass of tissue usually formed on the outside of the little toe, on the upper surfaces of other toes or between the fourth and fifth toes. Corns have a core, which thickens inwardly and causes acute pain upon pressure.

Corns are common in the aged and are

often caused by ill-fitting shoes, arthritic changes in the bones of the feet, and deterioration of the fat pad of the feet. Symptoms include pain and limping.

Since corns are usually caused by ill-fitting shoes, changing footwear can help. The use of various molds of felt, foam rubber, rubber, leather, or plastic and a properly fitted shoe that eliminates pressure or friction areas is important. Soaking feet daily in warm soapy water and scrubbing the corn with a pumice stone or emery board can also help. Occasionally steroid, whirlpool, and ultrasound treatments may be necessary for relief of inflammation. Over-the-counter corn removers are caustic and can cause severe burns, therefore should be used with caution. Analgesics or other pain medications may also be required. Surgery may be necessary in advanced cases.

See also BUNIONS.

Anderson, H. C. *Newton's Geriatric Nursing*, 5th ed. St. Louis: C. V. Mosby Co., 1971.
Shea, T. P. and Smith, J. K. *The Over Easy Foot Care Book*. Glenview, Ill.: Scott, Foresman and Co., 1984.

correspondence   Older individuals often live a considerable distance from family and friends. In these instances, when frequent visits are not possible, cards, letters, cassette tapes, and phone calls are very meaningful. These should be sent or made on a regular basis.

Letters written in a chatty fashion that tell of experiences or recall past shared events can awaken memories and give the older person vitality. Correspondence should be positive. Although the writer must occasionally include tragic or disappointing news, he or she should avoid irrelevant gloom and doom. Cards and notes from friends, and religious and social organizations are often appreciated.

The White House, with volunteer help, is now sending birthday greetings to people 80 years or older, and anniversary greetings to couples married 50 years or more. Requests can be sent with the older person's name and address, 30 days before the birthday or anniversary date, to:

Greetings Office
The White House
1600 Pennsylvania Ave.
Washington, DC 20500

See also CONSISTENCY; VISITING, TO HOMEBOUND AND INSTITUTIONALIZED ELDERLY.

Gillies, J. *A Guide to Caring for and Coping with Aging Parents*. Nashville: Thomas Nelson Publishers, 1981.

cosmetic surgery (plastic surgery)
Cosmetic surgery is a specialty that seeks to improve physical function or to minimize the scarring or disfigurement from accidents, birth defects and disease. Also called plastic surgery because the word *plastic* is derived from the Greek word meaning molding or giving form.

Cosmetic surgery can reshape facial and bodily features and is designed to improve an individual's appearance. Many elderly people seek cosmetic surgery to remove wrinkles and repair other unwanted cosmetic problems caused by a lifetime of exposure to sun and the natural aging process.

The following are the most common cosmetic surgical procedures.

• Rhytidectomy (facelift)—usually performed to remove excess or loose, sagging skin from the face and neck. The surgery can be done as an outpatient or in the surgeon's office.
• Submental Lipectomy—a procedure combined with a facelift to remove excessive fat from under the chin.
• Mammoplasty—breast alteration that can be either reduction or augmentation and is usually performed under general anesthesia.
• Liposuction (body fat reduction)—fat deposits on hips, thighs, buttocks, and abdomen are the prime areas for removal of excess fat. Fat deposits can also be removed from arms, knees, calves, upper

torso, neck, and under the chin. This procedure is not a substitute for weight reduction and is not a cure for obesity.

- Rhinoplasty—surgery that corrects deformities of the external nose. It is most common cosmetic surgical procedure and the most difficult.
- Blepharoplasty—a surgical procedure to remove excess skin and protruding fatty tissue from upper and lower eyelids.
- Direct or midforehead brow lift—designed to remove skin just above the brows and to elevate the muscles around the eyes to improve drooping of the eyebrows.
- Forehead lift—elevates the eyebrows and diminishes forehead wrinkles and frown lines.

American Society of Plastic and Reconstructive Surgeons, Inc. Pamphlets. Chicago, Ill.: 1984.

cost of living, regional ratings (see Tables 3, 4) Many elderly people on a fixed income feel motivated to change their lifelong residence when they retire because they are attracted by the amenities of some new location. The cost of living in the new location definitely needs to be considered when contemplating such a move.

Generally, the cost of living and taxes are highest in the Northeast. Costs and taxes are generally lower in the South and West due, in part, to the relatively mild weather of the Sunbelt. Homes in much of the South generally do not need central heating. Property taxes in southern states tend to be lower because some services paid for by taxes, like snow removal, are not usually needed.

Dickinson, P. *Retirement Edens.* Washington, D.C.: AARP, 1986.

crafts See HOBBIES.

credit Credit problems for older people have abated somewhat following the passage of the 1974 amendments to the Housing and Community Development Acts and the 1975 Equal Credit Opportunity Act. The credit status of women, however, requires particular attention because women are known to experience considerable income loss and difficulties in establishing credit if they become widowed.

These laws prohibit discrimination on the basis of sex, age and marital status in consumer and mortgage lending. Lenders cannot deny credit solely on the basis of marital status. If a woman is a good credit risk but is denied credit on the basis of a husband's past credit history, she can request to examine her credit status.

Credit bureaus gather and sell credit information about consumers and are a principal source of information about credit history. To obtain a credit history, make a request to a bureau for a report. The report may include what credit accounts one has, how one pays one's bills, if one has ever filed for bankruptcy or been sued. It is also a good opportunity to update one's credit report if one has credit accounts that were not reported.

When a woman is widowed, divorced, or wants credit in her own name, the credit bureau may report "no file" exists. She may have had a past credit history but in her husband's name. A newly married woman may have the same problem if she changes her name. Old accounts held in her maiden name may not have been transferred, and the credit history is lost. Women who do not have a credit history should start to build a good record at once. If they have credit under a different name or in a different location, they should make sure the local credit bureau has complete and accurate information about them in a file under their current name. Calls should be made to local credit bureaus to see what files they may have.

If a woman shared accounts with her husband or former husband, check with the credit bureau to see if the credit was reported in the wife's name as well as the husband's.

If one is married or divorced recently and has changed one's name on accounts, one should ask creditors to enter the name change for accounts. Each creditor should be notified that one wants accounts shared with one's husband reported in both names. Then check in a couple of months to see if the accounts are being reported as requested.

When applying for credit, one should list one's best accounts, including accounts shared with one's husband or former husband. If necessary assist the creditor in providing information verifying one's credit references. If one can show a credit history of one's own, even though it was in one's husband's or former husband's name, the creditor must consider it. If a previous credit history was unfavorable but did not reflect one's credit worthiness, clarify this with the creditor.

If one is married and wants to establish a credit history, one must write one's creditors and request it. Creditors are obligated to provide the history in both names when accounts are shared.

The Equal Credit Opportunity Act gives one the right to know the specific reasons for denial of a credit application. If the denial was based on a credit report, one is entitled to know the specific information in the credit report that led to the denial. After one has received this information from the creditor, one should contact the credit bureau to find out what information was reported. The bureau cannot charge for disclosure if one asks to see one's file within 30 days of being notified of a denial based on a credit report. One can request that the bureau investigate any inaccurate or incomplete information and correct its record.

In a community property state, a creditor may consider one's husband's credit history even if one is applying for one's own account. One still needs to make certain that one's credit bureau has a separate credit file in one's name.

Loewinsohn, R. J. *Survival Handbook for Widows*. Washington, D.C.: AARP, 1986.

crime   Fear of crime has been rated by older people as their most serious problem, according to a 1975 Harris Poll. This poll showed rather astonishing evidence—fear of crime even outstripped concern about health—23 percent of the elderly rated it as their top problem compared to 21 percent who rated health foremost.

The General Social Survey also shows that more than 50 percent of the 65 + population expresses fear about walking in their general neighborhood at night compared to 40 percent for the rest of the population. Researchers have yet to establish the reason why the elderly express above average fear of crime, but it is likely that concern over their ability to recover from criminal victimization may supply the motive. For the elderly, physical injury received in the course of a criminal attack may be more disabling and require a longer period of recuperation. Recovery from financial or property loss may be difficult at best, or impossible at worst. Fear of crime undoubtedly affects the quality of life of the elderly—it causes a greater sense of personal isolation and produces a sense of powerlessness that may lead older people to restrict their activities. Members of minority groups, especially African Americans, suffer most acutely from the problem of crime.

Considering the greater fear of crime among the elderly, it may seem odd that the young actually experience a higher rate of criminal victimization than the old—crime afflicts them much more frequently. U.S. crime statistics show that the young are three times more likely than the old to be targets of household larceny and burglary, five times as likely to encounter personal larceny (theft of property outside the home), four to five times more likely to have a vehicle stolen, and four to five times more likely to suffer assault and rape. Purse snatching, pickpocketing, and fraud represent the only areas where the elderly exceed the young in encounters with crime.

In a recent year criminal victimization (meaning violent crimes and larceny/theft) in the total population was 95.6 cases per 1,000, whereas for the elderly (65 +) it was 23 per 1,000. This represented a decline from 30 per 1,000 in 1980, the peak year for victimization of older people. Typical annual rates for personal and household crimes are as follows:

Rate of Crimes per 1,000 Persons

	Elderly Persons	Total Population
Violent Crimes		
Total crimes	4.5	28.1
Rape	—[1]	.7
Robbery	1.7	5.1
Assault	2.8	22.3
Larceny Theft		
Total Crimes	18.5	67.5
Purse snatching	.7	not given[2]
Pick-pocketing	1.8	not given[2]
Household Sector Crimes		
Total	78.2	170.0
Burglary	33.3	61.5
Larceny	40.6	93.5
Motor Vehicle Theft	4.3	15.0

[1] Too few cases to report.
[2] Not reported in the table.
SOURCE: *Sourcebook of Criminal Justice Statistics.*

Of all these crimes, fraud is most likely to cause personal devastation to the older individual because it may result in the loss of an entire lifetime of savings painstakingly built up to supply essential income during the late years. One example of a fraudulent swindle is perpetrated by criminals masquerading as bank examiners. In this instance a phoney bank examiner contacts an older individual with a request that he or she withdraw a large sum of money from a bank account to be used to trap a bank employee suspected of embezzlement. The victim is promised a reward and assured that the funds will be returned when the employee has been arrested. The person turns the funds over to the presumed examiner, receives a receipt and the reward, and then waits in vain for the funds to be returned.

Other frauds directed at the elderly include misrepresentation of health insurance information to solicit purchase of insurance already covered in Medicare supplementary policies, outright insurance fraud, real estate investment schemes in poor acreage or swampland, inducement to invest in worthless businesses or securities, diamond sales of artificial or overpriced stones, and so on.

Not infrequently, schemes that separate older people from their cash and lifelong savings may qualify as legal but be so risky as to have virtually no chance of success. Often investments in risky and marginal "get-rich-quick" projects, such as limited partnerships in oil well drilling programs or tax-sheltered real estate, are nothing more than a front for individuals who seek to gain sales commissions or capital for their own personal use rather than for serious business enterprise.

These risky investments are sometimes sold by apparently respectable people who are themselves elderly and move freely in retirement communities or organizations with large numbers of older members. They make their sales pitch under the guise of friendly financial advising, but they are, in reality, completely indifferent to the well-being of their clients and merely want the commission they will derive from the sale. Without conscience, these individual will induce financially inexperienced widows to mortgage mortgage-free homes, draw out lifetime savings, cash in annuities, etc. to invest in schemes so risky as to have virtually no chance of success.

The best guard against fraud and confidence schemes is to rely on reputable and conventional banks and brokerage houses and to review potential investments with certified public accountants and established attorneys.

Jamieson, K. M., and Flanagan, T. F., eds. *Sourcebook of Criminal Justice Statistics*. U.S. Department of Justice, Bureau of Justice Statistics. Washington, D.C.: U.S. Government Printing Office, 1987.

Schick, F. L., ed. *Statistical Handbook on Aging Americans*. Phoenix: Oryx Press, 1986.

U.S. Bureau of the Census, *Statistical Abstract of the United States: 1989*, 109th ed. Washington, D.C.: U.S. Government Printing Office, 1989.

CVA   See cerebral vascular accident.

cycling   Many older people prefer cycling to get their exercise because it places less strain on the joints, leg muscles, and tendons than jogging, yet it has positive aerobic value and muscle toning effects.

Some people who prefer to bicycle might choose to buy an adapter accessory to convert an ordinary bicycle into a stationary bicycle when the weather is bad.

Others prefer the large adult size tricycles (sometimes called tri-wheelers). No balance is required with these tricycles, and they are, therefore, safer than a bicycle.

Gillies, J. *A Guide to Caring for and Coping with Aging Parents*. Nashville: Thomas Nelson Publishers, 1981.

D

dating   Loving and being loved are meaningful parts of human existence, no matter what the age. After a period of grieving due to loss of a spouse by death or divorce, the older individual may decide to fill the void by initiating new intimate relationships.

Dating again after being married for a number of years can be a totally new experience. There is usually, but not always, a much freer attitude toward dating and sex now. The older person who decides to date again must determine his or her own values about becoming emotionally and/or sexually involved with a new partner. However, some people who have become widowed may feel that dating again would be betraying their deceased spouse. Others are afraid of becoming emotionally involved again because they want to protect themselves from experiencing another loss.

Before becoming involved in a new relationship, it is important that people should have had an adequate period of time to grieve a former relationship, whether terminated by death, divorce or separation. The required time of waiting varies from person to person, but studies show that grieving usually begins to subside anywhere from six months to a year.

A healthy attitude was expressed by one widow, who remarked, "When you are a caring person and you get involved with people, you do take chances. But to experience pain is better than to experience nothing."

Adult children may or may not approve of their parents' new emotional involvements, and when older people start dating they may encounter unexpected problems. They may face prejudice, ignorance about their needs, interference from their children, and even denials that they are competent to make independent decisions any longer. Adult children often feel they have the right to approve or disapprove their parents' choices, including friends, lifestyles, dating choices, and personal behavior.

A parent's decision to remarry may provoke an outburst of objections when children do not approach the matter with an open mind. These objections may stem from a variety of causes, including selfishness, overprotectiveness, jealousy, and most especially fear of losing an inheritance.

Adult children need to understand that the loss of one parent does not mean that the other remaining parent has surrendered his/her life simply because a relationship has been terminated by death. Most frequently it is the parents themselves who must take the initiative in explaining their new relationships to their children. When introduced tactfully over time, with reassurance of a continued commitment to existing family, parents' new personal relationships usually cause no difficulty.

Newly chosen partners also need to understand and accept the existing family obligations of their newly found intimate "other." They must be prepared to make former family relationships of a new spouse a part of their own lives, whether this involves visits from grandchildren, holiday get-togethers, or various forms of support and help typically provided in families.

See also RELATIONSHIPS WITHOUT MARRIAGE; REMARRIAGE; SEXUALITY.

Loewinsohn, R. J. *Survival Handbook for Widows*. Glenview, Ill.: AARP, 1984.
Seskin, J. *Alone Not Lonely*. Glenview, Ill.: AARP, 1985.

death, attitudes toward   Death is a reality of life, a condition of living. Today death is relegated to the closet and avoided as an unwanted intruder. While older people often address the subject openly in order to confront their own finitude, family members usually suppress it as morbid. Today death has been dismissed from the home to the nursing home and hospital, the places where two-thirds of the American population die.

In past times death usually occurred at home, and funeral events were generally community affairs. Now death and funeral events have become largely "privatized" in the respect that people die with only family present, and the succeeding ceremonies are often restricted to immediate family and kin.

Elaborate funeral rituals, which provide a means for expressing feelings of loss, coping with grief, and an appropriate communal means for addressing death have been attacked in recent years as mere exploitation and as being too expensive. Their ritual and psychological values have been obscured by a tumult of criticism.

Yet studies carried out by gerontologists reveal that negative and hush-hush attitudes toward death and its surrounding rituals are inappropriate for the elderly. Researchers have shown that older people have less fear of death, approaching it more openly, than their younger fellows. A survey of people aged 45 to 74 posed the question, "How afraid are you of death?" Almost two-thirds of the individuals answering the question said, "not at all," one-third some "somewhat," and only 4 percent said "very."

According to researchers in the field of thanatology (the study of death), older people have a more positive approach to death than other age groups—they are more aware of their own finitude, think about death more often, discuss it more openly, feel more capable of facing death, and accept it more peacefully. Researchers do not consider it morbid when older persons talk about their own passing, their plans for disposing of their property, or their funeral arrangements. Rather, they view openness about death as a psychological preparation, a means of squarely facing the close of life, and a way of taking charge of the surrounding events. Family members and friends may prefer to avoid the open discussion of death initiated by older people, but an accepting attitude would prove more helpful.

Elizabeth Kübler-Ross, probably the most popularly known authority on death, identified five stages that she believed typified the attitudes of people as they approach their own passing. While working as a psychiatrist in the cancer ward of the University of Chicago hospital during the 1960s, Kübler-Ross described these stages as beginning with a denial that death is inevitable, then moving on to anger, bargaining, depression, and finally acceptance.

Authorities today agree that her pioneering analysis helped to bring the subject of death out into the open, but note that later research has failed to consistently support her work. It appears that these stages do not occur invariably, nor that there is any "typical" way to die. Individuals die much as they have lived, in styles that fit with their own attitudes and personalities. The great value of Kübler-Ross's work is that it emphasized openness about death and acceptance of people who are dying. It also affirmed the importance of caring for dying people when the general tendency of health professionals has been to dismiss them because they seem beyond help.

The hospice movement, begun by Dr. Cicely Saunders at St. Christopher's Hospice in London in 1967 and introduced in the United States in Branford, Connecticut, near New Haven, in 1974, has created an outstanding model for an affirmative approach to death. Especially designed for people who are terminally ill (most frequently with cancer), the hospice plan aims to preserve the dignity of dying people so that they can remain in control of the final events of their lives.

The hospice method, whether it is rendered through home care or in an institutional residential setting, creates a warm, familial environment, provides psychologi-cal counseling, and gives physical assistance and medication as required for the relief of pain. Studies conducted at St. Christopher's showed the success of the plan—over three-quarters of the patients described St. Christopher's as having the atmosphere of a family.

But the dramatic advance of medical technology that have made it possible to prevent death even for those who are terminally ill and comatose, has also kindled debate over the issue of euthanasia. Specifically at issue have been the right of people to die, living will laws, and ethical issues concerning the termination of life. A number of states have passed living will laws that entitle individuals to direct physicians and family members to discontinue treatment when there is no reason to expect them to recover, and protect professional and family members from prosecution when they do permit death to takes its course. Opponents, however, argue that people sometimes survive seemingly hopeless illnesses, that new cures will come along, and that euthanasia under the guise of "mercy killing" can become legalized murder of unwanted older family members.

In the face of these debates public opinion surveys show growing acceptance of controlled forms of euthanasia, as recorded by the 60 percent "yes" response to a General Social Survey question worded as follows: "When a person has a disease that can not be cured, do you think that doctors should be allowed by law to end the patient's life by some painless means if the patient and his family request it?" Between 1972 and 1986 young and old differed in answering this question—whereas 70 percent of 18–24 year olds agreed, only 39 percent of those over age 85 did so. In recent years, however, older people have become somewhat more affirmative in their response to this question.

As to the experience of death itself, studies show that death usually takes place in a relatively short period of time—from 75 percent to 80 percent of deaths occur within three months of the onset of a terminal illness. Near the turn of the century Sir William Osler, the world famous Canadian physician, reported that most people do not suffer when experiencing death. Sixty percent of the deaths he had observed occurred during sleep, and most others took place when the individual was unconscious. Recent reports of near death experiences appear to confirm Osler's observations about the general absence of any psychological trauma during the process of dying. In these, individuals who have recovered after reaching a state of clinical death commonly report a pleasant psychological state of emotional warmth, being in the presence of loved ones, and sometimes seeing God or a god-like figure.

The crucial issue in regard to attitudes about death is the way that individuals feel about their own mortality, the way family members and health professionals deal with persons for whom death is an oncoming reality, and our social customs and behavior respecting death. While openness about death appears to be on the rise, we might all still benefit from sharing the attitude of the 93-year-old man who declared his own openness and mastery of the last event of his life by saying, "It's mine . . . don't belong to nobody else."

Kalish, R. A. "The Social Contest of Death and Dying," in Binstock, R. H., and Shanas, E., eds. *Handbook of Aging and the Social Sciences,* 2nd ed. New York: Van Nostrand Reinhold Co., 1985.

Kastenbaum, R. "Dying and Death: A Life-Span Approach," in Birren, J. E., and Schaie, K. W., eds. *Handbook of the Psychology of Aging,* 2nd ed. New York: Van Nostrand Reinhold Co., 1985.

Kübler-Ross, E. *Death: The Final Stage of Growth.* Englewood Cliffs, N.J.: Prentice-Hall, 1975.

Russell, C. H., and Megaard, I. *The General Social Survey, 1972–1976: The State of the American People.* New York: Springer-Verlag, 1988.

Ward, R. A. *The Aging Experience,* 2nd ed. New York: Harper and Row, 1984.

death causes of, and declining death rates   The leading causes of death after age 45 at this time are: heart disease, cancer, and stroke. The per-100,000 population rates of mortality from these diseases now stands at:

Death Rates at Various Ages from the Leading Causes

Age	Heart Disease	Cancer	Stroke
45–64	346	306	49
65–74	1,231	801	244
75 +	4,135	1,332	1,242

Because these illnesses stand as the three main killers, they have been the subjects of intense research and control efforts since the mid-1960s, when government, the medical profession, drug companies, hospitals, universities, and philanthropic foundations that fund biomedical research launched major research and publicity campaigns to control them. With the exception of cancer, the incidence of these diseases has dropped dramatically since the 1960s, the rates having fallen from 307.6 to 188.5 per 100,000 for heart disease, and 88.8 to 34.3 per 100,000 for stroke. Cancer rates have remained stubbornly high, rising from 125.4 in 1950 to 132.3 in the 1980s, partly because the risk of cancer increases as more people reach the advanced years of life, a time when immunity declines severely.

Causes of death that rank behind these three main killers vary somewhat with age. From 45 to 64 accidents stand fourth, with 43 deaths per 100,000, followed by cirrhosis of the liver at 37 per 100,000, and diabetes milletus with 18 per 100,000. At 65 to 74, diabetes ranks fourth, with 64 per 100,000, then pneumonia with 62 per 100,000, accidents at 61 per 100,000, and cirrhosis at 42 per 100,000. After 75 pneumonia takes over fourth position, at 264 deaths per 100,000, followed by accidents with 166 deaths per

100,000, then diabetes at 162 per 100,000, and, last, emphysema, causing 65 deaths per 100,000.

Overall, death rates have declined markedly in the past 50 to 60 years. Government statistics show, for instance, that in 1960 there were 7,786 deaths for every 100,000 people aged 65–74, but at present death rates for this age group are at 5,706 per 100,000—nearly a 27 percent drop in just 30 years. Although half of all people who enter their 75th year die before they reach 85, the average annual death rate declined 1.1 percent per year for men and 2.0 percent for women between 1940 and 1954. For a time thereafter there was no further reduction, but the decline resumed in the late 1960s, when the rate began to fall 1.5 percent per year for men and 2.3 percent per year for women.

Since the 1960s the gains in life expectancy have resulted primarily from more effective control of the three major diseases. People over 65 can now expect to live about six years longer than anyone over that age could expect to live in the 1960s. Control of stroke has added another 1.2 years of life, and, in spite of the increased proportion of late life deaths due to cancer, better management and cure of this disease has added another 1.4 years to life expectancy for the average person.

Much still remains to be done—diseases of the heart still remain the main killer. People who reach 65 have a 46 percent chance of eventually dying of heart problems, and the probability of such a death rises 10 times between ages 65 and 85.

Studies of accidental deaths show an increasing rate of mortality from this cause as age progresses. Older people actually have fewer accidents than younger people (see ACCIDENTS), but they experience more serious ill effects from this source. In a recent year people 65 and over had only 11 percent of all accidents in the nation (a percentage about equal to the proportion of older people in the population at the time), but nearly 23% of all fatal accidents occurred to the age group. While people age 1–44 die less frequently from accidents, during the teen years and early adult years accidental death claims the highest proportion of lives—from age 15–24 accidents account for five times as many deaths as the next leading cause.

It is probable that continuing reductions in the death rate over the next 50 years will depend as much on changes in lifestyle as on advances in biological and medical research. Diet, smoking, exercise, and use of drugs and alcohol directly influence health and therefore longevity. All of these factors are under the control of individuals. If those who wish to enjoy a high quality of life and to age successfully actually do modify their lifestyles, then, barring major wars or natural calamities, the decline of the death rate may well bring most people to live to the maximum biological human lifespan—120 years.

Brody, J. A., and Brock, D. B. "Epidemiological and Statistical Characteristics of the United States Elderly Population," in Finch, C. E., and Schneider, E. L., eds. *Handbook of the Biology of Aging,* 2nd ed. New York: Van Nostrand Reinhold Company, 1985.

Schick, F. L. *Statistical Handbook of Aging Americans.* Phoenix: The Oryx Press, 1986.

Sterns, H. L.; Barrett, G. V.; and Alexander, R. A. "Accidents and the Aging Individual," in Birren, J. E., and Schaie, K. W., eds. *Handbook of the Psychology of Aging,* 2nd ed. New York: Van Nostrand Reinhold Company, 1985.

U.S. Bureau of the Census, *Statistical Abstract of the United States: 1989,* 109th ed. Washington, D.C.: U.S. Government Printing Office.

death, child's or grandchild's   Probably the death of a grown child or grandchild is almost as painful a loss for an older person as the death of their spouse. The loss of a member of the next generation is becoming increasingly common today because the longer the years of life the more likely it is for a child to grow old and possibly die before its own parent. It would not be uncommon, for instance, for a 95-year-old woman to have a son or daughter, who was born when she was 19, who had died at age 75 when she was 94. When offspring or grandchildren die, feelings of loss, mourning, grief, anger, and sometimes a sense of guilt may well parallel those felt on the death of a spouse.

Death of a child or grandchild prior to one's own death seems contrary to the laws of nature. People who suffer such a loss may feel that they are being punished, or that they should not have to endure such a death. Because of these feelings, recovery from grief and mourning may be extremely difficult.

Most older people have had some preparation for the death of their parents, a spouse, or brothers and sisters because they will at least have thought about these possibilities. Not so with the death of a child or grandchild, unless the loss was preceded by a terminal illness. An unexpected death, therefore, can be devastating and accompanied by fear of being left alone in the world.

Today many support groups exist to help with the adjustment to death of a child or grandchild. Local hospital libraries, or the national organizations listed below often can provide information about chapters near the residence of individuals who have experienced this severe loss.

For more information write or call:

The Compassionate Friends
P.O. Box 1347
Oak Brook, IL 60521
(312) 323-5010

Dignity After Death
668 Monroe Ave.
Rochester, NY 14607
(716) 442-1150

Forum for Death Education and Counseling
P.O.Box 1226
Arlington, VA 22210

THEOS Foundation
306 Penn Hill Mall

Pittsburg, PA 15235
(412) 243-4299

Deedy, J. *Your Aging Parents*. Chicago: The Thomas More Press, 1984.
Gillies, J. *A Guide to Caring for Coping with Aging Parents*. Nashville: Thomas Nelson Publishers, 1981.
Lester, A. D. and Lester, J. L. *Understanding Aging Parents*. Philadelphia: The Westminster Press, 1980.

death, definition of   In the past it was customary to attribute death to "natural causes," which were thought to bring about a termination of life as if by unavoidable destiny—with no particular cause specified. Since the early 1900s, however, death has no longer been thought to happen unavoidably without specific cause. Today physicians who fill out death certificates usually must enter a specific disease or condition that caused the death, even though there has been some evidence very recently of a return to a generic term like "natural causes" when a variety of health problems led to a death.

In spite of the long precedent in recording a cause, or causes, for death, enormous advances of medical science in the last 30 to 50 years have made the medical meaning of the term *death* itself increasingly ambiguous. Death used to be signaled when the vital functions of a person, especially breathing and circulation of the blood, had ceased. Today, however, dramatic progress in the development of medical apparatus and treatments required to support life have made it possible to maintain body functions even after mental functions have ceased irreversibly. In order to deal with these problems, a Harvard University *Ad Hoc* Committee on the Examination of the Definition of Brain Death in the late 1960s proposed a new definition of death, which has obtained increasing acceptance: the criterion of death has been reached when the recorded brain function has ceased for a 24-hour period. In recent years an additional criterion has been added—death occurs when circulation within the brain, recorded by one of the modern medical techniques, has ceased.

Kart, C. S.; Metress, E. S.; and Metress, J. F. *Aging and Health: Biologic and Social Perspectives.* Menlo Park, Calif.: Addison-Wesley, 1978.

death, location of

Many terminally ill individuals or their families may have a choice of where the person will die. When medical intervention is not necessary, the dying person may prefer to be at home. Frequently, a family member can be taught to give pain medications or a home nurse may be employed.

It is a misconception in our society that death is a horrible event. In many situations it is quiet and peaceful. Dying at home may eliminate the fear of indignity and depersonalization that may occur in institutions. Many families find that sharing the last days of life with a loved one is a positive, rewarding experience.

Some families find it impossible to provide the necessary nursing care in the face of heavy feelings of responsibility and fears of the dying process. Hospice programs can provide for care both in institutions and at home. A hospice can provide help by teaching the family members or the person to give pain medications. They can also help the individual or their families to deal with their feelings about the dying process.

Most larger cities have an established hospice program. If not, the attending doctor may be willing to help with arrangements so that dying can take place at home.

Gillies, J. *A Guide to Caring for Coping with Aging Parents.* Nashville: Thomas Nelson Publishers, 1981.
Lester, A. D. and Lester, J. L. *Understanding Aging Parents.* Philadelphia: The Westminster Press, 1980.

death, premature   see PREMATURE DEATH REDUCTION.

death, spouse's

Some years ago psychologists Thomas Holmes and Richard Rahe conducted a survey that demonstrated that the death of a spouse ranks as the most severe of all problems that people experience. Death of a spouse was given the top value of 100 stress points, while divorce, the next most serious problem, was far down the scale with a score of 73. Both ranked ahead of separation, a jail term, death of a close family member other than a spouse, personal injury, loss of a job, and a multitude of other problems.

The problems of adjustment to widowhood occur to women more frequently than they do to men—by age 65 nearly 30% of all women have already become widows, while widowhood is a rarity for men; and, by age 75+, 67 percent of women are widowed compared to only 23.6 percent of men. The problems of widowhood may include learning to live alone; having a more limited social life; living on a reduced income; and performing responsibilities that the former spouse had assumed.

Women typically have to take on new financial responsibilities, such as paying mortgage and tax bills, reviewing cancelled checks and bill payments to maintain bank accounts, keeping track of investments, and undertaking routine automobile maintenance and care of lawns and landscapes. Widowers may have to learn how to become cooks, wash and fold the laundry, shop, and even do some sewing. Spouses who have shared in these tasks before the death of their marriage partner adjust most successfully, as do those who previously discussed funeral arrangements, and shared information on the location of valuable papers, bank accounts, and safe deposit boxes.

With respect to advice to a surviving spouse, it is preferable to postpone any major decisions for a year after the death of a mate because the grieving process, which often lasts a year or more, may cloud a survivor's judgment. Adult children usually can be called on for help in coping with adjustment tasks, but it is important to remember that a child may also experience severe grief over the loss of a parent and may need support following a parental death.

Appropriate mourning, even when intense, rarely creates mental or physical problems, but suppressed grief may break out into other forms of behavior—high irritability, restlessness, and depression. Children or other family members should allow a surviving spouse to recall and reminisce about the deceased even to the point of tears. Family members should help the widowed spouse to reach decisions about practical day-to-day affairs because the process of developing judgments fosters healthy and necessary independence. Family can also assist the survivor in resuming social activity when grief or depression might otherwise lead to social isolation.

Finally, though it is rarely perceived by others, one of the most devastating losses caused by the death of a spouse is the termination of physical intimacy—hugging, kissing, tender embraces, all exchanged with affection. While sexual activity may be nonexistent for the survivor, children and family can help to fill the void in physical contact by themselves embracing, hugging, and kissing the widow or widower. A touch, a quick pat on the shoulder, an affectionate squeeze, or a peck on the cheek all can communicate love and help to fill the need for affection.

Gillies, J. *A Guide to Caring for Coping with Aging Parents.* Nashville: Thomas Nelson Publishers, 1981.

Holmes, T. H., and Rahe, R. *Journal of Psychosomatic Research* 11 (1967).

Loewinsohn, R. J. *Survival Handbook for Widows.* Glennview, Ill.: AARP, 1984.

Lester, A. D., and Lester, J. L. *Understanding Aging Parents.* Philadelphia: The Westminster Press, 1980.

U.S. Bureau of the Census, *Statistical Abstract of the United States: 1989,* 109th ed. Washington, D.C.: U.S. Government Printing Office.

death rates and later life expectancy

Because advances in public health, medical sciences, nutrition, and public awareness of good health practices have brought about increases in life expectancy in the last 100 years, the likelihood of death has been pushed forward to the later years of life. In 1900 the average person died before age 50; today half of the newborn population can expect to live beyond age 75.

About 18 percent of the population—roughly 2½ million persons—dies before age 65, and 18 percent, therefore, represents the odds for dying by that age. By age 70 the estimate is that about 14.5 percent will die, bringing the odds of death by age 70 to about 32 percent. In the next five years, to age 75, another 16.6 percent die, bringing the odds of death by this age close to 49 percent. In five more years, to age 80, over 27 percent more persons will have died, bringing the odds of death by this age to about 76 percent. As the biological limit of human life is 120 years, the odds of dying by 120 are 100 percent.

In spite of the increasing likelihood of death as age advances, the foregoing figures do not show the surprising truth that *later life expectancy* remains considerable in the advanced years. Knowledge about later life expectancy is highly useful because it can serve individuals as the basis for a number of late-life decisions, such as: calculating payout plans from annuities and pension benefits; recognizing the time when it becomes essential to make a will; knowing when to think about making funeral arrangements and choosing a final resting place; and even deciding whether one is likely to gain a pay-off from a late life business venture or financial investment. Later life expectancy tables, of course, themselves represent averages (i.e., about half of the surviving population is likely to die before a year indicated and about half to die after it), but recently published figures are as follows:

Average Remaining Life Expectancy

Age	Remaining Years of Life Expectancy	Total Life Expectancy for Age
50	33.1	83.1
60	24.2	84.2
70	16	86
80	9.5	89.5
90	5	95
99	2.8	101.8

Myers, G. C. "Aging and Worldwide Population Change," in Binstock, R. H., and Shanas, E., eds. *Handbook of Aging and the Social Sciences,* 2nd ed. New York: Van Nostrand Reinhold Co., 1985.

Russell, C. H. *Good News About Aging.* New York: John Wiley and Son, 1989.

decubiti (pressure sores, bedsores)

Pressure sores are areas of soft tissue breakdown or skin ulceration usually occurring over bony areas, such as hip, heel, shoulder, or elbow, caused by occlusion of the capillary circulation. Since more elderly people have conditions that confine them to wheelchairs or beds, decubiti are a major problem for the incapacitated elderly.

Decubiti are caused by excessive or prolonged pressure produced by the weight of the body or limb. There are four factors that may contribute to their development; pressure, shearing, friction, and moisture. The prevention of a pressure sore is far simpler than treatment or care. Frequent changing of the position of an immobile person, thorough cleansing of the skin, gentle massage of the bony prominences to stimulate circulation, and use of sheepskin, antipressure padding, or water mattresses are all extremely helpful.

Treatment of pressure sores is directed at establishing a clean, moist environment that will encourage regrowth of skin. Another factor for improved healing is treatment of existing medical conditions such as anemia and diabetes mellitus. Topical agents are used to heal the infection. Simple saline dressings have proven to be a superior treatment of pressure sores since they are nontoxic to the tissues. Transparent adhesive dressings may be useful if placed over small, clean ulcers located in areas that are vulnerable to soiling from urine or feces. Physical agents such as infrared and ultraviolet light, ultrasound, hyperbaric oxygen, oxygen, heat lamp, and whirlpool are also used as treatment. Debridement (removal) may be necessary. The debridement may be surgical or chemical.

When all of these methods fail, skin grafting may be considered. This may not be successful, however, since the area of the pressure sore usually has a decreased circulation, causing a large percentage of skin graft rejections.

Treatment and prevention of pressure sores are extremely important because severe infections may develop, which may cause prolonged hospitalization or even death.

Ham, R. *Geriatric Medicine Annual—1987.* Oradell, N.J.: Medical Economics Co., 1987.

dehydroepiandesterone   See DHEA.

delirium (acute confusional states)

(see Table 7) Delirium is a transient disorder of cognition and attention that constitutes psychopathological manifestations of brain dysfunction. Delirium can occur at any age but is most common in the elderly.

Delirium can be caused by a wide variety of factors including:

1. Primary cerebral diseases, such as infection, neoplasm, trauma, epilepsy and stroke
2. Systemic diseases that affect the brain, notably metabolic, cardiovascular, and collagen diseases
3. Intoxication with exogenous substances, such as alcohol, poisons, and medical or recreational drugs

4. Withdrawal from substances of abuse in a person addicted to them, such as alcohol and sedative-hypnotic drugs

In the elderly, more than one causative factor is often implicated and may involve therapeutic doses of drugs such as diuretics, digoxin, antiparkinsonian, and antidepressants. Drugs with anticholinergic activity are especially liable to induce delirium. Other common causes of delirium of the elderly include congestive heart failure, pneumonia, urinary tract infection, cancer, dehydration, sodium depletion, and cerebral infarction.

Symptoms of delirium include disorders of awareness, consciousness, and attention; disruption of sleep pattern; anxiety; restlessness; drowsiness; insomnia; depression; tachycardia; sweating; elevated blood pressure; fear; and rage.

Once delirium is diagnosed on clinical grounds, its organic cause must be treated. In the elderly, all drugs are reevaluated. Polypharmacy should be avoided. A neurological and psychiatric evaluation may also be necessary.

Symptomatic and supportive therapy is important. Fluid and electrolyte balance, nutrition and adequate vitamin supply need to be ensured. Reality orientation is beneficial in reducing delirium.

It is important to recognize delirium because it is often the presenting feature of acute physical illness, such as myocardial infarction, pneumonia, or drug intoxication.

Lipowski, Z. J. "Delirium (Acute Confusional States)." *JAMA* 258:1789–1792 (1987).

dementia, acute reversible   See ORGANIC BRAIN SYNDROME.

dementia, presenile   See ALZHEIMER'S DISEASE.

denial (withdrawal)   Denial is a defense used by many older people to cope with the aging process. It is an unconscious process in which the person does not admit that a situation exists until the person is able to adjust. Denial is all right in moderation because it allows the person to continue to function and feel useful. Denial becomes negative only when it becomes damaging to the person's health.

Denial can keep a person from accepting reality. In such a situation, people may go to extremes to look younger with wigs, cosmetics, or youthful clothing and refuse to be involved with their peer groups.

Some individuals attempt to maintain control of their lives by avoidance. Sometimes this withdrawal is a way of handling the undesirable effects of the aging process. Isolation becomes the person's protection and keeps him or her secure in his or her own environment.

If denial or withdrawal becomes so extensive that it might jeopardize the older person's health, psychotherapy may be necessary.

Lester, A. D., and Lester, J. L. *Understanding Aging Parents*. Philadelphia: The Westminster Press, 1980.

dental care   See ORAL HYGIENE.

dependence   As a general rule older people maintain their independent living status and autonomous control over their lives as long as they are physically able to do so. For example, only a small proportion (probably not more than 7 percent or 8 percent according to statistics in the General Social Survey) of older people share homes with their children or people other than their spouse. Ten percent of the housebound and bed-ridden population over age 80 maintain a residence in the community rather than going to a nursing home.

Throughout life people successfully cope with and adapt to their circumstances, maintain their own homes, and do not depend on others. In age they do likewise, and extensive dependence on others is the exception, not the rule.

Yet it is also true that all individuals at some time in life rely on a social network for some measure of support, and age is no exception. Probably most people at some time have turned for help to parents, children, relatives, friends, churches, hospitals, nurses, physicians, and others, as well deriving support from the entire economic, political, and social community in which they live. In age this normal level of dependence may increase for individuals who become disabled.

Statistics show that there are approximately 22 million disabled persons in the United States, and that the elderly make up about 40 percent of this number, or approximately nine million persons. About 3.5 percent of those over 65 are severely disabled; and, although only about 5 percent of the population over 65 resides in a nursing home, the rate of nursing home residence rises to about 20 percent after age 85, when older people make up 85 percent of the population living in this type of facility. Not all nursing home residents are elderly however; young people with serious disabilities may also live in nursing homes.

Conditions that interfere with performance of major activities, such as going to work, keeping house, or performing an activity of daily living (known as ADL—dressing, bathing, feeding oneself, toileting, walking, and the like) are the most likely causes of dependency. Even though 39 percent of all people over 65 have a limitation in a major activity (most often due to heart or blood pressure problems), less than one million persons over age 65 living outside nursing homes need help with an activity of daily living.

Because most people feel constrained and frustrated when they must rely extensively on others for help, loss of independence can be a very difficult experience. Not only may an individual be unable to drive a car, go shopping, or get about the house, but performance of such routine self-care activities as bathing, cooking, shaving, and controlling bodily functions may require assistance. Irritability, depression, and withdrawal may accompany loss of independence.

Occasionally individuals lose their complete sense of competence when they become dependent on others. Researchers have proposed a way to reverse this condition by creating a "social reconstruction syndrome." The key to this form of therapy lies in providing environmental supports, which increase the individual's sense of competence. Recently this therapeutic approach has been applied to families that have suddenly faced problems of increased dependency of an older member. By supplying various "inputs," such as help through respite care, family members as well as dependent individuals themselves can adjust to and deal with the problems caused by dependency.

Older people who need help have sometimes been referred to as the frail elderly. Assistance provided to these individuals most commonly involves practical chores of daily living—shopping, doing errands, providing escort service and transportation, and managing of financial affairs. Yet, studies of the array of tasks performed for the frail elderly show that morale boosters, such as visiting, sitting and talking, keeping company, watching TV together, also represent important forms of support.

Most of the help provided to older people comes from a spouse or other close family members (according to Ethel Shanas, a leading gerontologist and co-editor of *The Handbook of Aging and the Social Sciences,* family members provide about 80 percent of all such assistance), and is given willingly, even under conditions of considerable stress. For frail people the amount of time of help in hours per week may range up to: 35 hours by spouses; 18 hours by children; five hours by relatives. From all sources together for all dependent people, the average time of help provided is about 11 hours per week.

These data show that though dependency is fairly common in late life, it is by no means universal nor is it usually disdained by family members as too burdensome. It is the family and, surprisingly, disabled individuals themselves who are the first line of support in cases of dependency.

For additional information write or call:

National Council on Aging
409 3rd St. SW 2nd floor
Washington, DC 20024
(202) 479-1200
Administration on Aging
Dept. of Health, Education and Welfare
Washington, DC 20402
(202) 619-0724

Cantor, M., and Little, V. "Aging and Social Care," in Binstock, R. H., and Shanas, E., eds. *Handbook of Aging and the Social Sciences*, 2nd ed. New York: Van Nostrand Reinhold Co., 1985.

Crichton, J. *Age Care Sourcebook*. New York: Simon & Schuster, Inc., 1987

Kemp, B. "Rehabilitation and the Older Adult," in Birren, J. E., and Schaie, K. W., eds. *Handbook of the Psychology of Aging*, 2nd ed. New York: Van Nostrand Reinhold Co., 1985.

Lester, A. D., and Lester, J. L. *Understanding Aging Parents*. Philadelphia: The Westminster Press, 1980.

National Center for Health Statistics, Dawson, D. A., and Adams, P. F. Current Estimates from the National Health Interview Survey; United States, 1986. *Vital and Health Statistics*. DHHS Pub. No. (PHS) 87-1592. Series 10, No. 164. Public Health Service. Washington, D.C.: U.S. Government Printing Office, 1987.

dependency ratio   Some social scientists and political figures have been concerned about the growing number and percentage of the population that is depending on people of working age for support. The idea is that one part of the population works, primarily those between 20 and 65, and supports the rest. If the proportions of the two groups get out of balance—that is, if there were too many dependent people in relation to the size of the working population—then it might become a burden on those who are still employed, and the prosperity of the entire population might suffer.

Recent discussions about the dependency ratio have actually focused more on the "old-age dependency ratio" rather than the total proportion of people who depend on the working population. A number of scholars and demographers have noted with concern that the proportion of old people in the U.S. population is increasing. They point out that the percentage of those over age 65 who are retired and drawing Social Security, now at about 12 percent, will almost double over the next 35 to 40 years. In consequence, a comparatively smaller work force will be supporting a larger group of retirees.

There are, however, flaws in looking at the dependency ratio only in terms of the size and proportion of the older population. Those who depend on others for support consist in two major groups—children and young people in school as well as older retired people. A perspective on these two categories—the young as well as the old—not only gives a more accurate picture of the size of the population that will require support in the future, but it shows that the dependency ratio is actually *falling* and will not reach its past high level even when the older population nearly doubles in size.

In 1970 young and old combined made up 43 percent of the population, but by the year 2000 this percentage will have fallen to 38 percent, a 5 percent fall since the peak. By 2030, at the height of the aging boom, the percentage, then 41 percent, will still not match the 1970 level. The reason for these changes is that the mass of the Baby Boom population, born between 1946 and 1964 and 75 million strong, will have moved from youthful dependence in 1970 to old age in 2030.

Some authorities express a sense of crisis even with these figures at hand. They point out, for instance, that in the year 2000 there will be 63.2 people in the dependent groups for every 100 persons whose work produces the school taxes and Social Security funds for nonworking people. In the year 2030, when the retired population will near its peak, there will be 73.8 dependent persons for every 100 workers.

These facts need not lead to a sense of crisis, however. The U.S. Congress has demonstrated its awareness of the growth of the older population by modifying the Social Security system to take into account the larger number of future retirees. One such change, the eligible age for full benefits, is closely geared to the major rise of the older population anticipated in the next century. It will go into effect in the year 2000, when the present age of eligibility for full benefits, now 65, will slowly increase to reach age 67 by 2027. Meanwhile the Social Security trust fund, now expanding at a rate of more than $40 billion per year, is expected to reach $12 trillion by 2030—an astronomical figure far beyond the three-month reserve that was on hand in the early 1980s when concern about the dependency ratio was at its height.

There are factors other than the growth of the Social Security trust fund that give reason for having confidence in America's ability to deal with the changing dependency ratio. The future solvency of the Social Security system, as well as of other pensions, depends on the will of the American public to put aside funds to assure its future financial security—and it appears that younger Americans are becoming increasingly aware of this need.

Some of those who express fears about the rising dependency ratio appear to imply that the older generation is not deserving of support. They disregard the past contributions of older people to the Social Security fund and to other pension savings that have helped to create the vast wealth the country has today. The high standard of living that Americans now enjoy and will continue to enjoy in the future rests on the introduction of numerous products—microchips, TVs, computers, microwaves, jet air travel, super highways and equally super cars, etc.—which were developed during the working lifetimes of both the people who are now reaching old age and the others who will achieve that status over the next 30 to 40 years. In fact, the very pension savings put aside by young and old become available for business investment and contribute to the growing of the wealth of the nation. By virtue of their contributions to the present high standard of living, members of the older generation fully deserve any support that future generations will provide for them.

The costs of health care for the older population have also been of concern. While it is evident that these costs are high, it is also true that less than half of these are paid for by the public through the Medicare program—the elderly themselves pay the rest.

Along with this is the fact that several European nations, including England, West Germany, the Scandinavian countries, France, and Italy already have higher proportions of older people in their populations than the United States. These range from 13 percent to 17 percent, while the U.S. now stands at about 12 percent. Six of these nations have proportions that exceed 14 percent and they are all managing quite successfully.

When these factors are taken into consideration they show that fears of a rising specter of an older population are unwarranted—the old have earned their keep and will continue to do so. America met the challenge of providing education on a massive scale for the Baby Boom population, and it will again meet the challenge of providing for future generations of the elderly.

These same elderly, which will shortly include the Baby Boomers, have created the wealth that made the nation prosperous. Like the generations before them, they should legitimately share in consuming the wealth of the nation when they have finished their working days. With intelligent social planning there is no reason to expect that the age wave will swell the dependency ratio to a point where it will swamp the nation when it crests in the next century.

Russell, C. H., and Megaard, I. *The General Social Survey, 1972–1976: The State of the American People*. New York: Springer-Verlag, 1988.

Soldo, B. J. "America's Elderly in the 1980s," *Population Bulletin*, Vol. 35, No. 4. Washington, D.C.: Population Reference Bureau, Inc., 1980.

dependent care credit   A person who pays someone to care for an elderly dependent while he or she works may be able to take a tax credit of up to 30 percent of the amount paid for such care.

To qualify, the person paying for care and his or her spouse must have income from work during the year. The expenses incurred for the dependent care must be incurred to allow that person and his or her spouse to work or look for work. The dependent must be physically or mentally incapable of caring for him or herself.

Work-related expenses are limited to $2,400 for one qualifying dependent or $4,800 for two or more dependents. The most the person paying for care can reduce his or her tax in any year is $720 if expenses are for one qualifying person or $1,440 if the expenses are for two or more dependents.

Department of the Treasury, Internal Revenue Service. Publication #503, 1987.

Friedman, D. E. "Eldercare: The Employee Benefit of the 1990's," in *Aging*, Goldstein, E. C., ed. Vol. 3, Art. 13. Boca Raton, Fl.: Social Issues Resources Series, Inc., 1981.

depression   Depression is a morbid sadness or melancholy often symptomatic of a psychiatric disorder, neurosis, or psychosis. It is distinguished from grief, which is a realistic and normal reaction to personal loss or tragedy.

Depression in the elderly is usually thought to be exogenous, or reactive, as opposed to endogenous in younger people. Exogenous depression arises in response to events that occur outside the individual such as loss of a spouse, retirement, poor health, or a change in lifestyle. (Endogenous depressions are thought to be related to intrapsychic, or internal, characteristics of the individual.)

Depression is probably related to the very high SUICIDE rate of older men. Thus, this disturbance is to be taken seriously when it occurs in an aged person and treated actively, with special emphasis on dealing with the environmental factors precipitating it.

Symptoms of depression may begin with physical signs such as weight loss, loss of appetite, severe fatigue, and sleep difficulties, especially early awakening or insomnia. The psychological indications of depression include sadness, low activity and interest levels, severe pessimism, and difficulty making decisions. Sometimes the person cries a great deal or experiences severe guilt or anxiety.

In diagnosing depression in the elderly, two additional possibilities should be evaluated as contributing factors. The first is whether medications the patient is taking may be causing a drug-induced depression. The second is whether the depression is associated with an illness.

A number of drugs may produce depression including Reserpine, Indomethacin, clonidine, propranolol, phenmetrazine, and amphetamines. Often, a drug-induced depression will require treatment with a tricyclic antidepressant.

The physical illnesses that appear to generate depression include hyperthyroidism, Addison's disease, Cushing's disease, Parkinson's disease, and cerebral arteriosclerosis.

In treating a secondary depression, proper attention to the primary illness is essential. Rehabilitation may be necessary if disability results from the effects of the illness.

Treatment for primary depression includes psychotherapy or counseling to determine the source of the depression. Antidepressant drugs may be needed. Involving the person in group activities or regular exercise programs may be helpful. The families of the older person need to be drawn into the treatment programs to lend their encouragement and support.

See also ALCOHOL ABUSE; ANXIETY; DRUG ABUSE.

Rossman, I. *Clinical Geriatrics,* 3rd ed. Philadelphia: J. B. Lippincott, 1986.
Steinberg, F. U. *Care of the Geriatric Patient,* 6th ed. St. Louis: C. V. Mosby Co., 1983.

DHEA (dehydroepiandesterone)   The blood levels of the hormone dehydroepiandrosterone (DHEA) are very high in young adults and decline dramatically throughout life. This dramatic decline leads scientists to speculate that DHEA may be involved in aging. The hormone appears to prevent breast cancer and to delay immune system disorders. In experiments, animals given DHEA weighed significantly less than the control group. This weight reduction could be the reason for the treated animals' longevity.

(see also AGING, BIOLOGICAL THEORY OF)

Kurz, M. A. "Theories of Aging and Popular Claims for Extending Life," in *Aging,* Goldstein, E. C., ed. Vol. 2, Art. 88. Boca Raton, Fl: Social Issues Resource Series, Inc., 1981.

diabetes mellitus   Diabetes mellitus is the inability of the body to oxidize, or break down, carbohydrates because of faulty pancreatic activity and disturbance of the normal insulin mechanism.

The symptoms of diabetes include polyuria (frequent urination), polydipsia (excessive thirst), polyphagia (excessive eating), fatigue, blurred vision, poor wound healing, and frequent infections. Diabetes is common in old age. Generally, diabetes that has an onset in old age is mild and frequently without symptoms.

Diabetes mellitus affects the entire body, therefore, a diabetic needs to be monitored closely. By classifying the diabetes' severity, the treatment may be determined. If the diabetes is mild, it may be controlled by a diet and exercise program. More severe cases need oral or parenteral medication.

Type II diabetes is adult-onset diabetes controlled with oral hypoglycemic medications. Type I is juvenile-onset diabetes, which is usually controlled with insulin. Type II diabetes is a disease that affects older people who frequently have other chronic diseases, physical limitations, and psychosocial and economic problems that complicate management and limit the ability for self-care. A major problem for most people with diabetes mellitus is obesity.

Several principles of management are important for Type II diabetes. The first is to provide the diabetic with initial education and therapy. One needs to allow at least three months for a trial of exercise and diet before beginning more therapy. If drug therapy is instituted at the beginning, an attempt should be made to reduce the medication once control is established. After the trial period, the physician will select a method of drug therapy—sulfonylurea or insulin.

The choice between sulfonylurea (oral hypoglycemic agent) and insulin depends on the patient's as well as the physician's preference. The choice also depends on the patient's physical condition as well as other factors. If a patient is obese, the physician should try to avoid insulin because peripheral insulin resistance may occur. When the patient has advanced neuropathy or retinopathy, insulin therapy is preferred over sulfonylurea. Elderly diabetics are at a great risk of stroke, myocardial infarction, or aspiration during hypoglycemia.

After the method of drug therapy has been chosen, the physician will develop the method and program for the patient's home glucose surveillance. The doctor will decide the technique, frequency of testing, and the manner or reporting. Other diabetes mellitus patients are less likely to have wide swings in blood sugar, therefore frequent measurement of urine sugars is not as important as it is with Type I diabetes mellitus patients.

Diabetes is a very serious disease, which, if allowed to go uncontrolled, could result in severe complications of the eye, kidney, and nervous system.

For additional information write or call:
American Diabetes Association
1660 Duke Street

P.O. Box 257757
Alexandria, VA 22314
1-800-232-3472
See also DIABETIC RETINOPATHY; FOOT CARE; SEXUALITY.

Davidson, M. B. *Diabetes Mellitus Diagnosis and Treatment.* New York: Wiley Medical Publication, 1981.

Rogers, C. S., and McCue, J. D. *Managing Chronic Disease—1987.* Oradell, N.J.: Medical Economics Co. Inc., 1987.

diabetic retinopathy Diabetic retinopathy is a retinal disease caused by DIABETES MELLITUS, which includes hemorrhages, overgrowth of blood vessels, scar tissue, and edema of the retina. Retinopathy usually appears 10 years or more after the onset of diabetes. Diabetic retinopathy can be detected in 65 percent of people who have had diabetes for 15 years and in 90 percent of people who have had diabetes for 30 to 40 years. Diabetic retinopathy is responsible for 10 percent of cases of newly reported blindness and 20 percent of blindness in people from 45 to 75 years of age.

The only symptom of diabetic retinopathy is a loss of central and/or side vision, which may occur gradually or abruptly.

Treatment for diabetic retinopathy may involve laser therapy. In photocoagulation of the retina by the xenon arc or argon laser, an intense beam of light is directed through the pupil of the eye into a small spot on the retina. The light is then transformed into heat thereby coagulating the new vessels, which helps to prevent a hemorrhage into the vitreous. This prevention is necessary because bleeding in the vitreous blocks the transmission of light and also allows fibrous tissue to form, which may cause a traction retinal detachment. To remove the diseased vitreous it is necessary to perform a vitrectomy. Hypophysectomy, surgical removal of the pituitary gland, was formerly used to treat diabetic retinopathy, but is rarely performed as diabetic retinopathy treatment now. Because of limited surgical methods, efforts are turned toward the prevention of diabetic retinopathy.

Currently there is no uniformly satisfactory treatment of diabetic retinopathy. However, good control of diabetes in the first years of the disease may minimize the amount of retinopathy. Panretinal photocoagulation in which a large amount of laser is used on the retina will help to decrease the incidence of diabetic retinopathy.

Scherer, J. C. *Introductory Medical-Surgical Nursing,* 3rd ed. Philadelphia: J. B. Lippincott Co., 1982.

Steinberg, F. U. *Care of the Geriatric Patient,* 6th ed. St. Louis: C. V. Mosby Co., 1983.

diarrhea Diarrhea is a series of loose, watery stools that is a result of a change in the fecal contents or an increase in intestinal transmit time so that less fluid is reabsorbed. Diarrhea may be caused by the intake of certain foods, stress, or an infectious or inflammatory process. Specific drugs such as iron and digitalis may also cause diarrhea.

Diarrhea is often severe in the elderly and can be life-threatening. Thirty-four percent of diarrhea in the elderly is caused by viruses and 14 percent by bacteria.

Viral diarrhea has an abrupt onset and tends to be short-lived (one to five days). In diarrhea caused by bacteria, bloody stools and a sharp rise in temperature is found. Dehydration can occur quickly in the elderly.

About 75 percent of all diarrhea cases will subside within 7–14 days. Outbreaks in nursing homes, however, can last 4–6 weeks. Scrupulous hygiene and isolation procedures are necessary to curb the spread of this problem.

Symptoms of diarrhea include abdominal cramping or distention, and fatigue. Dehydration can result from diarrhea, causing low sodium and potassium and other electrolyte problems.

Treatment of diarrhea usually consists of correcting the underlying cause, allowing the bowel to rest, and obtaining electrolyte balance. Drugs used for decreasing intestinal motility are opium derivatives, such as paregoric. Lomotil is commonly prescribed. Providing bulk, such as Metamucil, to decrease the fluidity of stools may be helpful. If diarrhea occurs primarily after meals, antidiarrheal medications should be given 30 to 60 minutes before the meal for maximum effect.

Dietary restrictions decrease stimulation of the intestinal tract, thereby allowing the bowel to rest. With severe diarrhea food may be withheld for 24 to 48 hours, with a gradual progression to a low fiber/high protein and calorie diet.

Frequent watery stools cause perineal irritation. The perineal area must be kept dry and clean to prevent skin breakdown.

Phipps, W. J., *et al. Medical Surgical Nursing.* St. Louis: C. V. Mosby Co., 1983.
Scherer, J.C. *Introductory Medical Surgical Nursing.* Philadelphia: J. B. Lippincott Co., 1982.
Steinberg, F. U. *Care of the Geriatric Patient,* 6th ed. St. Louis: C. V. Mosby Co. 1983.

diet, anti-aging   See ANTI-AGING DIET.

dignity in late life   Researchers who emphasize study of the "self" have developed important theories about humans' inner beings and inward experiences as they go through the various stages of life. Researchers observe that each person is conscious of having an inner being, and, although this inner being is stable and to a large extent under one's own control, it changes throughout life under the influence of outside forces—including the way others treat one and the situations one is in.

Psychological research on happiness and self-esteem has consistently shown that older people maintain above average ratings in both areas, but is is obvious that an older individual's sense of dignity, or self-esteem, could be fragile. This is especially the case for individuals who become physically dependent or senile. Their circumstances may bring on seemingly childlike behavior, but in fact they remain adults inwardly and, barring extensive mental breakdown, they look back on lifetimes as independent, self-responsible, and autonomous beings.

Consequently, people who relate to older individuals, and especially to those who are dependent, need to maintain respect for the rights of the old to the fullest extent possible. When decisions respecting the welfare of older dependent people must be made, the reasons for actions need to be given to them; matters should be explained; and their ideas and opinions should be solicited. Professionals who care for the elderly need to listen to them, and to address them personally rather than simply to communicate with family members. By making efforts to support the self-esteem of the old, both professionals and family members can assist them to experience life with dignity.

Bengtson, V. L.; Reedy, M. N.; and Gordon, C. "Aging and Self-Conceptions: Personality Processes and Social Contexts," in Birren, J. E., and Schaie, K. W., eds. *Handbook of the Psychology of Aging,* 2nd ed. New York: Van Nostrand Reinhold Company, 1985.

diphtheria immunization   See IMMUNIZATION ELDERLY.

direct or mid-forehead brow lift   See COSMETIC SURGERY.

disability and dependence prevalence   Disability is a state in which existence at home without help is considered impossible. Dependence is defined as a disability that prohibits self-care. In a study done on people who were disabled and over the age of 65, it was found that: 48 percent had a neurological disorder, 22 percent had a functional psychiatric disorder, 38 percent had a cardiorespiratory disease, 25 percent joint disease, 16 percent were obese, 11 percent had visual impairment, and 3 percent were persistently incontinent. When the dependent subjects were studied, it was found that 77 percent of them had dementia and 33 percent were persistently incontinent.

Brocklehurst, J. C. *Textbook of Geriatric Medicine and Gerontology*. New York: Churchhill Livingstone, 1985.

disc degeneration of the spine   The discs of the spine are layers of fibrocartilage between the vertebra consisting of a pulpy center enclosed by a fibrous capsule. The discs act as a cushion between the vertebrae. With the aging process, the pulposus nucleus becomes brown and compressed. Splits or tears in the fibrous capsule can result causing degenerative changes, especially in the lumbar area.

Men are affected more often than women, indicating a correlation with heavy manual work. Other factors leading to disc degeneration are postural disorders, kyphoscoliosis (humplike curvature of the spine often associated with a heart disorder), and ochronosis (deposits of brown-black color in connective tissue and cartilage).

The majority of patients with degenerative disease of the spine are symptom free. When pain or symptoms occur, conservative treatment should be started. Bed rest and the use of analgesics to relieve discomfort are the first line of treatment. Traction, steroid injections, and surgery are only rarely used. Heat therapy and exercise can also be beneficial.

See also BACKACHE.

Brocklehurst, J. C. *Textbook of Geriatric Medicine and Gerontology*. New York: Churchhill Livingstone, 1985.

disciform degeneration, macular   See MACULAR DEGENERATION.

discounts, senior citizens'   Many businesses offer discounts to senior citizens, which older individuals can take advantage of to help stretch their budgets. Banks often make no monthly charge for checking accounts of people over 65. Buses, theaters, department stores, drug stores, restaurants, museums, airlines, and others offer senior citizen discounts also. This can represent a substantial savings, if one takes advantage of it. Sources that provide information on such discounts include AARP publications and newsletters like the *United Retirement Bulletin* edited by Bostonian Edith Tucker.

Deedy, J. *Your Aging Parents*. Chicago: The Thomas More Press, 1984.
Gillies, J. *A Guide to Caring for and Coping with Aging Parents*. Nashville: Thomas Nelson Publishers, 1981.

diverticulitis   Diverticulitis is inflammation of the small blind pouches that form in the lining of the colon trapping bacteria and fecal material. Weakness of the muscles of the colon may be produced by chronic constipation.

Diverticulitis is caused by perforations of the diverticula. An erosion occurs and the contents of the bowel escape into the surrounding tissue. In a small perforation the infection and inflammation are confined to a small area. The intestinal contents are prevented from entering the abdominal cavity by a small abscess that seals the leak. A large perforation can result in severe complications including peritonitis (swelling of the membrane that covers the wall of the abdomen).

Diverticulitis is very common in older people and is frequently asymptomatic. Symptoms of diverticulitis include constipation, diarrhea, fever, blood in the stool, tenderness of the left lower abdomen, abdominal cramps, and flatulence.

Intestinal obstruction or a perforation leading to peritonitis can also result from the inflammatory process.

Diverticula that are asymptomatic require no treatment. During acute episodes, however, the person may be placed on intravenous fluids with no oral intake for several days. Antibiotics are started and as the inflammation subsides oral foods and fluids are resumed. Efforts should be made to avoid constipation by encouraging good fluid intake and regular evacuation. A stool softener may be helpful. If the condition does not respond to treatment or if complications occur, such as perforation, intestinal obstructions, or severe bleeding, surgery is necessary. The portion of the colon containing the diverticula is removed. Depending on the location and extent of the disease, a temporary colostomy may need to be performed. At a later operation the continuity of the bowel is restored and the colostomy is closed.

See also BOWEL OBSTRUCTION; PERITONITIS; ULCERATIVE COLITIS.

Bockus, H. I. *Gastroenterology.* Philadelphia: W. B. Saunders, 1985.
Goldberg, M. and Rubin, J. *The Inside Tract.* Washington, D.C.: AARP, 1986.

divorce Divorce among older people remains a rarity—only 1 percent of all divorces in the United States involve people over 65. People from age 50 to 64 account for only 4 percent of all divorces while people aged 25 to 29 account for about 22.5 percent of all divorces. The lifetime experience with divorce among older people is also far below that of the younger population. Experts predict that late life divorce will continue to remain a rarity—primarily because those who remain married in late life are people who have already successfully weathered the storms of marriage for many years.

Even though divorce will remain comparatively rare among the old, it is also true that the termination of marriage after age 65 has increased. While the divorce rate for the entire population was growing five times, it doubled among the elderly. Further, more people in the future will enter their advanced years as divorcees, so that the status of being a divorced person will become more common among the older generation in the years ahead.

When divorce does occur in late life, the problems are certainly as serious, and possibly more serious, than in early life. Research shows that women suffer a severe impairment to their financial situation, and men experience difficulty in their personal lives. Divorced people report less satisfaction with family life, lower rates of personal happiness. Mortality records show that divorced people have a higher death rate than the rest of the population.

Because divorce in late life may result from stress caused by illness of one or the other of the marital partners, the difficulties of coping with a new life situation may be even more acute than for younger divorcees; and relationships with kin, children, and grandchildren may suffer. Successful divorce in late life requires careful provision for the financial well-being of both parties, candid discussion and resolution of personal and emotional conflicts, and efforts to maintain good relationships with family and friends.

Uhlenberg, P., and Myers, M. A. P., "Divorce Among the Elderly." *The Gerontologist:* 21, 276–282 (1981).

divorce, children's and grandchildren's Because divorce has become a common occurrence, many older individuals will be faced with a divorce of their children or grandchildren.

Several guidelines may be helpful when dealing with a child involved in divorce. The older person should not blame him or herself for the failure of the child's marriage. During a divorce the child will need understanding. The older person should avoid giving advice or telling the child "I told you so." What is beneficial for one couple may not be for another. Finally, the older person should never withdraw his or her moral support. Hurt people need to heal and not to be judged.

Adhering to these guidelines may be difficult. However, trying not to interfere with an adult child's life may be the best way to provide a genuinely loving and caring atmosphere.

Deedy, J. *Your Aging Parents.* Chicago: The Thomas More Press, 1984.

dizziness　See VERTIGO.

driver's license renewal　The U.S. has
more than 146 million drivers, and over 21
million (about 15 percent) of them are 60
and over. Statistics about California drivers
are of special interest because that state has
one of the highest rates of automobile usage
and miles driven in the world. California
reports that 64 percent of its population over
age 65 is licensed, about one in three persons
over 80 holds a license, and some 3,500
people over 90 have valid licenses.

Several studies have compared the rate of
accidents for older people with those of
younger people, but the results are contradictory. Although no firm generalizations
can be made at this time, it appears possible
that older drivers may have accident rates
more like those of people under 25 than
people aged 25–65.

Requirements for renewal of driver's licenses vary from state to state. Inquiries
should be made at each state office concerning their regulations, particularly when moving to a new area.

Forty-one states or jurisdictions have some
type of retesting or re-examination program,
which may include vision screening, knowledge, or sign recognition. Five require a
medical report. In New Jersey, 10 percent
of drivers have random vision checks.

Ten states and the District of Columbia
require special testing based on age. In Maine,
vision is tested at ages 40, 52, and 65.
Oregon checks vision at age 50. Pennsylvania begins checking vision at age 45 and
conducts random medical testing at age 45.

Knowledge and road testing are conducted
in Illinois every three years starting at age
69 and in the District of Columbia, Indiana,
and New Hampshire beginning at age 75. In
New Mexico, drivers over age 75 must have
their licenses renewed annually. Iowa and
Rhode Island retest drivers 70 years of age
and older every two years, and in Hawaii,
drivers over age 65 must renew their licenses
every two years.

Sterns, H. L.; Barrett, G. V.; and Alexander, R.
A. "Accidents and the Aging Individual," in
Birren, J. E., and Schaie, K. W., eds. *Hand-
book of the Psychology of Aging.* 2nd ed. New
York: Van Nostrand Reinhold Company, 1985.

driving and old age　As a group elderly
drivers have fewer accidents on a per-drive
basis, according to a 1982 National Public
Safety Research Institute Report. However,
annual mileage traveled by elderly drivers is
much less than other drivers. On a per-mile
basis, elderly drivers have a higher accident
rate than other drivers.

Older drivers tend to be responsible for
the accidents in which they are involved.
The likelihood of an older individual being
injured or killed in an accident is greater.
These accidents usually occur on clear days,
on straight, dry pavements, and at intersections within 15 miles of the driver's home.

Driving in the United States is considered
to be a person's right. It is the only mode
of transportation available in many areas. It
maintains a sense of independence allowing
people to continue to meet their daily needs
and overcome a sense of isolation.

Aging has a definite effect on driving
ability. Changes first begin to occur in basic
sensory and cognitive functions. These
changes are so gradual older adults are unaware of them. These age-related problems
can significantly affect an individual's driving performance.

Government studies have found a link
between poor vision and poor driving that
increases among drivers 50 years and over.
More than 95 percent of all information
processed by drivers is through one's eyesight. Day and night, the amount of illumination that reaches the retina at the age of
60 is only one-third of that of a 20-year-old.

Declining physical ability, the mental state
of the driver, and the use of medications
affect the elderly. One out of every five

people over the age of 55 has impaired hearing, and one out of three over the age of 65. Hearing loss particularly affects older men's ability to hear high-pitched sounds.

Several states use mandatory retesting of senior citizen when their licenses expire. According to the Federal Highway Administration the number of states with these requirements has declined from 11 states and the District of Columbia in 1977 to three states and the District of Columbia in 1984.

The American Association of Retired Persons (AARP) has opposed mandatory retesting. They began a driver education program called "55 Alive." The program is offered in all 50 states. To date 220,000 people have taken "55 Alive." The eight-hour course emphasizes defensive driving skills.

Seniors are encouraged to have regular eye examinations. Depth perception and other problems are treated by emphasizing positive steps to correct the situation. A refresher course over the state driver manual to update knowledge of the rules of the road may be offered.

"55 Alive" is being recognized as an effective driving course for senior citizens. Recent studies have shown a trend toward accident and violation reductions among graduates. Some states and insurance companies are offering economic incentives for people to sign up.

As the population ages, more programs will be needed to help senior citizens learn new skills to compensate for the aging process.

Thiernes, J. "Old Age and Driving Don't Always Mix," in *Aging*, Goldstein, E. C., ed. Vol. 2, Art. 91. Boca Raton, Fl.: Social Issues Resource Series, Inc., 1981.

drug abuse   The abuse of drugs in the elderly is mainly in the misuse of prescription or over-the-counter drugs, often unknowingly. "Street drugs" are not generally a problem with the elderly.

Some older people become excessively dependent upon hypnotic drugs to induce sleep or relieve tension. Such people often cite severe insomnia or pain as justification for the use of such drugs. Often patients will combine over-the-counter drugs with prescription medicines and experience adverse effects.

Symptoms of drug abuse include dizziness, confusion, disorientation, hypochondriasis (unjustified belief that one has a physical illness), insomnia, lack of energy, accident-proneness, incontinence (inability to control the urine flow), and lack of concentration. Often the person may request refills on prescriptions out of proportion to his or her needs. If this request is not granted, the individual may seek another doctor.

Treatment should include patient and family education on interactions of their prescribed drugs, over-the-counter drugs, and alcohol. Psychotherapy or a drug abuse program may be useful. Care should be taken to make sure that the older person understands exactly how to take his or her prescribed medications and to be aware of any limitations with its use.

See also ALCOHOL ABUSE.

Reichel, W. M. *Clinical Aspects of Aging*. Baltimore: The Williams & Wilkins Co., 1979.
Steinberg, F. U. *Care of the Geriatric Patient*, 6th ed. St. Louis: C. V. Mosby Co., 1983.

drug interactions   A drug interaction is defined as the effect of one drug altering the known effects of another drug. Interactions can occur between different drugs, between drugs and laboratory tests, and between drugs and food consumption. The elderly are affected by drug interactions because they often take many different drugs at one time.

Drug-drug reactions may occur by changes in the absorption, distribution, metabolism, or excretion of medications.

Drugs may interfere with clinical laboratory test procedures by physical or chemical means. The color of body fluids can be altered, for example, by riboflavin. False positive readings can be obtained by ascorbic acid or nalidixic acid when urine glucose levels are determined by copper-reduction methods.

Ingestion of food with drugs may alter both the extent and the rate of drug absorption. Food changes the amount of secretion of gastric acid, digestive enzymes, and bile, thus altering the rate of absorption. Drug metabolism can be affected by charcoal broiled foods, for example. Urinary pH can alter the effects of a drug. Acidic drugs are excreted more rapidly in a basic urine and more slowly in an acid urine. Conversely, the excretion of basic drugs is enhanced in an acid urine and delayed in a basic urine.

See also DRUG REACTIONS, ADVERSE.

Covington, T., and Walker J. *Current Geriatric Therapy*. Philadelphia: W. B. Saunders, 1984.

drug reactions, adverse   Adverse drug reactions occur more frequently in the elderly. In one survey, 15.4 percent of hospitalized patients over age 65 suffered reactions compared to 6.3% of those patients under age 60. This higher incidence in the elderly may be due to a greater use of drugs in this age group, increased sensitivity to drug effects, impaired homeostatic mechanisms (steady state of body functions) and decreases in renal (kidney) and hepatic (liver) function.

Adverse reactions may be classified as pharmocologic, allergic, or idiosyncratic. Toxicity occurs from over-dosage but can also be present in an elderly patient on normal dosages because of increased sensitivity to drugs as well as decreased renal and hepatic elimination. Another pharmocologic reaction is that of side effects, the undesirable secondary actions that are inseparable from the desired action of the drug. For example, the induced sedation that occurs from the use of antihistamines is a generally unwanted side effect. Both the toxic effects and the side effects can be minimized with reduction in the dosage.

Allergic reactions are the result of antigen-antibody interaction (the process in which white blood cells produce substances to respond to a foreign body) and require prior exposure to the antigenic agent (drug). Reactions range from a mild rash to anaphylaxis (severe reaction resulting in swelling and even shock) and death. Careful documentation of previous drug experiences will help avoid such medication in the future. Health-care personnel should be prepared for the necessity of resuscitation.

Idiosyncratic reactions are rare, unpredictable, often severe, and are not related to dosage. Drugs that precipitate hemolysis (breakdown of red blood cells) in glucose-6-phosphate dehydrogenase deficiencies (such as primaquine) and acute intermittent porphyria (barbituates) are examples of idiosyncratic reaction.

To prevent such adverse reactions, several precautions should be followed. A careful history of current medications and past medication experiences is necessary so that repetition of bad reactions can be avoided. Patients at greatest risk, including the elderly and those with impaired renal function, should be started at lower dosages that can be gradually increased as tolerance is determined.

It is also necessary to be aware of possible toxic reactions associated with a particular drug.

The most significant way to prevent adverse reactions is to avoid unnecessary drug exposure. Prescriptions should be limited to only those instances where drug therapy is clearly indicated and should be discontinued as soon as possible.

Covington, T., and Walker, J. *Current Geriatric Therapy*. Philadelphia: W. B. Saunders, 1984.

dry eyes   See KERATOCONJUNCTIVITIS SICCA.

dumping syndrome   Dumping syndrome is the rapid entrance of food directly into the jejunum (portion of small intestine).

The hypertonic solution in the gut draws fluid from the circulating blood volume into the intestine, thereby reducing the blood volume and producing syncope (fainting).

The onset of symptoms may occur during the meal or from five to 30 minutes after the meal. The attack can last 20 to 60 minutes. Symptoms include weakness and faintness, accompanied by profuse perspiration and palpitations. This reaction appears to be greater after the ingestion of sugar. Sugar is the most quickly processed food and thus should be avoided with the dumping syndrome. These symptoms are also attributed to the sudden rise in blood sugar (hyperglycemia).

People who experience the dumping syndrome should eat a low-carbohydrate, high-fat, high-protein diet; drink fluids only between meals; avoid eating large amounts of food at one time; and rest after meals for 30 minutes. Sometimes anticholinergic (antispasmodic) drugs may be prescribed to be taken before meals.

See also ULCER PEPTIC.

Rossman, I. *Clinical Geriatrics,* 3rd ed. Philadelphia: J. B. Lippincott Co., 1986.
Scherer, J. C. *Introductory Medical-Surgical Nursing,* 3rd ed. Philadelphia: J. B. Lippincott Co., 1982.

dysequilibrium See VERTIGO.

dyspareunia Dyspareunia is a physically painful sexual experience. In the elderly man, dyspareunia involves painful erection, painful intromission, and painful ejaculation. In the elderly woman, dyspareunia involves uterine cramping or vaginal irritation.

Male dyspareunia is usually caused by prostatic pain secondary to infection, benign prostatic hypertrophy, or carcinoma. Female dyspareunia can be attributed to decreased sexual opportunity, decreased hormone production, urinary tract infections, and extended periods of intercourse due to delayed ejaculation. Dyspareunia can often be the first symptom of an infection or an inflammatory condition.

Treatment for male dyspareunia usually involves administering testosterone replacement therapy. Treatment for female dyspareunia includes systemic or topical hormone replacement combined with increased fluid intake, better hygiene, and taking urinary antiseptics (such as Septra) to help control urologic infections. Applying a lubricant (such as K-Y gel) to the penis before intercourse may also be beneficial.

See also SEXUALITY.

Rossman, I. *Clinical Geriatrics,* 3rd ed. Philadelphia: J. B. Lippincott Co., 1986.
Steinberg, F. U. *Care of the Geriatric Patient,* 6th ed. St. Louis: C. V. Mosby Co., 1983.

dysphagia Dysphagia is difficulty in swallowing. In the elderly, dysphagia is frequently caused by extraesophageal disease. The most common example of this is pseudobulbar palsy due to cerebrovascular disease. Intrathoracic lesions, like bronchial carcinoma or lymph nodes that are enlarged by metastatic spread, may press on or invade the esophagus. More than one possible cause can exist in a patient. A mild or severe stroke may bring on dysphagia.

See also CANCER, ESOPHAGEAL; ESOPHAGEAL STRICTURE.

Brocklehurst, J. C. *Textbook of Geriatric Medicine and Gerontology.* New York: Churchhill Livingstone, 1985.

dysuria Dysuria is a condition of painful or difficult urination. Bacterial infection is a primary cause, but vascular problems, especially hypertension, can be contributing factors. Patients with diabetes and cardiac failure are also subject to dysuria. Nursing home patients and those who are primarily bed-ridden are prone to dysuria. In men, an enlarged prostate is frequently the main contributing factor.

See also URINARY TRACT INFECTION.

Brocklehurst, J. C. *Textbook of Geriatric Medicine and Gerontology.* New York: Churchhill Livingstone, 1985.

E

ears, ringing in   See TINNITUS.

ectropion (outward turning lid)   Ectropion is the turning outward of the margin of the eyelid, resulting in the exposure of the bulbar and palpebral conjunctiva (white of the eye). Ectropion is most frequently seen in the elderly due to a decrease in muscle tone and loss of fat around the eye.

Symptoms result from exposure of the conjunctiva and cornea. When the lower eyelid is involved, the inferior punctum (entrance to tear duct) is not adjacent to the lacrimal lake and tearing may occur. Other symptoms include a foreign body sensation and an increased incidence of chronic infection. Ectropion occurs in several forms: atonic, cicatricial, spastic, and conjunctival. Atonic ectropion is caused by a lack of tone in the eyelid; whereas cicatricial is from scar tissue from a previous infection or inflammation. Spastic ectropion results from a tightness of the eyelid muscles around the eye. Conjunctival ectropion is caused by a previous infection. The lower lid is involved in the atonic type, but the cicatricial and conjunctival types may involve either the upper or lower eyelid.

Treatment for ectropion is surgery usually done on an outpatient basis. Between diagnosis of the condition and surgery the person with ectropion should be encouraged to wipe the tears with an up and inward movement and to use artificial tears as needed for comfort.

Newell, F. W. *Ophthalmology Principles and Concepts,* 6th ed. St. Louis: C. V. Mosby Co., 1986.

Slatt, B. J., and Stein, H. A. *The Ophthalmic Assistant Fundamentals and Clinical Practice,* 4th ed. St. Louis: C. V. Mosby Co., 1983.

eicosapentaenoic acid   Eicosapentaenoic acid is found in high concentration in marine fish such as mackerel. Unlike arachidonic acid, eicosapentaenoic acid does not cause platelet aggregation. High levels of eicosapentaenoic acid may protect humans from blood clots. Eicosaentaenoic acid is currently being marketed in the United States.

Studies done on the Eskimos of Greenland reveal little change in weight, blood pressure, and cholesterol levels as the population aged. The incidence of ischemic heart disease was also low. Their diet contained a high content of eicosapentaenoic acid.

See also AGING, BIOLOGICAL THEORY OF.

Brocklehurst, J. C. *Textbook of Geriatric Medicine and Gerontology.* New York: Churchhill Livingstone, 1985.

elder abuse   In spite of the considerable publicity given to elder abuse, the prevalence of this problem is not well established scientifically. One study gave an estimate of a 4 percent abuse rate in the elderly population in the United States, but this was done in a single city, Washington, D.C., and only 16 percent, or 73, of the people surveyed answered the question on abuse. Another study done in New Jersey found a much lower rate—15 cases per 1,000 older persons, or 1.5 percent.

The most statistically valid study was done in Boston in 1987. It produced estimates of 32 cases per 1,000, or a 3.2 percent rate of abuse. The study reported the following rates of types abuse: physical violence in 20 cases per 1,000; chronic verbal aggression in 11 cases per 1,000; and neglect in 4 cases per 1,000. (These figures are as given in an article by Pillemer and Finkelhor; discrepancy in figures may be due to the presence of more than one type of abuse in a single case.) A city like Boston does not represent the entire

U.S. statistically, but if the 3.2 percent figure were to hold nationally it would represent close to one million cases of abuse.

Instances of abuse generally fall into the categories found in Boston. Physical abuse is most common, and involves shoving, hitting, physically restraining, or sexually abusing the victim. A second type of abuse is psychological, and it may include neglect of the older person's presence or needs, treating the older person as a child, or inflicting verbal abuse—swearing, screaming, and verbal cruelty. Another type is monetary, and arises when family members steal or manage older people's financial resources without proper consent. Outright neglect constitutes yet a fourth type of abuse, and includes: failure to provide bodily care and toileting; allowing bedding to become filthy; or withholding of food, medications, eyeglasses, access to medical treatment, and other necessities.

Publicity about abuse has laid the blame, falsely in most cases, at the door of adult children who are financially pinched and overburdened by the obligation to care for an older parent. According to the Boston study this stereotype is highly inaccurate—58 percent of the cases of abuse were committed by a spouse and only 24 percent by adult children. The fact is that elders are most likely to be abused by people with whom they live, and those who are not living alone most often reside with their spouse, not with their children. Further, cases of abuse often involve alcoholism and drug use by the abusers.

Though frail and dependent older women are portrayed as the main victims, the Boston study found that it was husbands who were most often abused—52 percent of the victims were males compared to 48 percent females. The probable reason for this is that older women more often live alone so are not exposed to people who might abuse them. Older men, on the other hand, are often married; and, ill and dependent, they

may be living with a spouse who is herself old and under stress due to the problems of caregiving.

It is possible that some abused elders fail to report that they are experiencing problems out of fear of reprisal, concern about the legal consequences for the abuser, or to avoid the risk of being removed to an institutional setting. Currently, 41 states have laws that mandate reporting cases of elderly abuse and neglect. Many of these laws, however, provide no penalty for perpetrators.

Efforts to control abuse have extended to the federal level, where legislation to create a national center to conduct research and disseminate information on abuse has been introduced in Congress annually since 1981. Authors of this legislation and critics of federal inaction predict that incidents of abuse will increase as the longevity and numbers of older people continue to grow.

Beck, C. M., and Phillips, L. R. *Abuse of the Elderly. J. of Gerontological Nursing.* 9: 97–102 (1983).

Pillemer, K., and Finkelhor, D. "The Prevalence of Elder Abuse: A Random Sample Survey." *The Gerontologist:* Vol. 28, No. 1, 51–57 (1988).

Quinn, M. and Tomita, S. *Elder, Abuse and Neglect.* New York: Springer Publishing Co., 1986.

emphysema Pulmonary emphysema is characterized by changes in the lung tissue with distention of the alveolar sacs (lining of lungs), rupture of the alveolar wall, and destruction of the alveolar capillary bed. This loss of elasticity results in the trapping of air that should be expired. Emphysema is found more frequently in men. In those over 60, it occurs in 60 per 1,000 persons. Mortality from emphysema increases with age from approximately 200 per 100,000 for those between 65 and 70 years of age to 450 per 100,000 for those over age 75.

One of the earliest symptoms is exertional dyspnea (labored breathing). As the disease progresses, shortness of breath may be present even when resting. A chronic cough with productive yellowish white sputum is present. Inspiration is difficult because the accessory muscles of respiration are used and expiration is prolonged and often accompanied by wheezing. The patient may appear anxious and pale. During expiration the veins in the neck are distended.

In advanced pulmonary emphysema the patient may have a loss of memory, drowsiness, confusion, and loss of judgment. These changes are due to a marked reduction in oxygen reaching the brain and an increased amount of carbon dioxide in the blood. If untreated the level may reach toxic levels resulting in lethargy, stupor, and coma.

The diagnosis is made by physical examination, X-ray films and fluoroscopy (exam that shows shadows of X-ray as they pass through the body). Pulmonary functions and blood gas studies are useful. Bronchospasm (spasmodic contraction of the smooth muscle of the larger air passages of the lungs) may be reduced by epinephrine and aminophylline. In the advanced stages of the disease bronchospasms may be responsive to bronchodilator therapy.

See also ASTHMA.

Rogers, S. C., and McCue, J. D. *Managing Chronic Disease*. Oradell, N.J.: Medical Economics Co., 1987.

Scherer, J. C. *Introductory Medical-Surgical Nursing*. Philadelphia: J. B. Lippincott Co., 1982.

endocarditis   Endocarditis is an inflammatory alteration of the heart valves and of the membranes lining the heart. Infective endocarditis includes all presentations (acute, subacute) and causes (bacterial, fungal) of infectious complications of cardiovascular disease.

Depending on the virulence of the infecting organism, the symptoms of endocarditis may be insidious (as in subacute) or fulminant (as in acute). Typical symptoms are fever, which may be low grade, sweating, weakness, weight loss, complications of infarcts, arthralgias (joint pain), skin lesions such as petechiae (pinpoint, intradermal, or submucous hemorrhage), Osler's nodes (tender areas found in the pads of fingers, toes, or soles of feet), and splinter hemorrhages. Acute bacterial endocarditis may have sudden onset of chills, fever, and congestive heart failure. Endocarditis is frequently seen in intravenous drug users and patients undergoing hemodialysis (the artificial filtering of impurities from the blood).

Examination shows signs of heart disease, fever, skin lesions of mucosal surfaces and the distal extremities, splenomegaly (enlargement of the spleen). Laboratory testing may reveal anemia, an elevated sedimentation rate, gross or microscopic hematuria (bloody urine), pyuria (pus in urine), proteinuria (protein in urine), elevated gamma globulin levels, and renal dysfunction. Blood cultures are positive in 85 percent to 90 percent of patients.

In the last 20 years there has been an increase in the number of elderly cases of endocarditis. Because of the nonspecific nature of the symptoms, this illness tends to be overlooked in the elderly. Also, fever is less prominent in this age group and heart murmurs may be absent in as many as 30 percent of the cases. The mortality rate is over 60 percent in those over age 70.

Antibiotics are the primary mode of treatment in infective endocarditis. When possible, bactericidal drugs (penicillins, cephalosporins, vancomycin) should be used because bacteriostatic drugs (tetracyclines, sulfonamides, chloramphenical) usually fail. Because of decreased renal function in the elderly, these regimens may produce more toxicity.

The patient with congestive heart failure may require immediate surgery with valve replacement. In infections of prosthetic devices, surgical debridement, or replacement is usually indicated.

Covington, T., and Walker, J. *Current Geriatric Therapy.* Philadelphia: W. B. Saunders, 1984.

entropion (inward turning lid)   Entropion is the turning inward of the margin of the eyelid caused by a decrease in muscle tone and loss of fat around the eye in the elderly. This condition causes the lashes to irritate the eye, producing corneal epithelial defects (corneal scarring), conjunctival injection and tearing, which sometimes leads to a secondary infection of the cornea or conjunctiva. An entropion usually involves the lower lid. In the elderly this problem occurs as atonic, cicatricial, or spastic types.

Symptoms of entropion include tearing and a foreign body sensation caused by the eyelashes rubbing against the eye.

In minor cases temporary relief may be obtained by drawing the skin of the outer eyelid down by means of a strip of adhesive tape or by pulling the lashes. These methods have little long-term value. Surgical correction is often necessary and the procedure is usually performed on an outpatient basis.

Newell, F. W. *Ophthalmology Principles and Concepts,* 6th ed. St. Louis: C. V. Mosby Co., 1986.

environment   As individuals grow older they find themselves more confined to their homes. Growing older and retiring strips away reasons for getting out of the house, and makes motility more difficult. Sometimes poor health confines the older person to his or her home. Whatever the reason, when a person stays at home every effort should be made to make that home enjoyable.

See also LIVING SPACE, SECURITY, ADVICE ON.

Gillies, J. *A Guide to Caring for and Coping with Aging Parents.* Nashville: Thomas Nelson Publishers, 1981.

epistaxis (nosebleeds)   In older adults nosebleeds are more often found to originate in the posterior part of the nose rather than in the anterior part as occurs in children and younger adults. The cause is usually spontaneous rupture of a hardened vessel. The bleeding is worse if the patient is hypertensive.

Epistaxis is often an early warning sign in many blood diseases such as anemia, leukemia, and various coagulation defects.

Treatment of nosebleeds first involves applying firm pressure on the nose for several minutes. A calm environment to reduce the level of anxiety is essential. If the bleeding does not stop quickly medical treatment should be obtained.

Control of bleeding from posterior epistaxis is complicated by the inaccessibility of the bleeding site. Hospitalization is not unusual. Postnasal packing is frequently necessary as is cauterization of the bleeding site. If lesser measures are not successful ligation of the vascular supply may be indicated.

Probably the best treatment for nosebleeds is prevention. It is important to maintain adequate humidification, especially during the winter months, and use Vaseline or lanolin ointment to moisten the nasal membranes. The person should also refrain from traumatizing the nose with the finger or other objects, avoid forceful blowing of the nose, limit the use of aspirin, and control high blood pressure.

Ballenger, J. J. *Diseases of the Nose, Throat, Ear, Head and Neck,* 13th ed. Philadelphia; Lea & Febiger, 1985.

Eskimos   The Eskimo diet consists mainly of fish, seals, whales, and other aquatic animals. The Eskimos have a very active lifestyle, and often have to travel vast distances to find food. Eskimos do not age prematurely despite the harsh environmental and difficult conditions under which they live. Weight, skin-fold thickness, and blood pressure do not increase between the ages of 20 and 54. Cholesterol levels do not increase with age. Between the thirties and the fifties a decline in vital capacity and hand-grip has been found.

The fish and meat they consume are rich in polyunsaturated fatty acids. Their diet is also very low in carbohydrates, and the combination of low sugar and high protein content has necessitated a large number of metabolic adaptations. For example, plasma lipids and plasma lipoproteins do not increase much between the ages of 31 and 61 in either sex.

The incidence of ischemic heart disease is low. The fact that the blood lipid pattern of Eskimos living in Danish areas resembled that of the Danes points strongly towards an environmental determinism of the low lipids levels and related age changes in this population.

See also CLIMATES, EXTREME.

Brocklehurst, J. C. *Textbook of Geriatric Medicine and Gerontology.* New York: Churchhill Livingstone, 1985.

esophageal cancer (See CANCER, ESOPHAGEAL.

esophageal stricture Esophageal stricture, or narrowing of the esophagus, is frequently encountered in the elderly. It is a serious manifestation not only because of the diseases that underlie it but also because of its implications as regards nutrition and aspiration.

Benign esophageal stricture is about one-third as common as carcinoma of the esophagus. The diagnoses of benign esophageal stricture should be made only after carcinoma has been completely excluded. Esophageal stricture usually occurs as a complication of reflux esophagitis, a penetrating peptic ulcer, a motor paralysis (usually due to stroke), or following the swallowing of a corrosive substance. A biopsy is essential to rule out malignancy.

The treatment for this condition is either the progressive dilation with bougies or the use of dilators, and correction of the cause

if possible. The development of the esophageal balloon dilation catheters, used in conjunction with endoscopy to examine, will allow stretching of benign strictures under direct vision and in a controlled manner without surgery.

See also CANCER, ESOPHAGEAL.

Brocklehurst, J. C. *Textbook of Geriatric Medicine and Gerontology.* New York: Churchhill Livingstone, 1985.

estate planning Even modest property holdings call for final disposition through a will, though it is only when property holdings are large enough to meet requirements for federal and state estate taxes (over $600,000 to require federal taxes and varying amounts from state to state) that cash expenditures for assistance with estate planning are necessary. For many people a will drawn up with the use of a self-help guide purchased from a bookstore, or with advice from a Legal Aid Society or local area agency on aging, may be sufficient. People with taxable property, however, need to retain the services of an attorney who has specialized knowledge of estate planning. For such people, failure to consult an estate planner can deprive heirs of their legal inheritance as a result of overpayment of taxes.

A national survey showed that even though 80 percent of the public thought that it was better to make plans for death, only 25 percent had drawn up a will. A great many people die without leaving a will (intestate), apparently under the mistaken notion that their property will automatically pass on to their spouse—but it is not quite that simple. To die without a will is to invite battles in the family. Children's inheritances also may be reduced when one's spouse dies unless there is a will that states, in language specified in the tax law, the intent to make use of the federally approved marital deduction.

Because of the complexity of estate planning, and the need to tailor plans to personal circumstances, only the most basic elements of estate planning can be outlined here. First, an attorney should be consulted when drawing up a will, or to determine if an existing will meets current federal and state law. Second, the beneficiaries should be decided upon—spouse, children, relatives, charities, churches, colleges and schools, museums, public art galleries, musical foundations, etc. Third, the information needed for making a will should be organized: beneficiaries' names and addresses, Social Security numbers, birthdates; a list of assets and obligations should be compiled; property that is held jointly or individually should be specified; life insurance companies, policy types, and value of policies should be identified. Fourth, the possibility of using trusts for taxes as well as to assure the safety and security of funds left to others should be considered. Fifth, an attorney should be consulted to determine if joint ownership of property, like an automobile, home, or boat makes sense— generally it does, but not always. Sixth, an executor should be named. Seventh, specific items, such as jewelry, antiques, and art works, should be willed. If necessary, an inventory of specific bequests to individuals or institutions should be drawn up. Last, instructions for final matters—arrangement for the funeral, cremation or interment, or other important considerations—should be left.

Russell, C. H. *Good News About Aging*. New York: John Wiley and Sons, 1989.
Weaver, P., and Buchanan, A. *What to Do with What You've Got: The Practical Guide to Money Management in Retirement*. Washington, D.C.: American Association of Retired Persons, 1985.

euthanasia   The word *euthanasia* refers to a positive or passive act of allowing someone to die, or assisting them to death. According to the General Social Survey, young people are far more willing than the old to consider euthanasia as an acceptable act. When asked the question, "When a person has a disease that cannot be cured, do you think doctors should be allowed to end the patient's life by some painless means if the patient and his family request it," 71 percent of the 18–24 year olds answered "Yes" compared to only 39 percent of those in the 85+ age category.

The survey also showed that men in all age groups are more willing to approve of euthanasia than women—for instance, at 18– 24, 75 percent of the men approved compared to 68% of the women, and at 85+, 46 percent of the men approved compared to 36 percent of the women. In general, there has been growing acceptance of the idea that euthanasia may be appropriate, especially with reference to the idea of "death with dignity" under conditions of hopeless illness when the patient is unconscious.

The practice of euthanasia, however, is still laden with difficult personal, medical, legal, and ethical problems. Oddly, these problems have been provoked in part by the outstanding progress of medical science and technology; progress that now makes it possible to support life by means of breathing, nutrition, and blood circulation apparatus, when an individual has become, or remained, brain dead for weeks or months.

By 1968 the medical capacity to take "heroic measures" to maintain life when the patient was in a coma had made the issue of euthanasia so persistent that Joseph Fletcher, writing in *Ethical Issues in Medicine,* defined four types of "elective death." One type, which he identified as "voluntary and indirect," depended on the individual's own instructions to discontinue extraordinary measures to support his/her life. Such instructions are often given by means of a "living will" in which individuals protect professionals and family members from prosecution by directing them to discontinue treatment when their recovery from an illness is out of the question. Over half of the states have adopted living will laws.

A second form of elective death is involuntary as well as indirect, and may be chosen when a person has fallen into a permanent coma without any form of a living will. Under these circumstances relatives must direct physicians to discontinue extraordinary efforts to maintain the individual's life. It is not uncommon for the children or spouse of an older person to confront the need to decide to carry out an act of "passive" or "negative" euthanasia. Though the legal status of such decisions remains uncertain in a number of states, prosecutions for them are rare.

Two other types of elective death are highly questionable legally and even more so ethically. The first form, known as *voluntary* and *direct*, is equivalent to suicide, and applies when an individual consciously chooses to induce his or her own death. Family members and medical personnel who may be asked to assist in this process risk legal liability. The second, known as *involuntary* and *direct*, involves a positive act by someone to terminate a patient's life, as by administering a deadly drug overdose, without the patient's consent. This is considered illegal, liable to prosecution, and tantamount to murder.

People who object to the first two types of euthanasia (voluntary and indirect, and passive and negative death) make several arguments in opposition, the two principal ones being that: New medical discoveries may lead to the patient's survival with a meaningful life; and legal acceptance of the right to terminate life may lead to actions taken for the benefit of others—notably prospective heirs—rather than the patient.

Those who argue in favor of these two forms of euthanasia point out that extraordinary efforts to support life may simply prolong death rather than support life; and, secondly, that individuals have a right to die a "good death"—one that is peaceful, painless, and proceeds naturally without human interference. Whatever point of view one may have on the issues involved, it is likely that growing public acceptance of the first two types of euthanasia will eventually lead

to effective resolution of the personal, ethical, medical, and legal questions at stake.

See also RIGHT-TO-DIE LAWS.

Russell, C. H., and Megaard, I. *The General Social Survey, 1972–1976: the State of the American People.* New York: Springer–Verlag, 1988.

Ward, R. *The Aging Experience,* 2nd ed. New York: Harper and Row, 1984.

exchanges between generations   Studies of relationships between older people, their children, and other family members have repeatedly shown that help flows both ways between the generations. Older parents help their adult children with babysitting; take over child care when their daughters or sons travel away from home on vacation or business trips; help out in the household and with nursing when family members become ill; do daily chores involving housekeeping, preparing meals, and paying bills; and are called upon for advice. A national survey showed that 67 percent of the elderly population had recently provided assistance to children and family members. Help provided by children and family to older people is by no means meager—the same national survey showed that two-thirds of the elderly say that they have received support from family members in the past month.

When it comes to the important and morale boosting matter of visiting between the elderly, their children, and family, quite contrary to what many people think, the vast majority of older people are by no means isolated or neglected. About 80 percent of the older population have living children; over three-fourths of the older population live within a half hour's travel from at least one child; almost 90 percent of the elderly with children have seen a child in the past month; three-fourths see a child at least weekly and more than half do so every day or two. Besides this, three-fourths of grandparents see a grandchild weekly, while anywhere from one-third to one-half get together with a brother or sister every week.

See also CAREGIVER; ROLE REVERSAL.

Ward, R. *The Aging Experience*, 2nd ed. New York: Harper and Row, 1984.

exercise   Until recent years there was little positive scientific proof that exercise had any great effect on aging or its underlying biological processes. The most affirmative idea about exercise was the observation of many physicians that it made people "feel better," a respectable judgment even though it rested on clinical observation rather than survey or experimental evidence.

Until recently scientific research focused primarily on the decline of physical capacity as age advanced rather than any positive benefits of efforts to maintain capacity. The typical research study compared the young and the old, and showed, for example, that young men could achieve a heart rate of 200 beats per minute compared to a maximum of 70 to 90 beats for men aged 70 to 90. The question of whether it might be good for the older men to raise their heart beats to these or any other levels got little attention.

Today studies of aging increasingly ask questions phrased in this fashion: does exercise have any direct and measurable effect on physiological, neurological, and endocrine factors that underlie the process of aging? Can exercise improve physical capacity, bone strength, heart function, oxygen uptake and use, mental function, and possibly even personality processes? Can exercise retard the onset of typical indicators of age, and can it moderate their effects and perhaps reverse them? These are bold and challenging questions that are beginning to receive affirmative answers.

One interesting and somewhat exotic piece of research of this kind concerned the cardiovascular adjustments and maximum oxygen consumption of Somali herdsmen engaged in long-distance running. The subjects were 15 male tribe members between 14 and 64 years of age. Many of the members of the tribe outperformed athletes of Olympic standards. Balanced and sustained physical training allows adults such as these to make the best use of their physical abilities. Sustained exercise also prevents the accumulation of fatty deposits during adulthood and helps decrease the cholesterol level.

Even these elderly herdsmen, with their high caloric and fat intake, did not have elevated serum cholesterol levels. Furthermore, their body weight and beta-lipoprotein levels did not increase significantly with age. There was a moderate rise in blood pressure in those up to 70 years of age but no signs of clinical symptoms suggestive of ATHEROSCLEROSIS were shown.

Closer to home, the first positive and highly dramatic evidence of the effect of exercise came from a study of 17,000 Harvard graduates published in the *New England Journal of Medicine* in March 1986. This study showed that death rates were 25 percent to 33 percent lower for men who had engaged in mild as well as strenuous exercise. The specific activities performed by the longer surviving members of the research group included simple walking, climbing stairs, and everyday physical exertions such as that recommended by one exercise physiologist—carrying a bag of groceries from the car into the house from time to time— as well as more strenuous aerobic exertions.

While current research confirms the positive benefits of exercise, experts strongly caution against unwise and suddenly instituted, stressful regimens. The body's physical capacities do in fact decline with age, and sudden deaths like that of runner Jim Fixx can occur. Strenuous aerobics programs popularized by actress Jane Fonda are unsuitable for those who have not maintained or do not enjoy good physical condition. Walking, gentle stretching, and bending typical of Yoga style exercises, and ordinary physical activity all have value. Any decisions to start a new exercise program should, like dieting, include prior consultation with a physician.

Russell, C. H. *Good News About Aging*. New York: John Wiley and Sons, 1989.

exercises, Feldenkrais   Moshe Feldenkrais, an Israeli physiologist with a considerable background in Judo, developed several hundred unusual exercises to enhance body function and movement. These exercises are beneficial to the elderly in that they help increase the ease of body movement. Some examples of these exercises include autogenic training, biofeedback training, group breathing, Hatha Yoga, meditation, self-image exercise and Tai Chi Chuan.

See also AUTOGENIC TRAINING; BIOFEED-BACK TRAINING; HATHA YOGA, MEDITATION; SELF-IMAGE EXERCISE; TAI CHI CHUAN.

Fields, S. "Sage Can Be a Spice in Life," in *Aging*, Goldstein, E. C., ed. Vol. 1, Art. 26. Boca Raton, Fl.: Social Issues Resource Series, Inc., 1981.

exercise, self-image   See SELF-IMAGE EXERCISE.

exophthalmic goiter   See HYPERTHY-ROIDISM.

external otitis   External otitis is inflammation of the external auditory canal. This disorder may be classified as infectious (inflammatory), eczematoid, or seborrheic and may be acute, recurrent, or chronic. Although external otitis can affect all age groups, the elderly are more susceptible.

The symptoms common to all forms are itching, edema, pain, and discharge from the ear canal. Heat and humidity lower the canal skin's resistance to infection. This accounts for an increased frequency of infection during the summer months.

In inflammatory external otitis the infecting organisms are usually staphylococcus (for acute localized), *Pseudomonas aeruginosa* (for acute diffuse) and *Aspergillus ni-ger*, actinomyces, or yeasts (for chronic diffuse). Topical and systemic antibiotics are used in treatment followed by dilute alcohol solutions to keep the canal dry and clean.

The major causes of eczematoid external otitis are topical antibiotics or ear vehicles (as in dermatatis medicamentosa); allergy to chemicals or metals used around the ear, such as hair sprays or earrings (as in contact dermatitis); or atopic reaction due to ingested antigen (as in atopic dermatitis). Eczematoid external otitis is most difficult to treat because causative agents often remain undiagnosed. Corticosteriods combined with antibiotics in an otic solution produce rapid healing and are usually used for five days. Any ear preparation used for more than 10 days may itself produce an eczematoid reaction.

Skin testing may be necessary in contact dermatitis. Atopy (hypersensitivity) is detected by a family history of allergy plus manifestations of asthma and hay fever. Each of these types represent a distinct form of allergy and are characterized by histamine release in the tissue. Because of its allergic nature, eczematoid external otitis tends to be recurrent. Each episode tends to make the ear more susceptible to future attacks.

Control of seborrheic dermatitis of the scalp is necessary to control seborrheic external otitis. The best agent for this is a selenium sulfide shampoo once a month. Silver nitrate and diluted alcohol are used on the canal and concha to keep them clean and dry.

Malignant external otitis is a special form of acute diffuse external otitis typically occurring in elderly diabetic patients. This infection is usually unilateral and begins with itching, which is followed by painful discharge and swelling.

Topical therapy is ineffectual and the disease progresses to involve the surrounding tympanic bone. Intense pain develops, and profuse granulation blocks the ear canal. Facial nerves may become involved causing peripheral paresis or paralysis. Temporizing treatments are contraindictated as the disease will extend to involve the surrounding areas of the temporal bone: the mastoid squamous and petrous portions. Sequestration (isolation) of the temporal bone and even death have occurred in a number of these patients, thus the ominous name—malignant external otitis.

This pathology is a progressive osteomyelitis (inflammation of the bone and bone marrow) with *Pseudomonas aeruginosa* as the usual infecting organism. Standard treatment is hospitalization of the patient together with the use of high doses of antibiotics specific for *Pseudomonas* for an extended length of time.

Special attention to diabetic management and to proper aural hygiene is indicated to prevent recurrence of the problem.

See also OTITIS MEDIA.

Ballenger, J. J. *Diseases of the Nose, Throat, Ear, Head and Neck,* 13th ed. Philadelphia: Lea & Febiger, 1985.

eyelid, droopy   See PTOSIS.

eyelid, excessive skin   See BLEPHARO-CHALASIS.

eyelid, inward   See ENTROPION.

eyelid, outward   See ECTROPION.

F

facelift   See COSMETIC SURGERY.

fainting   See VERTIGO.

falls   People over 65 constitute the age group most affected by home accidents, accounting for 9,900 fatalities per year and 43 percent of all accidental fatalities in the home. As people age, falls become an increasingly significant cause of death. They overtake motor vehicle accidents by age 75–79, when the mortality rate from falls reaches 36.9 per 100,000 compared to 30.5 for motor vehicle accidents. At age 80–84 the death rate from falls climbs to 79.2 per 100,000 compared to 32.3 for motor vehicles, and by 85+ it reaches 186.3 per 100,000 compared to 24 for motor vehicles.

Women and men about equal one another in deaths caused by falls, with stairs the most prominent place of injury. Misuse of alcohol and acute and chronic health problems are also factors in 42 percent of these deaths but it is estimated that environmental hazards enter the picture in 45 percent of the cases.

Physical disorders that often appear to produce falls include recently acquired gait disorders (such as learning to walk after hip replacement, leg muscles weakened after a bed stay, and imbalance produced by drugs and alcohol). In terms of environmental causes, stairways represent the most serious danger because visual control of movements is vitally important at top steps where lighting is often not adequate. Remedies for stairway problems include proper lighting, installation of handrails, efficient stair design (suitably deep treads and a gradual rather than steep incline), and removal of stairwell features that may distract the walker's attention. Other factors causing home falls include loose and slippery rugs, poorly secured carpets with edges that can cause tripping, and raised thresholds in doorways that cause stumbling. Loose slippers and robes may appear comfortable and suitable for scuffing about, but these too can be a hazard.

An excellent discussion of the causes and ways of avoiding falls written in nontechnical language for the lay person appears in an article in the *Harvard Medical School Health* for December, 1989, (Vol. 15:2). Here the author makes an important concluding observation: There is some evidence that remaining in good physical condition, including graded exercise and gait training for those who need it, maintains the leg muscle strength and good balance that can help to prevent falls.

Sterns, H. L.; Barrett, G. V.; and Alexander, R. "Accidents and the Aging Individual," in Birren, J. E., and Schaie, K. W., eds. *Handbook of the Psychology of Aging,* 2nd ed. New York: Van Nostrand Reinhold Company, 1985.

far-sightedness See HYPEROPIA.

fear See ANXIETY.

fecal impactions Fecal impaction is stool that has remained in the colon until it becomes exceedingly hard. Constipation and fecal impaction is prevalent among the elderly due to lack of body mobility caused by stroke, depression, senility, and other chronic debilitating diseases.

Symptoms of fecal impaction include abdominal pain, decreased appetite, headache, and watery diarrhea-like stools with intermittent constipation.

Fecal impactions usually can be softened and removed by oil and cleansing enemas. If these treatments are not effective digital removal may be necessary.

For the hospitalized patient, efforts should be made to identify the causes of the impaction and make changes in lifestyle and diet. Improving intake of fiber foods such as fruits and whole grains, and fluids, eliminating constipating drugs, encouraging ambulation, and providing privacy promote normal bowel elimination. For paraplegics (paralysis of both lower extremities), digital stimulation may be necessary. Stool softners, laxatives, and enemas may also be necessary on a regular basis to prevent an impaction.

See also CONSTIPATION.

Scherer, J. C. *Introductory Medical-Surgical Nursing.* Philadelphia: J. B. Lippincott Co., 1982.
Steinberg, F. U. *Care of the Geriatric Patient,* 6th ed. St. Louis: C. V. Mosby Co., 1983.

fever See HYPERTHERMIA.

fever of undetermined origin Patients who maintain a temperature of 101 degrees Fahrenheit or greater for more than three weeks and have undergone screening evaluation with no firm diagnosis are said to have fever of undetermined origin. In general the elderly person with fever of undetermined origin is more likely to have a serious illness than a younger individual.

The most common etiologies encountered in fever of undetermined origin are infectious, neoplastic, and inflammatory. The infectious illnesses include intra-abdominal (liver, gallbladder), endocarditis, and tuberculosis. Neoplastic diseases such as lymphoma (neoplastic disease of lymphoid tissue), nephrocarcinoma and metastatic tumors to the liver may also cause fever. Those illnesses frequently found in the inflammatory category are lupus erythematosus (systemic subacute skin lesions, usually chronic), polyarteritis nodosa (inflammation and necrosis of arteries), and giant-cell arteritis. For 5 percent to 15 percent of cases an etiology is never found.

Symptoms are extremely varied. Generally, however, the person does not manifest the usual symptoms of the disease in question. Every patient with an unexplained fever should have a thorough medical history and careful physical examination, which should be repeated at frequent intervals. A systematic approach to laboratory testing should be employed with follow-up of any leads. Specific abdominal tests may be necessary as well as bone marrow examination and liver biopsy. Abdominal exploration may be indicated in selected patients.

Covington, T., and Walker, J. *Current Geriatric Therapy.* Philadelphia: W. B. Saunders, 1984.

FGP See FOSTER GRANDPARENT PROGRAM.

finances Older individuals should carefully plan their financial assets. It is important to discover and secure all the resources that are available. It is also important to know the legal ways to transfer financial responsibilities in the event that the older person should become mentally incompetent or physically unable to manage his or her own affairs.

See also INFLATION; LEGAL REPRESENTATION; MEDICAID; MEDICARE; SOCIAL SECURITY; SUPPLEMENTAL SECURITY INCOME.

Gillies, J. *A Guide to Caring for and Coping with Aging Parents.* Nashville: Thomas Nelson Publishers, 1981.

fitness See EXERCISE.

flatulent dyspepsia syndrome A frequent cause of dyspepsia (impairment of digestion) and abdominal pain without any organic cause has become increasingly recognized in recent years. This condition is usually called flatulent dyspepsia syndrome and is characterized by upper abdominal pain usually in or radiating from the left hypochondrium (abdomen) and is often accompanied by a feeling of fullness, with nausea and frequent eructation (belching) of air. Flatulent dyspepsia syndrome is seen frequently in the elderly and is thought to be caused by excessive swallowing of air, which is secondary to stress or anxiety. The condition is often worse after meals and in the evening. There may also be a sensation of churning in the stomach. This condition is usually precipitated by anxiety or stress.

The treatment of this condition is symptomatic. A treatment that is used often is five to 10 mg of metoclopramide given before meals. Treatment of the underlying psychological upset may also be necessary.

Brocklehurst, J. C. *Textbook of Geriatric Medicine and Gerontology.* New York: Churchhill Livingstone, 1985.

fluid intake Fluid intake is often inadequate in older individuals. If incontinence (inability to control urinary flow) is a prob-

lem, the older person may believe that by limiting his or her fluid intake control will be possible. Others simply do not get thirsty due to inactivity and therefore do not take in adequate fluids. For whatever reason, an elderly person can quickly become dehydrated, which can lead to very serious consequences.

The older person needs to be reminded to drink sufficient fluids. Some older individuals find that it is easier to remember to drink fluids if they routinely drink a glass of fluid each time they take medicines. By carefully choosing fruit and vegetable juices and soups, additional nourishment, as well as additional fluid intake, can be provided.

Water is an essential component of nutrition. Older individuals should drink approximately 1.3 quarts (7 glasses of 8 ounces each) of water daily unless they are on a specific restricted-fluids diet.

See also INCONTINENCE.

Scherer, J. C. *Introductory Medical-Surgical Nursing,* 3rd ed. Philadelphia: J. B. Lippincott Co., 1982.
Steinberg, F. U. *Care of the Geriatric Patient,* 6th ed. St. Louis: C. V. Mosby Co., 1983.

folic acid deficiency Folic acid deficiency is generally caused by nutritional deprivation. In the elderly, nutritional folic acid deficiency is seen in those who have poor access to an adequate diet, those who are chronic alcoholics, and those who use certain medications that inhibit the enzyme involved in normal absorption of folic acid through the intestinal wall. Other disorders of the small bowel may also be associated with folic acid deficiency.

Symptoms of folic acid deficiency include fatigue, dizziness, pallor of the skin, diarrhea, dementia, neurologic symptoms, and weight loss.

Treatment of folic acid deficiency is usually oral folic acid and a well-balanced diet. In the alcoholic with folic acid deficiency, the simultaneous administration of folic acid with alcohol may inhibit the response to folic acid.

Ham, R. J. *Geriatric Medicine Annual—1987.* Oradell, N.J.: Medical Economics Books, 1987.
Phipps, W. J., *et al. Medical Surgical Nursing.* St. Louis: C. V. Mosby Co., 1983.
Reichel, W. *Clinical Aspects of Aging.* Baltimore: Williams & Wilkins Co., 1979.

food groups, basic   People need the same nutrients throughout their lives yet the amount needed varies with age, health, and activity level. The main nutrients in food are proteins, carbohydrates, fats, vitamins, and minerals. An elderly person's body tends to increase in fat and decrease in muscle mass and metabolic rate. Physical activity may also decrease. Thus, elderly people need to decrease their caloric intake and consume adequate amounts of calcium and fiber.

The basic four food groups should be included each day;

1. Four or more servings of fruit and vegetables.
2. The equivalent of two glasses of milk
3. Four or more servings of breads or cereals
4. Two servings of a meat group

The older individual may find it easier to chew and digest fruits and vegetables that are chopped or dried. Stewed fruits, especially prunes, can help constipation, which is a major problem among the elderly.

The dairy product requirement may be met with milk, cheese, yogurt, or other dairy products. Milkshakes, ice cream, and custards are often enjoyed by older people since they pose no problem in chewing, but they may be high in fat and thus not the best choice. Skimmed milk and buttermilk are frequently preferred because of lower fat and caloric content.

An adequate amount of the bread group helps to form necessary bulk in the older person's diet and also helps to eliminate constipation.

The meat group is the most expensive and the most difficult to chew. Because of this it is the one most commonly omitted from the older person's diet. Older people should be encouraged to buy a variety of meats and to broil or boil them. Frying meats adds more fats and calories without increasing the nutritional value. Fish and poultry have become increasingly popular due to the low fat and caloric content.

Eggs, beans, nuts, and peanut butter are also excellent sources of protein and can be substituted for some of the meat requirement.

See also CONSTIPATION.

Scherer, J. C. *Introductory Medical-Surgical Nursing,* 3rd ed. Philadelphia: J. B. Lippincott Co., 1982.
Steinberg, F. U. *Care of the Geriatric Patient,* 6th ed. St. Louis: C. V. Mosby Co., 1983.

food stamps   The food stamp program is a program designed to help qualified people who live independently or in certain home-care situations.

The food stamp program is a function of the U.S. Department of Agriculture but is usually administered in individual states by welfare or human resources departments.

People who qualify for the food stamp program may also be eligible for the surplus food program. This is a program in which qualified recipients are given surplus foods such as cheese, eggs, milk, etc.

Many elderly people may qualify for this type of assistance because of the effect of inflation on their fixed income. Interested individuals should inquire about food stamps and surplus food programs at their local Social Security office.

See also MEDICAID; SOCIAL SECURITY.

Deedy J. *Your Aging Parents.* Chicago: The Thomas More Press, 1984.
Gillies, J., *A Guide to Caring for Coping with Aging Parents.* Nashville: Thomas Nelson Publishers, 1981.

foot care   Foot care is of utmost importance in older individuals because of the need for ambulation and mobility.

Circulation to the lower portions of the body tends to decrease with age. Decreased circulation, coupled with diminished sensation, can lead to skin breakdown and infections.

Older individuals are less agile and may experience difficulty in maintaining good hygiene of the feet. These individuals may experience shortness of breath or dizziness while bending over or may be unable to reach their feet due to arthritic changes or muscular weakness. Diabetics may have more difficulty with their feet.

It is extremely important to keep the feet thoroughly dry to prevent cracking, which can lead to ulceration and infection. If physical disabilities prevent proper drying, the use of a hair dryer held 15–18 inches away from the foot may be a good alternative.

Toenails should be clipped. Long jagged nail edges may lead to a laceration that can lead to infection. If the person is unable to clip his or her toenails, a family member or friend can do it. Soaking feet 15 minutes once a day for four days prior to clipping will help soften the toenail and cut down on the chance of injury. In addition, cutting the nail straight across rather than curving the nail will reduce the incidence of the nail embedding in the adjacent tissue.

People should also be instructed to inspect their feet, toes, and between their toes daily. The use of a mirror can aid in seeing the bottom of the feet. It is also important to wash the feet daily and avoid extremes of temperature; inspect the shoes daily for foreign objects, nails, and torn linings; wear properly fitted footwear, not to go barefooted; and to have the feet examined at each doctor's visit.

The ability of an individual to remain ambulatory may be the only dividing line between institutionalization and remaining an active and viable member of society.

Therefore, good foot care is essential in remaining independent.

Gillies, J. *A Guide to Caring for and Coping with Aging Parents.* Nashville: Thomas Nelson Publishers, 1981.

foot massage   Foot massage can be performed as self-massage or by others. Elderly people enjoy foot massage because it is an unthreatening form of body stimulation. Another benefit of foot massage for the elderly is stimulation of blood circulation, which is often a problem of the elderly.

See also FOOT CARE.

Fields, S. "Sage Can Be a Spice in Life," in *Aging,* Goldstein, E. C., ed. Vol. 1, Art. 26. Boca Raton, Fl.: Social Issues Resource Series, Inc., 1981.

forehead lift   See COSMETIC SURGERY.

forgetfulness (memory loss)   As people age, forgetfulness becomes more common. Learning little strategies to deal with this difficulty eases the problem and can help avoid embarrassing situations. The following is a list of such strategies.

• Recalling a name is usually the most frequent type of memory loss. To recall someone's name, a person should review everything he or she knows about that person. The elderly person should slowly and deliberately go through the alphabet and try to pronounce the name. If that person will be in a setting with a large group of people, it helps to review in advance the names of the people who will be there. When an elderly person is introducing someone and cannot recall that person's name, it may help to pass it off lightheartedly by saying that he or she always forgets the names of those he or she most wants to remember or joking about how often one can forget one's own name.

- When something occurs to a forgetful person that he or she wants to be sure to remember, it may help to do some physical thing to help remember: for instance, hanging an umbrella on the doorknob as a reminder to take it if rain is predicted.
- If one needs to take pills at a certain time, it may be useful to connect it to something else one does at that time—brushing one's teeth, for example. A pill case can be attached to your toothbrush with the correct number of pills for the day. Or a quarter of the day's calendar could be blackened each time one takes medicine that is needed four times a day.
- Appointments are easier to remember if a large wall calendar is hung in a prominent place and entries made promptly.
- To remember events or duties within the framework of a few hours, the use of a timer may be helpful.

Developing corrective strategies will enable an individual to lead a more enjoyable life.

Skinner, B. F. and Vaughan, M. E. "When the Words Won't Come Back," in *Aging*, Goldstein, E. C., ed. Vol. 2, Art. 59. Boca Raton, Fl.: Social Issues Resource Series, Inc., 1981.

foster care (group care)   One alternative to nursing home care is that of "sheltered" living where supportive and safe care is provided for the aged.

A foster home can be established in which a family or a couple will provide room and board for several older people, receiving compensation through welfare agencies for their services in much the same way as in foster homes for children.

Candidates for such a living arrangement would preferably be those who require an intermediate level of medical and custodial care but do not require the 24-hour services offered by nursing homes. In some instances, nursing care might be provided at the foster home through a public health service or some other provider of home health care.

As a rule the cost of the care provided in a foster home is far below the cost of nursing home care. Even more important, elderly residents of foster homes continue to live in a family setting where they can interact with others in a less structured and institutionalized environment commonly found in nursing homes.

See also LIVING ALONE; LIVING WITH ONE'S CHILDREN; NURSING HOMES, HOW TO SELECT MONITOR, AND EVALUATE; RETIREMENT RESIDENCE CENTERS.

Deedy, J. *Your Aging Parents*. Chicago: The Thomas More Press, 1984.
Gillies, J. *A Guide to Caring for and Coping with Aging Parents*. Nashville: Thomas Nelson Publishers, 1981.

Foster Grandparent Program (FGP)
Over two decades old, the Foster Grandparent Program (FGP) is staffed by individuals 60 years of age and older who meet federal and state low-income standards. The program is offered under the auspices of the federal service agency, ACTION.

Foster Grandparents receive 40 hours of pre-service orientation and training. They are supervised by child-care teams in their assigned agencies and give four hours of in-service training monthly. Volunteers receive a tax-free stipend, a transportation allowance, hot meals on service days, accident and liability insurance, and an annual physical examination. Service is usually four hours a day, five days a week.

Volunteers act in the capacity of grandparent figures and work in cooperation with schools, hospitals, juvenile detention centers, Head Start, shelter for neglected children, state schools for the mentally retarded, and drug rehabilitation centers.

See also ACTION.

For more information write:
Foster Grandparent Program
c/o ACTION

806 Connecticut Avenue, N.W.,
Washington, DC 20525
(202) 678-4215

free radical theory of aging   The free
radical theory proposes the existence of small
molecules, or free radicals, each with an
unpaired electron, which are formed as a
byproduct during normal metabolism. The
free radicals are very reactive and bounce
around inside a cell causing damage to DNA,
RNA, proteins, and lipids, which can lead
to cellular death. Free radical damage may
account for a number of diseases, such as
cancer, arthritis, and certain cardiovascular
problems. A diet that includes compounds
known as antioxidants, or free radical scav-
engers, could prolong life by as much as 10
years by protecting cells from the free radicals. These antioxidants include vitamins A
and C, selenium, cysteine, and the food
preservative BHT.

See also ANTIOXIDANTS; AGING, BIOLOG-
ICAL THEORY OF.

Kinney, T. "Living Longer," in *Aging,* Goldstein, E. C., ed. Vol. 3, Art. 10. Boca Raton,
Fl.: Social Issues Resource Series, Inc., 1981.

friends (convoy of social support)   Although friends usually do not substitute for
family among old people, researchers have
developed the term *convoy of social support*
to describe the network of social relationships that people rely on as they go through
life. Viewed in this light, friendships do
become a source of help, and they may be
especially important in strengthening an individual's self-image as age advances. For
example, they offer individuals an opportunity to rebuild roles that they have abandoned as life has progressed (i.e., giving up
a job at retirement) by offering substitute
networks and activities that act as a buffer
against the individual's sense of aging. Because friends tend to accept one another,
they help individuals to remain themselves
and to maintain a sense of self-esteem.

As in earlier life, friends in age tend to
be like oneself and drawn from among people who are alike—similar in age, interests,
locale, economic circumstances, and the like.
When asked to describe the elements of their
friendships, men often describe "instrumental roles" of their companions, saying that
they engage in activities like playing golf or
cards, bowling, fishing, or working on home
painting and construction together. Women
are more likely to mention "confidant" relationships, such as intimacy, self-disclo-
sure, and emotional closeness, when they
describe friendships.

No one has satisfactorily answered the
question of whether these differing perceptions of friendships reflect a social destiny
that casts men into instrumental relationships
in life and women in more personal relationships, or whether the differences derive from
inner biological forces that shape the experiences of the two sexes. Interestingly, however, some studies show that men look to
their wives for exchange of confidences,
whereas women look to their friends. Women
as a rule appear to participate more in personal social relationships and to derive more
from them than men do.

Whatever the reason for such differences,
each sex needs to maintain friendships in
age. Statistics clearly show that friendships
play a major part in later life for most people. According to a Harris poll conducted
for the National Council on Aging, 60 percent of the U.S. population over 65 recalled
having seen a close friend within the past
day or two. The General Social Survey also
showed that 70 percent or more of people
over age 65 expressed a great deal of satisfaction with their friendships.

Social skills of meeting, greeting, and
chatting with people are needed to maintain
friendships, and these may require some
effort in late life, especially so for people
with diminished eyesight or hearing. Joining
groups, reaching out to others, being a part
of the social stream, and belonging to a

social milieu may place demands on older people, but the return in stimulation and personal reinforcement make the effort worthwhile.

Russell, C. H., and Megaard, I. *The General Social Survey, 1972–1976: the State of the American People.* New York: Springer-Verlag, 1988.
Ward, R. *The Aging Experience,* 2nd ed. New York: Harper and Row, 1984.

funerals Consumerism has dominated much of the publicity about funerals ever since Jessica Mitford published *The High Cost of Death* some years ago and has produced a point of view that masks the important personal and social functions of funeral rituals. At the root, funerals are one of the major social ceremonies of life, and whether people acknowledge the similarity or not, funerals fall in the same class as the ceremonies that initiate children into the world (baptisms, namings, confirmations, Bar Mitzvahs, Bas Mitzvahs, etc.) and ceremonies that mark other important occasions, including weddings, birthday parties, and retirement events.

Like these, funerals provide a way of marking a transition in life that has important social as well as personal meaning. Probably the first record of some sort of a ceremony to compassionately and tenderly put someone to rest dates from some 50,000 years ago when a group of Neanderthal cave dwellers (a human group that may be ancestral to modern humans) scattered quantities of flowers over the body of a young man laid to rest in a shallow grave in the floor of a cave. Archeologists deduced that the flowers were spread over the body of the young man because an unexpectedly large quantity of flower pollen suffused the soil that surrounded the skeleton. While it is not certain just what sort of ceremony might have been involved, this evidence of interment along with the pollen suggests that people at the dawn of modern humanity had a way of marking the passage from life to death.

Funerals provide people with a way to deal with death. Unlike other animals, the human species does not abandon its dead, but rather gives meaning to the life of a person in death. Humans memorialize the individual, providing an appropriate way to set the person to rest and to bid him or her farewell. By means of funeral and burial ceremonies, and the social events represented by wakes and visiting hours, people come together in a fashion that symbolizes their social continuity. By these means they overcome the finality of death—death may be an end, but through their celebrations and memorials it is a continuation and perhaps even a beginning of a new state of life.

For the dying person, knowledge of funeral events can serve as a means for overcoming death by understanding—and sometimes personally arranging—the events surrounding their own passing. Individuals can anticipate and manage their own death by making a will to dispose of their property, purchase a cemetery plot, provide for the perpetual care of the surroundings in which they and their loved ones will rest, anticipate family visits to grave sites, select their own casket, clothing, and jewelry for their funeral, and even create the character and tone of their final ceremony by selecting prayers to be said, songs to be sung, and who will speak parting words.

Some individuals have even provided for the refreshment of their families and friends by prepaying the expenses of a meal. Often younger family members consider such preparations morbid, and discourage or even dismiss the subject of arrangements. Older family members, however, often initiate conversations about such matters with enthusiasm. In fact, anticipation of the final events of one's life can have the important function of making one psychologically comfortable about death. It also provides the possibility of remaining in control—independent, autonomous, individualistic—to the end. People who make their own funeral arrangements never become nonentities—they remain in charge even in death.

For family members, especially widows, widowers, and children, funerals provide a way of expressing and dealing with grief and bereavement. While they do not wipe these away, nor necessarily relieve a sense of loss, emptiness, loneliness, and despair that may accompany the death of a loved one, they provide a means for receiving support from family and friends and for confirming the presence of a social network that can make life bearable. Funerals and funeral ceremonies provide a structure, a plan action for what to do, a way of bringing a past relationship to a close, and beginning a transition to the future. At best they can provide comfort and a strong psychological support for those left behind by sanctifying the life and relationships of the one who has passed on.

Kalish, R. A. "The Social Context of Death and Dying," in Binstock, R. H., and Shanas, E., eds. *Handbook of Aging and the Social Sciences,* 2nd ed. New York: Van Nostrand Reinhold Company, 1985.
Kastenbaum, R. A. "Dying and Death: A Life-Span Approach," in Birren, J. E., and Schaie, K. W., eds. *Handbook of the Psychology of Aging,* 2nd ed. New York: Van Nostrand Reinhold Company, 1985.

funerals, planning arrangements and expenses of   A funeral can be one of the larger expenditures of a lifetime. Some surveys identify funerals as people's third highest investment, ranking behind a home and a car, and equaling a wedding.

Those older individuals who plan their own funerals may do so because they wish to convey particular meanings about themselves or about death; they may wish to spare family members the burden of the arrangements during a time of grief; or, they may simply consider themselves in the best po-

sition to avoid excessive funeral costs. These individuals take the responsibility for choosing a type of service, musical selections, who will preside, whether to have an underground burial or a cremation, and so forth.

Because space near cities may be scarce and burial plots quite distant and expensive, people in some areas are buried in tiers in above-ground vaults. Ground burial in most cemeteries now requires additional expense for a concret tomb liner to provide the solid surface necessary for perpetual care and mowing of grass by heavy equipment.

Rules vary by state, but embalming is generally required when: a person's body is to be transported for some distance; death is from a contagious disease; a body is to be placed on view; or, burial can not take place within 72 hours.

Some individuals will their bodies to medical schools for purposes of research, or donate their body organs for the benefit of other people. If an older individual has specific wishes of this type, they should be written down and put in an agreed upon place so that family members will be able to locate and execute them when needed.

Many older people do not preplan their funerals, and in such cases the bereaved family may be forced to make decisions and purchase merchandise and services while undergoing emotional distress. It is perfectly normal for the bereaved in such circumstances to experience feelings of guilt and confusion about planning the funeral. Because decisions are numerous, detailed, and can have costly consequences, a clear-thinking friend can sometimes assist and so help to relieve these problems.

There are a few fundamentals to keep in mind when making funeral arrangements.

• Although the person making the funeral arrangements may be experiencing profound emotion and a lowered capacity for good judgment, it is essential to remember that funerals are a business and must be approached in a businesslike way. In fact, business considerations offer an important reason to plan funerals before the event of an older person's death, at a time when one is less likely to exercise poor judgment or be influenced by emotion. As a general rule, a funeral is like a big wedding—it should be planned well in advance.

- There are lower cost alternatives, such as cremation, rental of a casket for viewing purposes only, and burial in a less expensive coffin.
- There is misinformation about embalming. Embalming does not prevent decomposition of the body over a period of time. Not all states require it, but people commonly believe it is mandated by law.
- Airtight and watertight caskets do not prevent decomposition.
- Funeral homes that are unwilling to make price information available are required to present it if asked—and it makes sense to ask and perhaps even do some shopping.

Memorial societies offer another type of lower cost funeral alternative. These are nonprofit membership groups organized and run by volunteers who seek contracts with cooperating funeral services to arrange set prices for members. Traditionally, memorial society members have preferred cremation, but some now offer a choice of a simple traditional funeral in place of cremation. Most memorial societies prefer people to join in advance, but some accept enrollment of a deceased person by family members after a death has occurred.

Traditional funerals involve several expenses. In addition to the costs of caskets and burial vault, these may include honoraria for clergy and sacred music, and charges for obituary notices, the death certificate, a cemetery plot, opening and closing of the grave, flowers, and funeral home charges for staff, use of facilities and funeral coaches and limousines. Costs for each of these items should be obtained when planning a funeral. If quoted prices seem too high, one needs to make a specific request for alternatives, because some funeral directors will describe options only if asked. Quoted prices may include extra charges, such as family cars, flower cars, motorcycle police escort, and a host of other items that can be eliminated without loss of dignity and meaning in a funeral event.

Means of payment are important matters to consider when making funeral arrangements. Financial assistance for funeral expenses are available under some circumstances. One such is a Social Security payment of approximately $250, available to a surviving spouse or entitled child. This can be paid directly to a funeral home or to the eligible dependent. Another form of assistance is the veteran's burial benefit available to veterans who were receiving, or were entitled to receive, a Veterans Administration pension. This benefit may include a $300 funeral allowance and a $150 burial allowance for a non–service connected death.

Payment of veterans' benefits are made to the person who pays the funeral expenses, and for this reason the benefit is not available for completely prepaid funerals. To ensure collection of the full benefit, the custom is to prepay a veteran's funeral expenses up to, but not including, the amount of the death benefit. Because the full expense has not been paid, the benefit can be collected by family members who pay the balance when the veteran dies.

Veterans and their immediate families are entitled to burial in a national cemetery or in the nearest veterans' cemetery—space permitting. Families of deceased veterans may also obtain a flag to drape over the casket during the ceremonies and may keep the flag after the event.

The funeral expenses of qualified indigent people are often covered by death benefits available from state or local government and social service agencies. Death benefits may also be available from certain companies, railroads, civil service departments, and fraternal organizations.

Deedy J. *Your Aging Parents*. Chicago: The Thomas More Press, 1984.

Gillies, J. *A Guide to Caring for Coping with Aging Parents*. Nashville: Thomas Nelson Publishers, 1981.

Nelson, T. C. *It's Your Choice*. Glenview, Ill.: AARP, 1983.

G

gallbladder disease (cholelithiasis, gallbladder stones, gallstones, biliary Colic, cholecystectomy)   A gallstone is a concretion formed in the gallbladder. Gallstones are the most common abnormality of the biliary system. They occur in 20 percent of people over 40 years old. This increases progressively with age. Gallstones occur four times more often in women than men, especially with a history of pregnancy, diabetes, or obesity.

Acute cholecystitis is a common complication of gallstones. Symptoms are secondary to blockage of the outflow of bile due to stones or spasms of the ductal system. Symptoms usually flare up after a meal containing fried, greasy, spicy, or fatty foods. The patient may have belching, nausea, and discomfort in the right upper abdominal area. This discomfort ranges from cramps to very severe pain. Very severe pain is called biliary colic. This pain may radiate to the back and shoulder. Vomiting may occur with biliary colic (intense pain felt in the right upper quadrant of abdomen from impaction of a gallstone in the gallbladder or liver.

In addition to the subjective symptoms the diagnosis is confirmed by a cholecystogram (gallbladder series). The evening before the test, special dye-containing tablets are given to the patient and foods and liquids are withheld. After ingestion the dye reaches the liver and is excreted into the bile and passes into the gallbladder, making it radiographically visible.

Usually removal of the gallbladder (cholecystectomy) is advised. Surgeons prefer to operate electively rather than in an emergency situation as complications are reduced.

People who are admitted with an attack of biliary colic are treated with rest, bland liquid diet, and sedation. If vomiting occurs nasogastric suction and parenteral fluids may be needed. Meperidine or other narcotic analgesics may be used to relieve severe pain. These drugs can cause spasm of the common bile duct and the sphincter of Oddi and should be used sparingly.

People whose attacks continue to worsen are usually treated surgically. Cholecystectomy is performed under general anesthesia.

Scherer, J. C. *Introductory Medical-Surgical Nursing*, 3rd ed. Philadelphia: J. B. Lippincott Co., 1982.

Steinberg, F. U. *Care of the Geriatric Patient*, 6th ed. St. Louis: C. V. Mosby Co., 1983.

gallbladder stones   See GALL BLADDER DISEASE.

gallstones   See GALLBLADDER DISEASE.

gambling and games   A great many older people resort to gambling for a touch of excitement. Although no one has ever actually estimated the numbers of seniors who participate in gambling, bingo, and lottery playing, they have long been approved pastimes for the elderly.

Then too, social groups and recreation agents sponsor day trips for seniors to Atlantic City and other gaming centers. There the senior participants eagerly flock to the slot machines and throng the gaming tables. Wisely, these sponsored trips usually caution their members to limit their pocket money ("bring only $30" is typical advice), so that losses are not usually disastrous, outings are stimulating and fun, and the few who come away cheerful winners receive the good humored jibes or plaudits of their friends.

Some people might dismiss gambling by elders as senseless and perhaps even sinful because many elders have limited incomes. A pair of researchers, Ken Stone and Richard Kalish, found positive values in gambling when they studied men who attended a legal poker club. They learned that these men enjoyed the hope of winning even if they did not really expect to; they like testing their skill and luck against that of others; they benefitted from socializing with friends and acquaintances; and they were stimulated by the excitement. As gerontologist Russell Ward concluded when reviewing this research, gambling offered these men "the possibility for social, emotional, and psychological engagement in an interesting activity."

Communities, churches, and nursing homes appear to recognize the positive values of gambling, and are frequent sponsors of bingo games, game nights, and other activities that involve some degree of chance and luck. Many individuals who have been active in playing competitive forms of gambling— chess, bridge, set-back, cribbage, and poker— continue to play as they grow older. Dominoes, checkers, Monopoly, Scrabble, and Mah-Jong all have their elderly enthusiasts whose expertise may even defeat young challengers. State lotteries and even bets on horses add zest to life. Older people do not necessarily gamble because they expect to win, but because they enjoy the excitement and unpredictability of the process. One might not expect it, but outcome of gambling is mental stimulation that may help older people retain their mental agility.

Fromme, A. *Life After Work*. Glenview, Ill.: AARP, 1984.
Gillies, J. *A Guide to Caring for and Coping with Aging Parents*. Nashville: Thomas Nelson Publishers, 1981.
Ward, R. *The Aging Experience*, 2nd ed. New York: Harper and Row, 1984.

gangrene   Gangrene is the deterioration and death of tissue associated with loss of the vascular supply followed by bacterial invasion. In old age, most cases of gangrene are caused by blockage in the circulation in either the arteries or the veins. It may occur acutely after an arterial embolus (detached clot) or be the culmination of a progressive arteriosclerotic obliteration (narrowing and occlusion of arterial lumen) of limb vessels.

A history of sudden onset of pain and paralysis, in conjunction with signs of a mottled, cold, pulseless limb is sufficient to diagnose embolic occlusion. A history of coronary thrombosis and an irregular pulse would explain the source of the embolus (heart) and confirm the diagnosis.

If the condition is recognized and treatment initiated early enough, the limb can be saved. When gangrene is established, the only course is to amputate.

See also ARTERIOSCLEROSIS.

Brocklehurst, J. C. *Geriatric Medicine and Gerontology*, 3rd ed. New York: Churchill Livingstone, 1985.

gardening   Many older individuals who are physically able are avid gardeners. Preparing the soil, planting, and watching things grow gives a person a great sense of accomplishment, and the older individual is no exception. Gardening not only can offer enjoyment, but can also provide fresh vegetables and fruits.

If an older person's health fails so that he or she cannot cultivate a garden as in the past, he or she may consider a miniature garden plot, which may be the size of a flower bed or even a window box.

Growing flowers, shrubs, and houseplants can also provide an interesting activity. Some older individuals may get so involved with flowers and houseplants that they will expand into a greenhouse.

Deedy, J. *Your Aging Parents*. Chicago: The Thomas More Press, 1984.

gastritis   Gastritis, inflammation of the lining of the stomach, is a common stomach disorder in the elderly. Causes of gastritis include foods, drugs, poisons, toxic chemicals, corrosive substances, and bacterial or viral infections. Chronic gastritis may be secondary to stomach cancer, gastric ulcer, or pernicious anemia.

Gastritis is frequently asymptomatic, and if symptoms are present they are vague. They may include complaints of epigastric fullness and pressure, nausea, heartburn, anorexia (loss of appetite), and flatulence (gas). Gastritis due to a bacterial or viral infection may include symptoms of diarrhea, fever, and abdominal pain. Drugs, poisons, toxic substances, and corrosives can cause gastric bleeding. Symptoms of chronic gastritis may be similar to acute gastritis.

Treatment is symptomatic. Nothing is given by mouth until the symptoms subside except clear liquids as the person tolerates them. If vomiting or diarrhea is severe, intravenous fluids may be necessary to correct dehydration and electrolyte imbalances. Ingestions of poisons, toxic chemicals, or corrosive substances require emergency treatment. For example, a chemical that is acidic is treated with an alkali to neutralize the substance.

Chronic gastritis is usually treated with an ulcer regimen, which consists of bland foods, antacids, and avoidance of foods that aggravate the condition.

See also CANCER, STOMACH; ULCER, PEPTIC; VITAMIN B$_{12}$ DEFICIENCY.

Phipps, W. J. *Essentials of Medical Surgical Nursing*. St. Louis: C. V. Mosby Co., 1985.
Steinberg, F. U. *Care of the Geriatric Patient*, 6th ed. St. Louis: C. V. Mosby Co., 1983.

gender gap The "gender gap" is the gap between the life expectancies of males and females. Currently women are expected to live 7.1 years longer than men. Many theories have been proposed as possible explanations of why women live longer. However, experts agree on four major areas of male-female differences: hormones, genetic makeup, natural immunity, and behavior. The female hormone estrogen gives women an advantage over men as far as heart disease goes. Women usually develop heart disease 10 years after men because of the presence of estrogen. Many personality characteristics, determined partly by genetic makeup, partly by hormones and partly by socialization, causes different behaviors in men and women. Men drink more, smoke more, and more often expose themselves to risks at work and play, thereby increasing their chances of death. Some researchers believe the "gender gap" is slowly closing because women today expose themselves to the stresses of work, smoke, and have adopted many behaviors typical of men.

"Closing the Gap," *AARP News Bulletin*. 28: 8–9 (1987).

geriatrics Geriatrics is the specialized branch of medicine that deals with older people. As a form of specialization, it has received increasing attention from the medical community in the past 10 years. Recently the American Board of Internal Medicine and the American Academy of Family Physicians established a certifying examination to establish competence in this new specialization. Over 2,000 physicians nationwide took and passed the exam and now have certification as geriatricians. The Accreditation Council For Graduate Medical Education, which is concerned with the education of physicians once they have acquired their basic medical degrees and licenses, has taken applications for advance training in internal medicine in the geriatic area and is in the process of accrediting educational programs.

The value of medical specialization in geriatrics rests in part with the unique health care requirements of people in later life. Some diseases, such as osteoporosis, are not entirely unique to the advanced years, but their effects and treatment become far more significant as life advances. Likewise, certain diseases that get major attention and are highly publicized with reference to younger people have been overlooked or neglected in later life. One such disease is breast cancer; it has been learned that less than 6 percent of women over 60 have ever had mammograms and breast examinations even though the risk of cancer increases throughout life.

Another value of medical specialization in aging is that it tends to stimulate research related to the specialty. Refering to cancer again, new studies have found a paradoxical situation among older patients. Here the presence of decreased immunity appears to *reduce* the rate of tumor growth. This occurs because the lymphokines, which are produced by the body's defense mechanisms against diseases such as cancer, *promote* tumor growth. Through knowledge of this type, people achieve not only better understanding of fundamental processes of biology in the presence of disease, but of how to take advantage of the body's own reactions to make medical treatment more effective. The progress of specialization in geriatrics, then, will help to continue the advance of medicine that has done so much to reduce illness and death and to improve the quality of life for everyone.

See also AGING, BIOLOGICAL THEORY OF.

Cohen, H. J., and Lyles, K. W. "Geriatrics." *Journal of the American Medical Association.* Vol. 261, No. 19, May 1989, p. 2847–2848.

gerontology Gerontology, a field that is defined as "the scientific study of the processes and phenomena of aging," originated as a unique area of research and service at the end of World War II. The cause of this development rested in part with the growth of the older population, which increased almost 60 percent, from 7.8 million persons over 65 to 12.4 million, in the brief span of 15 years between 1935 and 1950. The growth of the Social Security system and the increasing recognition of elderly people's need for support services further strengthened consciousness about the subject of aging. As

early as 1945 researchers and providers of professional aging services came together to form the Gerontological Society of America, and the following year this organization launched the *Journal of Gerontology.*

The federal government's commitment to aging, which began with passage of the Social Security Act in 1935, was boosted to a new and higher level by the White House Conference on Aging of 1951 and 1961. Another White House Conference was held in 1971, but in the meanwhile Congress had adopted the Older Americans Act that provided for the establishment of a U.S. Department on Aging, introduced the Medicare system to provide health insurance for the elderly under the umbrella of the Social Security system, and passed the Age Discrimination in Employment Act. Following the 1971 White House Conference, Congress indexed Social Security benefits to the cost of living, and later approved the Employees Retirement Security Act. All of these events greatly strengthened America's awareness of aging as a new factor in society and brought the field of gerontology to full maturity.

A distinctive feature of gerontology is its broad inclusion of the wide range of specialties engaged in research and service to the aged. Whereas most professional societies focus narrowly on one particular field (for example, law, or medicine, or nursing, or psychology, or history), the leadership in gerontology has insisted on an interdisciplinary approach that encompasses four areas: the physical (including biological research and medicine), the psychological, the social psychological, and the social (human services as well as sociological research).

As a consequence, the annual meetings of the Gerontological Society of America include a pleasing diversity of subjects and attract social workers, psychologists, sociologists, physicians, physiologists, scholars in literature and the humanities, operators of nursing homes and retirement communities and other services for older persons, and personnel at all levels of government. The annual meeting of this society provides an exceptionally diverse arena for thought and action on behalf of aging.

The root idea that animates this broadly representative organization is that a simple "maturation-maturity" model of aging, one that merely concentrates on physical change to describe later life, cannot adequately cover the full range of human experience in the advanced years. Psychological aspects of aging, for example, go beyond neurological changes in the structure of the brain to include the way that people think and feel and how the personality develops as one grows older. Besides this, people in society carry certain attitudes about aging, and there are specific social definitions, such as the one in Social Security, which has established 65 as the age for full retirement benefits, that define the characteristics, experience, and process of growing old. All of these factors must be considered if one is to understand aging and to create a satisfactory quality to late life.

Gerontologists recognize, also, that there is great variability in the way that people age. Physically, for example, diastolic blood pressure in men can vary from 45 to 105, and when one takes this type of variation into account along with other factors and experiences in life (i.e., being rich or being poor, divorced or married, living in a family or alone, etc.) it is obvious that no two persons can age in exactly the same way. Research clearly shows that most people age comfortably and enjoyably, but the way that each individual ages is unique.

Along with the uniqueness of the experience of aging, it is also true that the life of older people has improved markedly in the last 30 to 50 years. Not only are people living longer, remaining more healthy, and having a more financially secure old age, but according to a national poll conducted by Louis Harris and Associates, the old realize that things are better now than they were for past generations. For the future, the wide-ranging activities of gerontologists

will help to combat stereotypes and misinformation, increase fundamental knowledge of life processes, and help to establish an even higher quality of life for oncoming generations of older people. Gerontology stands out as a key agent in the effort to bring about a satisfying future for the growing older population.

Atchley, R. C. *Social Forces and Aging*, 4th ed. Belmont, Calif.: Wadsworth Publishing Company, 1985.
Ward, R. A. *The Aging Experience*, 2nd ed. New York: Harper and Row, 1984.

gerovital (GH3)   Gerovital is still popular as an anti-aging remedy despite more than 30 years of use during which no scientific evidence for its effectiveness has been established. Its main ingredient is the local anesthetic Novocaine.

Gerovital was first introduced in Romania in the 1950s by Dr. Ana Aslan. Gerovital has been claimed effective against practically every illness and physical change associated with aging. However, in controlled scientific studies it has not produced benefits in elderly patients. Gerovital's main ingredient (Novocaine) can produce side effects in some patients, although these are rarely severe. These side effects may include nervousness, dizziness, blurred vision, tremors, and convulsion.

See also AGING, BIOLOGICAL THEORY OF.

Meiter, K. A. "The 80's Search for the Fountain of Youth Comes Up Very Dry," in *Aging*, Goldstein, E. C., ed. Vol. 2, Art. 76. Boca Raton, Fl.: Social Issues Resource Series, Inc., 1981.

Gestalt dream analysis   In the Gestalt process patients are asked to focus on the present and to assume responsibility for their actions, predicaments, perceptions, and beliefs. Dreams are considered an expression of a person's state of being. All characters and relationships are considered expressions of feelings in the process. Elderly people

104   GH3

benefit from the process by having a way to express their feelings to a group without fear of ridicule. A negative self-image among the elderly can result in a general resignation to a continued decline. Group consciousness may become a powerful tool for rebuilding simple emotions of trust and sharing common concerns about life and death.

See also AUTOGENIC TRAINING; BIOFEEDBACK TRAINING; HATHA YOGA; MEDITATION; POSITIVE ATTITUDE; SELF-IMAGE EXERCISE; TAI CHI CHUAN.

Fields, S. "Sage Can Be a Spice in Life," in *Aging,* Goldstein, E. C., ed. Vol. 1, Art. 26. Boca Raton, Fl.: Social Issues Resource Series, Inc., 1981.

GH3   See GEROVITAL.

ginseng   Ginseng is an herb sometimes promoted as an anti-aging remedy. Ginseng is most often sold as an aphrodisiac or an antidote to the effects of stress. There is no scientific evidence that shows that ginseng has any health benefits. Ginseng, like many herbs, can be harmful in large doses. Possible side effects include nervousness, insomnia, gastrointestinal disorders, and elevation of blood pressure to an extent that might be dangerous to individuals who have hypertension.

See also AGING, BIOLOGICAL THEORY OF.

Meister, K. A. "The 80's Search for the Fountain of Youth Comes Up Very Dry," in *Aging,* Goldstein, E. C., ed. Vol. 2. Art. 76. Boca Raton, Fl.: Social Issues Resource Series, Inc., 1981.

glaucoma   Glaucoma is an ocular disease characterized by an increase in intraocular pressure, excavation and degeneration of the optic disk, and nerve fiber bundle damage producing defects in the visual field. The rate of aqueous production by the ciliary body and the resistance to the outflow of aqueous humor at the angle of the anterior chamber determines the height of the intraocular pressure. Clinically this pressure is

estimated by tonometry; an instrument designed to check the pressure. A definite diagnosis of glaucoma cannot be made unless the increased intraocular pressure has produced damage to the optic nerve. The chances for developing glaucoma increase as a person ages. Three out of every 100 people over age 65 have the disease, an estimated 722,000. Glaucoma is one of the leading causes of blindness for people over age 65, accounting for almost 20% of known cases. Women run a higher risk of developing glaucoma than men do. Although glaucoma cannot be prevented, the resultant blindness can be prevented through early detection and appropriate medical treatment.

The primary glaucomas are generally bilateral (both-eye) diseases, which are in part genetically determined. The term "secondary glaucoma" refers to pressure rises caused by some known ocular disease and is usually unilateral.

Glaucoma may be classified into angle-closure glaucomas, open-angle glaucoma and a mixed group in which both angle-closure and trabecular mechanisms may be contributory.

Angle-closure glaucoma occurs typically in hyperopic (farsighted) eyes, which have shallow anterior chambers. The resulting forward displacement of the peripheral iris covering the trabecular meshwork (filter controlling aqueous flow) with dilation of the pupil can lead to closure of the angle. Tension elevation tends to occur abruptly, causing typical symptoms of halos, hazy vision, and ocular pain. Laser iridotomy (hole made with laser in iris for better aqueous flow) usually bypasses the pupillary block and normalizes the outward flow of fluids if the trabecular meshwork is not damaged.

Secondary angle-closure glaucoma may be caused by a swollen lens, posterior synechiae (adhesion of iris to front of lens) to the lens, or lens subluxation. Each entity is treated according to its underlying cause.

With open-angle glaucoma, the most common type, the iris is not in contact with the trabecular meshwork; the sieve that allows aqueous to drain outside the eye. The reduced outflow of fluid is caused by an increase in the resistance in the trabecular meshwork and other portions of the outflow passages to the venous system. Symptoms are usually negligible until extensive ocular damage has occurred. The treatment of open-angle glaucoma is mainly medical. Topical eye drops are first used, then oral medication can be added if necessary. Laser treatment of the trabecular meshwork may help lower the pressure. Surgery is indicated if the intraocular pressure is persistently high or if there is progression of optic disk or visual field changes.

Secondary open-angle glaucoma may be caused by trauma, inflammation, and tumors.

Newell, F. W., *Opthalmology Principles and Concepts,* 6th ed. St. Louis: C. V. Mosby, Co., 1986.

gold-collar worker   Gold-collar workers are those workers in the labor force who are over age 50. Many companies are hiring, rehiring, and retaining older workers. Some firms are hiring workers over 50 because they possess particular skills that are in short supply, they experience less turnover and fewer sick days, and they relate better to older customers. One main problem encountered by "gold-collar workers" is that most of the jobs available to them are temporary or part-time clerical positions that have low pay and benefits.

See also HIRING AGE.

"The Advent of the Gold-Collar Workers." *Modern Maturity.* (October–November, 1986).

golf   Golf is one of the few sports that is not too physically demanding for the older individual. It involves many muscles through walking, bending, pulling, and swinging, as well as the additional benefits of fresh air and sun. This competitive exercise can heighten one's zest for life. There are tournaments for seniors, including the National

Senior Open, Senior Amateur, and Senior Women's Amateur.

Gillies, J. *A Guide to Caring for and Coping with Aging Parents.* Nashville: Thomas Nelson Publishers, 1981.

Gotu Kola   It has been claimed that the herb Gotu Kola can retard aging and cure senility. Dr. Frederick Sherman of Mount Sinai Medical Center reviewed this for the House Committee on Aging and reported that there is no clinical or theoretical support for the claims that Gotu Kola slows aging or is good for senility.

See also AGING, BIOLOGICAL THEORY OF.

Meiter, K. A. "The 80's Search for the Fountain of Youth Comes Up Very Dry," in *Aging,* Goldstein, E. C., ed. Vol. 2, Art. 76, Boca Raton, Fl.: Social Issues Resources Series, Inc., 1981.

gout   Gout is a metabolic disorder characterized by recurrent attacks of arthritis due to deposits of uric acid in the joints and other tissues. The big toe is the most common site of initial involvement in over 50 percent of cases. Later, other joints that are frequently affected include the finger joints, wrists, and elbows.

The great majority of patients have primary gout, which appears to be due to an inherited disorder of metabolism. Secondary gout is due to overproduction of uric acid or a retention of uric acid. In primary gout, over 90 percent of the patients are male with the peak period of onset during the fifth decade. Women are affected after menopause. In secondary gout, the average age of onset and the frequency with which women are affected are both greater than in primary gout.

Onset of acute gout is very rapid with maximal pain and swelling usually reached in several hours. The affected joint is exquisitely painful and tender and the patient may suffer chills and low-grade fever. After recovery from the initial attack, the patient can remain free of symptoms for months or years. However, subsequent attacks tend to occur with greater severity and at more frequent intervals.

Anti-inflammatory agents are prescribed for controlling the symptoms of gout. Lowering the level of body uric acid with the use of uriosuric agents is necessary to prevent urate deposition. These agents should be avoided during acute attacks of gout because they exaggerate the symptoms. If the joint is severely destroyed surgical joint replacement may need to be considered.

Reichel, W. M. *Clinical Aspects of Aging.* Baltimore: The Williams & Wilkins Co., 1979.

grandchildren, relationships with   Relationships between grandparents and grandchildren are normally rich and rewarding, and they have been officially recognized as such in the federal FOSTER GRANDPARENTS PROGRAM. Interviews with grandchildren have been carried out in a number of studies, and these show that grandchildren look to their grandparents as a source of love, help, understanding, and friendship. Grandchildren do not expect their grandparents to spoil them, and they do not consider them old-fashioned. They do not view them as "old people" but rather as friends.

Teenagers, who might be expected to rebel against their grandparents as well as their parents, also have favorable attitudes about their grandparents. Many grandchildren believe that they should go to visit their grandparents, they want to offer them love, and they willingly help them when necessary.

For their part, grandparents create an informal, easy-going relationship with grandchildren. They may even allow them privileges of disrespect that they would not have permitted to their own children, the people who have now become the parents of their grandchildren. Studies show that grandparents keep to the side as loving family members, and usually avoid interfering in the relationships between the grandchildren and their parents.

Deedy, J. *Your Aging Parents.* Chicago: The Thomas More Press, 1984.

Russell, C. H. *Good News About Aging.* New York: John Wiley and Sons, 1989.

Granny flat   "Granny flats" have a long history as a type of residence for widowed older women, and the name may have originated in England or Ireland. Typically, these have been apartments adjoining a family home or another apartment, but some may be trailers or prefabricated homes set on a property near the residence of the widow's children.

Recently "Granny flats" have gained official recognition in such nations as France and Australia, where the type of residence involved is a prefab, one-bedroom unit that can be put in the yard adjoining the nearby home. The French government is now providing price subsidies to help develop, promote, and sell Granny flats.

James, T. M. "The Elderly in America," in *Aging,* Goldstein, E. C., ed. Vol. 2, Art. 81. Boca Raton, Fl.: Social Issues Resource Series, Inc., 1981.

Grave's disease   See HYPERTHYROIDISM.

gray crime   Contrary to some highly sensationalized and widely publicized reports, there has been no outbreak of a crime wave among the elderly in recent years. The reason for the outburst of publicity about gray crime appears to be that people interested in hyping such stories have taken miniscule changes in elderly crime, calculated percentage increases, and then distorted their meaning to gain media attention.

The table below presents information for a typical set of years that shows one possible source of distorted reports about "gray crime." If one compares these three columns, one can see that various kinds of calculations could supply copy for almost any sort of story one might wish to promote. Sex offenses, for example, increased 100%— they doubled—over this period. Yet, sex offenses remain a miniscule part of elderly

Arrests by Offenses Charged and Age

	Age 18	Age 40–44	Age 65+
All offenses	480,368	487,908	91,709
Percent	4.7	4.7	0.9
Murder	674	896	226
Forcible rape	1,289	1,671	225
Robbery	8,405	2,304	203
Aggravated assault	9,876	14,425	2,442
Burglary	29,017	6,260	508
Larceny-theft	66,126	40,177	15,265
Motor vehicle theft	8,744	2,140	199
Arson	677	620	90
Forgery and counterfeiting	3,728	2,928	198
Prostitution and commercial vice	3,375	2,536	360
Gambling	427	2,916	1,091
Driving under influence	33,338	110,499	19,411
Drunkenness	19,530	69,322	17,391

criminal behavior (1.6 percent of elderly personal offenses at their highest point), and the higher percentage may reflect only the drop in the proportion of other kinds of crime (gambling decreased by nearly 100%) rather than an actual growth in the number of sex offenses. The second table shows that sex offenses (prostitution and commercial vice) among the elderly are far below the rate for other ages.

Percentage Distribution of All Arrests of Persons in the Age 55+ Group: Index Offenses and Misdemeanors

	1971	1976	1981
I. Property Crime Offenses			
Burglary	7.7	3.5	1.5
Larceny-theft	89.0	95.0	92.0
Auto theft	3.3	1.5	5.5
II. Personal offenses			
Sex offenses	.8	1.4	1.6
Drug abuse violations	.4	.6	1.9
Gambling	4.2	3.5	2.5
Drunkenness	71.1	57.8	43.3
Driving under influence	15.0	29.5	39.0
Disorderly conduct	8.5	7.2	11.7

According to the U.S. Department of Justice, the elderly commit less than 1 percent of all crimes, a far smaller proportion than might be expected considering that they make up 12 percent or more of the population. The rate of total arrests is only four per 1,000 population at age 65+, but 78 from ages 40–44, and 167 at 25–29.

A sampling of data from a recent FBI report on crime in the United States shows the comparatively low rate of crime among the older American population.

Atchley, R. C.. *Social Forces and Aging,* 4th ed. Belmont, Calif.: Wadsworth Publishing Co., 1985.

Schick, F. L., ed. *Statistical Handbook on Aging Americans.* Phoenix: Oryx Press, 1986.

U.S. Department of Justice, Federal Bureau of Investigation, *Crime in the United States, 1985.* Washington, D.C.: U.S. Government Printing Office, 1986.

Green Thumb Program   The Green Thumb Program, along with Foster Grandparents and other government sponsored projects, was designed to enhance the quality of life of older people by encouraging their participation in worthwhile community services. It has given several hundred thousands of older workers opportunities to earn and contribute to the well-being of their communities.

The program was created as a result of the Equal Opportunity Bill of 1965 and was spearheaded by the National Farmers Union. To be eligible for the Green Thumb Program a person must be 55 years of age or older and be economically disadvantaged. The program is now under the direction of the Senior Community Service Employment Program (SCSEP).

Participants have to come from rural districts. Their tasks have included beautifying parks and roadside areas, working as seamstresses, and performing clerical duties and relief work. They usually work 20 hours per week, with a limit of 1,300 hours yearly, normally at the minimum wage. Most of the job openings are with nonprofit organizations, but private businesses have participated with increasing frequency in recent years. Congressional hearings held in 1988 recognized the strong bipartisan support for the program and the increasing appropriations—from $10,000 in 1974 to $343,000 in 1988—that have followed upon its success.

House of Representatives, Select Committee on Aging. *The Senior Community Service Program: Its History and Evolution.* Comm. Pub. No. 100–695. December, 1988. Washington, D.C.: U.S. Government Printing Office, 1989.
Wallworth, J. "New Adventures for Seniors in World of Work," in *Aging,* Goldstein, E. C., ed., Vol. 1, Art. 67. Boca Raton, Fl.: Social Issues Resource Series, Inc., 1981.

grief   Elizabeth Kübler-Ross coined the term *grief-work* to describe the overwhelming emotional and psychological process of dealing with a severe personal loss. Grief is a normal inner experience that follows bereavement and in most cases is overcome with time. When the loss of a very close intimate, such as a spouse, is unexpected, the experience of grief appears to be totally unavoidable and overwhelming—so much so that it is difficult to describe it to anyone who has not had the experience. (See, for example, *A Song for Sarah,* written by Paula D'Arcy, which records the devastating pain experienced by a pregnant young mother when her one-year-old daughter and husband were killed at her side in a car accident caused by a head-on collision with a drunken driver who had crossed a median divider).

A most revealing account of grief was published by C. S. Lewis, the distinguished British scholar and author, professor at Oxford and later at Cambridge University, who late in life married the American poet Joy Davis. A committed Christian of strong religious faith, Lewis is sometimes called "the apostle to the skeptics" for his books that addressed a variety of difficult religious problems for the benefit of persons who have doubts about religion (e.g., *The Screwtape Letters*—letters from a senior devil to a junior devil with instructions on how to capture a young man's soul).

His late-life marriage to Joy Davis, not only American but a former member of the Communist Party and Jewish in religious origin, seemed most improbable, but turned out to be a perfect match—Lewis loved her with all his heart. Within a few years after their marriage Joy contracted cancer, and after a period of remission that gave them both hope, she died. Lewis was devastated, but, always the writer, he kept a diary to record, and perhaps relieve, his inward pain. He eventually published a book based on the diary under the title, *A Grief Observed,* to serve as an aid to others who might be engulfed by a similar devastating loss.

Lewis found that his grief overwhelmed his religious convictions; they were not able to assuage his pain even though he prayed for relief. At one point in *A Grief Observed,* Lewis compared his unremitting agony to the inner state that arose when he had felt fear as an officer in trench warfare in France during World War I. His description is not unlike the account of grief given by psychiatrist Erich Lindeman in an article written for the *American Journal of Psychiatry* in 1944, which reads:

> . . . sensation of somatic (bodily) distress occurring in waves lasting 20 minutes to an hour at a time, a feeling of tightness in the throat, choking with shortness of breath, need for sighing, and an empty feeling in the abdomen, lack of muscular power (weakness), and an intense subjective (inner) distress described as tension or mental pain. [parentheses added]

And, of course, for many people, grief includes uncontrollable sobbing and weeping.

A number of specialists have described the phases of normal grief that reveal certain broad characteristics:

1. A period of intense grief, lasting from a few weeks to several months, when the bereaved are unable to control their feelings, sometimes crying without ceasing for hours at a time, when a strong effort just to carry on with life is essential
2. An intermediate period of sadness, with occasional reversion to periods of overwhelming emotion, relieved by the gradual reconstruction of life
3. establishment of a new life, wherein the lost intimate companion is not forgotten but is remembered lovingly, where the bereaved person has reached a new state and sense of competence

The experience of grief is unavoidable. The task of filling the emotional gaps are indescribably painful. The difficulties of developing the competence to perform the tasks (often financial ones for widows) formerly carried out by the loved one are difficult. Yet, Helen Znaniecki Lopata's monumental studies of widowhood show that over 60 percent recover from their bereavement experience within a year. She also observed that the recovery period may take more than two years for 16 percent of widows, but that nearly everyone does recover.

Death rates for men increase following bereavement, and for both sexes it is quite common for distress to reach a level of clinically observable depression. For the rare instances of pathological grieving there are, fortunately, a variety of therapies. These include the use of psychotropic medicines (to assist with sleep, to overcome depression, and to improve appetite), and psychological approaches, such as grief counseling, cognitive therapy, and behavioral counseling.

Studies of grieving people show that those who experience an "on-time" loss (such as the death of a spouse in late life) may experience a somewhat less intense and also briefer period of grieving than those who go through losses earlier in life. Lopata's studies also showed that help, especially from close family and kin, is usually available to the bereft. Daughters generally provide emotional support to widows, and sons supply instrumental help by performing yard work or making repairs around the house.

Other research shows that those who anticipate a loss, as in the death of a spouse that follows several months of serious illness, may go through considerably milder forms of grieving because they have had more time to anticipate the loss. The results of anticipating death are not universally beneficial, however—extended periods of waiting, especially when accompanied by a heavy burden of caregiving, can wear the waiting individual down. The death under such circumstances becomes a positive relief.

Perhaps the most significant finding of studies of grieving is that other people, especially non-family members, may be unaware of, or insensitive to, the inner pain of the bereaved person. Since we have abandoned the ritual symbols of mourning—widows' weeds for women and black armbands for men—in the 20th century, there is no way for strangers and acquaintances to recognize that a person is bereaved and may be carrying a massive internal psychological wound.

Today, however, a variety of self-help books may offer some support to the bereft, as do organizations like Widow-to-Widow, Compassionate Friends, and others. Both friends and family in contact with bereaved persons need to realize that the aftermath of death brings on a period of grieving that can be overwhelmingly intense. Affection, kind words, and consideration are essential during this time.

La Rue, A.; Dessonville, C.; and Jarvik, L. F. "Aging and Mental Disorders," in Birren, J. E., and Schaie, K. W., eds. *Handbook of the Psychology of Aging,* 2nd ed. New York: Van Nostrand Reinhold Company, 1985.
Lopata, H. Z. *Widowhood in an American City.* Cambridge, Mass.: Schenkman. 1973.
Ward, R. *The Aging Experience,* 2nd ed. New York: Harper and Row, 1984.

group care   See FOSTER CARE.

guardianship   See LEGAL REPRESENTATIVE.

gum disease   See PERIODONTAL DISEASE.

H

hair care (scalp care)   Shampooing should be done at least weekly. Oils build up on the scalp and may cause scalp irritation. Long, unclean hair gives one an unkept appearance. If hair is long it should be kept in a braid, bun, or cut when older individuals are confined to bed. For women not confined to bed, a regular visit to the beauty shop could become a highlight of the week or month.

Elderly women tend to have an increase in facial hair, especially on the chin and upper lip. The excess hair is very distressing to many women, and these hairs can be removed by tweezers or professionally with an electric needle. A mild bleach can be used by many women to lighten the hairs and make them less noticeable. The drug

Spironolactone, which inhibits testosterone, may also be used. The usual dosage is 25 mg two times a day.

Men should visit the barber shop regularly. If they are not able to be out, family members may want to purchase an inexpensive barbering kit and cut the person's hair themselves.

See also HAIR, EXCESSIVE.

Gillies, J. *A Guide to Caring for and Coping with Aging Parents.* Nashville: Thomas Nelson Publishers, 1981.

hair, excessive (hirsutism)   Hirsutism is excessive body hair in a masculine pattern as a result of heredity, hormonal imbalance, porphyria, or medication.

Elderly women frequently have an increase in facial hair, especially on the chin and upper lip. This may be caused by postmenopause hormonal changes, adrenal tumors, or congenital disorders. This excess hair is very distressing to many women.

Treatment of hirsutism includes removal of hair by tweezers or professionally with electrolysis. A mild bleach can be used by many women to lighten the hair color and make it less noticeable. Currently, Spironolactone is being used to inhibit testosterone and therefore reduce facial hair growth. The usual dosage is 25 mg two times a day.

Steinberg, F. U. *Care of the Geriatric Patient,* 6th ed. St. Louis: C. V. Mosby Co., 1983.

hair transplants (baldness)   Baldness in men appears as early as the twenties, but 65 percent of Caucasian men by the age of 50 have some degree of vertical as well as bitemporal baldness. Sixty-four percent of women age 40–70 show bitemporal recession, and 20 percent of these have obvious vertical thinning.

Hair transplantion is a minor surgical office procedure in which hair from normal areas of the scalp, such as the back and sides, is moved to the bald areas. New surgical procedures to correct male pattern baldness include punch autografts, micro-grafts, strip grafting, scalp reduction, use of hairbearing flaps, and various combinations of these techniques.

- Autografts—Donor areas from the lateral and posterior portions of the scalp are implanted, beginning anteriorly at the desired hairline and continued in a fanning pattern posterior.
- Micrografts—Small, full-thickness graft units of one to eight hair follicles are implanted into "stab" incisions to soften edges of established graft hairlines and to fill areas that are unsuitable for conventional grafts.
- Strip grafting—Implantation of a strip of hair-bearing skin four to eight mm wide and several cm long. However, overall results are inconsistent and this procedure has only been used by a few doctors.
- Scalp reduction—"Instant hair" effect is created by this technique in those cases of baldness of the vertex or anterior vertex regions. Depending on the laxity of the scalp, the amount of tissue excised ranges from 2.5 to 5.0 cm in width and 12 to 22 cm in length. Not only is the amount of bald area reduced but the lateral hair margins are raised, resulting in a greater concentration of hair in the balding area.
- Flap procedures—The ideal candidate for a flap procedure is the balding person with finely textured, sparse hair or the patient with limited donor hair area who wants frontal coverage in the shortest period of time. The types of flap procedures are the preauricular flap, lateral flap, postauricular flap, Juri flap, and temporoparietal-occipital flap. Most of these procedures are done in two or three stages and have excellent success rates.

Stough, D. B., *et al. Surgical Procedure for the Treatment of Baldness.* Cutis, Vol 24: 303–305, 1979.

Stough, D. B., and Cates, J. "Contemporary Techniques of Hair Replacement." *Postgraduate Medicine,* Vol. 69: 1981.

happiness and self-esteem in age A 1975 national poll conducted by Louis Harris and Associates for the National Council on Aging produced conclusive evidence that the American public looks on age as a deprived time of life. (The Harris Polls are classics and have not been repeated in recent years but the data is still valid.) The majority of Americans see age as a time of low income, ill health, loneliness, and boredom. Recognized figures, like the distinguished French writer Simone de Beauvoir, have observed that people view age with aversion, and much of the research on aging concentrates on decline rather than the positive aspects of being old.

It may come as a surprise, then, to learn of studies about happiness and self-esteem that show that age is a period of richness of spirit, and that it may in fact be the greatest time of contentment in life. One source of evidence for this statement is the General Social Survey, a national poll of public opinion carried out annually by the National Opinion Research Center at the University of Chicago.

The General Social Survey question about happiness is addressed to a scientifically selected representative sample of Americans living in the general community (people in the army, hospitals, nursing homes, and jails are not surveyed), and asks: Taken altogether, how would you say things are these days—would you say that you are very happy, pretty happy, or not too happy. While someone might wonder if a question this simple can accurately report the feelings of the American public, research using more elaborate and philosophically worded types of questions does not change the overall picture of how Americans respond when asked about their happiness.

The results, which appear as percentages in the table on page 112, show that the largest proportion of persons at every age describe themselves as "pretty happy."

The percentages of people who describe themselves as "pretty happy," however, are

How Americans Rate Their Happiness

Age	Very Happy	Pretty Happy	Not Too Happy
18–24	27.3	57.3	14.3
25–34	31.2	57.6	10.7
35–44	32.5	55.5	11.5
45–54	34.8	51.4	13.3
55–64	35.2	50.7	13.4
65–74	38.6	47.4	13.2
75–84	36.5	49.5	13.4
85 +	33.5	50.0	15.4

highest among the younger age groups—up to age 44 at least 55 percent describe themselves in terms of this category. By comparison, the age groups from 55 and up stand at 50 percent or less. This suggests that one needs to look at the other columns to see if differences between age groups show up there also.

When one looks at the first column—the "very happy" column—one discovers an astonishing difference between the groups— the highest percentages of "very happy" persons appear among the seniors. In fact, the peak of happiness comes at age 65–74, and the low point comes at age 18–24.

Doesn't this suggest that the American public is wrong? What one sees in this table is that older people on the whole are just about as happy as everyone else, and that they may even be happier than people at earlier ages of life.

To test the general observation that old people are as happy as anyone else, look at the last column, the one labelled "not too happy." Here one notices that the percentages of people who say that they are "not too happy" are quite low at all ages, clustering around 13 percent. This tells us that the great majority of Americans (about 85 percent or more) do *not* see themselves as being "not too happy."

Besides this, the range of differences between the age groups is small—less than 5 percent. This means that Americans at all ages are quite alike when it comes to this quality. Contrary to what one might expect if the general opinion were true—that the old were lonely, bored, etc.—one sees here that there is no major increase in the proportion of "not too happy" people as age advances.

Notice, too, that the age groups from 45 to 84 are practically identical. There is scarcely any difference among them, and, in fact, only one-tenth of 1 percent more of the population aged 75–84 says it is "not too happy" than the middle aged group of 45–54-year-olds.

Finally, when one compares the percentage of "not too happy" people over age 85 with the other age groups, one sees that they most closely resemble the 18–24 year olds. The percentages here are 15.4 for the 85+ and 14.3 for the young people 18–24. Only 1.1 percent separates these two groups, so for all practical purposes they are alike. Add to this the fact that 6 percent more of the 85+ population in column reports itself as "very happy" as compared to the 18–24 year olds and you have an even more remarkable picture.

One can conclude, then, that the American public has been laboring under a misapprehension about the state of mind of the older population. Contrary to being bored and lonely, the majority are as happy as anyone else, some are even happier, and only a small proportion is not happy. How can we explain this unexpected truth?

Another study supplies the answer: Older people are more composed and at ease with themselves than the young. As a result, they are quite happy on the whole—far more so than we might expect.

This other study was also a national survey of a sample of the American population. The survey in this case was an adjective checklist that consisted of a series of descriptive words; individuals were asked to select which of the words applied to themselves. The respondents went through the list and checked each word that applied to them. How did the older population describe itself in comparison to the younger population?

First, the old thought of themselves as competent—they chose adjectives like hard-working, well-organized, tough, strong, intelligent, and able to get things done when describing themselves—and they chose these terms more often than the young did. Surprisingly, the young were more likely than the old to describe themselves as absent-minded, lazy, restless, and disorderly. The old also had a greater sense of self-control, self-reliance, and independence.

Second, in social situations the old were less likely to describe themselves as timid, indecisive, and helpless. The young expressed more discomfort in social situations, using terms like *shy, nervous,* and *embarrassed.*

Third, the young more often used negative terms to describe their inner feelings and behavior toward others—they felt frustrated and vulnerable, manipulative, and were more likely to say that they misrepresented situations. Overall, the old revealed a greater sense of comfort about life, about other people, and concerning themselves. They felt more effective in achieving their goals.

In another study, Carol Ryff, psychologist specializing in the field of aging at the University of Wisconsin, held interviews with 171 adults and elderly to determine how these individuals defined psychological well-being among their age groups. When reporting her interview results, Ryff observed:

More interesting . . . were older people's frequent reports that they were not really unhappy about anything and were not interested in changing their present lives. This rather optimistic assessment underscores the growing evidence that old age is not a time of great unhappiness, dissatisfaction, low self-esteem, or low morale.

Further, Ryff found that her middle-aged and elderly subjects both emphasized having an "others orientation" as part of their definition of well-being—that is, of being caring and compassionate, and of having good relationships with other people. When defining well-being, middle-aged people were more likely to stress self-confidence, self-acceptance, and self-knowledge, whereas older people considered acceptance of change and positive functioning as important. Both groups also considered having a sense of humor and enjoyment of life as good indicators of well-being.

The studies reported here are only a few among many that are beginning to document a generally happy and affirmative state of mind among older people. It is not that older people do not have difficulties—they certainly do, and ill health is one of the more prominent. These studies, however, show that the disposition of older people is positive. Americans need not fear the aging process. Rather, if they reach out and grasp age firmly with the intent to live it well, they have an excellent chance to achieve success.

Breytspraak, L. *The Development of the Self in Later Life*. Boston: Little, Brown and Co., 1984.

Russell, C. H. *Good News About Aging*. New York: John Wiley and Sons, 1989.

Russell, C. H., and Megaard, I. *The General Social Survey, 1972–1986: The State of the American People*. New York: Springer-Verlag, 1988.

Ryff, C. D. "In the Eye of the Beholder: Views of Psychological Well-Being Among Middle-Aged and Older Adults." *Psychology and Aging*. Vol. 4: 2, 195–210, 1989.

Hatha Yoga   Hatha Yoga is a system that is several thousand years old, which involves postures known as asemas. Asemas are balanced exercises for deep relaxation, toning, and revitalizing the mind and body. The meditative practices are sound for both relaxation and assisting elderly to take stock of their lives and face the prospect of death in a way that promotes growth. Such techniques are used by senior citizens in preventive mental health groups and in nursing and convalescent homes. They are intended to restore vitality to the elderly.

See also AUTOGENIC TRAINING; BIOFEED-BACK TRAINING; GESTALT DREAM ANALYSIS; MEDITATION; POSITIVE ATTITUDE; SELF-IM-AGE EXERCISE; TAI CHI CHUAN.

Fields, S. "Sage Can Be a Spice in Life," in *Aging,* Goldstein, E. C., ed. Vol. 1, Art. 26. Boca Raton, Fl.: Social Issues Resource Series, Inc., 1981.

hearing   Approximately one-third of the people over the age of 60 show some signs of hearing loss.

There are various types of hearing aids that are available. It should be impressed upon the individual with the hearing loss that too much hearing-aid volume can do further damage to his or her ears. Hearing aids also permit the individual to treat the world as a television, turning off the commercials and anything else he or she does not want to hear.

The individual who has a hearing loss should make that fact known to the person that he or she is speaking to. It is dangerous for the individual to pretend that he or she has heard when this is not the case. Ask people to repeat their statements or have a companion who knows the problem quickly repeat the statements. Individuals who do not hear well may find that by initiating conversation all the key words will be familiar and easier to understand.

See also HEARING AIDS; HEARING REHA-BILITATION, PRESBYCUSIS.

Steinberg, F. U. *Care of the Geriatric Patient,* 6th ed. St. Louis: C. V. Mosby Co., 1983.

hearing aids   The development of modern hearing aids has been a primary factor in the correction of hearing handicaps. Through the use of these devices even severe hearing losses may be helped.

There are four styles of hearing aids:

1. in-the-ear types, effective only for mild hearing loss
2. behind-the-ear types, for moderate to severe hearing loss
3. those contained in the eyeglass frames as an in-the-ear type
4. the type worn on the body

Other treatments for people with PRESBY-CUSIS include auditory training, lip reading training, and external noise reduction. If the older person is involved in a job or hobby with a loud environment, ear plugs may be suggested to prevent any further hearing loss.

Cox-Gedmark, J. *Coping with Physical Disability.* Philadelphia: The Westiminster Press, 1982.

hearing loss   See PRESBYCUSIS.

hearing rehabilitation   Education of the person with a hearing loss, as well as the family members, is important. Many ways exist to improve communication with people who have hearing disabilities. Touching the person and then speaking directly to him or her is helpful. Speaking louder and slower is beneficial. Eliminating noises, such as the television or radio helps with participation in conversation. The telephone company can provide amplification devices that make hearing much easier on the phone. These amplified phones also are available in many public phone areas now. If hearing the phone ring is a problem, it might be helpful to have a flashing light installed. Trained dogs are now available that dash about or bark when someone is at the door or the phone rings.

Help is there for the older person with a hearing loss if only he or she will acknowledge that the problem exists. Family members and friends need understanding and patience in dealing with these people.

See HEARING AIDS.

Lester, A. D., and Lester, J. L. *Understanding Aging Parents.* Philadelphia: The Westminster Press, 1980.

heart attack   See MYOCARDIAL INFARC-TION.

heart failure   See CONGESTIVE HEART FAILURE.

heat cramps   See HEAT INDEX.

heat exhaustion   See HEAT INDEX.

heat index   The heat index is the combined effect of high temperature and humidity on exposed skin. When temperatures are in the 90s and the humidity is also high, the apparent temperature, or how it feels, is well over 100 degrees. If the heat index is in the 90- to 105-degree range, sunstroke, heat cramps, and heat exhaustion are possible with prolonged exposure or physical activity, especially in the elderly or those in other high-risk groups. The elderly are highly susceptible to a rise in central temperature because of their inability to sweat readily. This is probably the main factor of increased mortality among the elderly during a heat wave. Mortality rates increase with the rise of body temperatures. The average rectal temperature on fatal cases of heat-related deaths has been reported as 106.4 degrees F. When the heat index is over 105 degrees, sunstroke, heat cramps, and heat exhaustion are very likely to occur and heatstroke is possible.

The most common heat-related illness is heat exhaustion. It is caused by the loss of fluid and salts through excessive sweating. Symptoms include fatigue, weakness, dizziness, blurred vision, nausea, muscle cramps, and possible vomiting and fainting.

Treatment for heat exhaustion consists of moving the victim to lie down in the shade, loosening clothing, and elevating the feet eight to 12 inches. Place a cool, wet cloth on the victim's forehead and body and move him or her to an air-cooled room as soon as possible. If the victim is not vomiting, give clear juice or sips of cool water every 15 minutes for one hour. Stop liquids if vomiting occurs. If symptoms become severe or last longer than one hour seek medical help.

Heat cramps occur in the group of muscles under stress. The first muscles affected are those in the stomach and legs. Cramps results from a loss of salt. The victim will experience painful cramping, spasms, heavy sweating, and possible convulsions. The affected muscles should be gently massaged with firm hand pressure and liquids should be administered slowly if no vomiting occurs.

Heatstroke is the most serious heat-related illness and is a life-threatening emergency. Body temperature may be as high as 106 degrees and the victim may be confused or unconscious and have a rapid pulse rate. A physician should be called immediately.

See also HYPERTHERMIA.

Brocklehurst, J. C. *Textbook of Geriatric Medicine and Gerontology*, 3rd ed. New York: Churchill Livingstone, 1985.
Coverage. Blue Cross and Blue Shield of Arkansas Publication, 18:1987.

heatstroke   See HEAT INDEX.

hemorrhoids   Hemorrhoids are an enlargement of otherwise normal veins in the anal area. They are primarily caused by excessive pressure at the time of defecation and are more common with constipation or obesity. Occasionally, liver disease, such as cirrhosis, can be a contributing factor because of excessive pressure in the veins of the intestines. Hemorrhoids are more commonly found in middle age but can also occur in the elderly.

Pain and bleeding from the anus usually occurs. Treatment consists of an increase of liquid intake to prevent the stool from getting too hard, the use of stool softeners, and warm baths to soothe the anal area. Creams and suppositories are generally used under a physician's supervision. Weight loss should be encouraged to help reduce straining. If hemorrhoids do not respond to medical treatment, various types of surgeries have proven effective.

Columbia University College of Physicians and Surgeons. *Complete Home Medical Guide*. New York: Crown Publishers, 1985.

hepatitis Hepatitis is an inflammation of the liver usually from a viral infection but sometimes from toxic agents. There are two major forms of viral hepatitis, hepatitis A and hepatitis B.

Hepatitis A occurs mainly in children and young adults. When it occurs in elderly patients, especially women, it is a more severe and prolonged form. Common features include anorexia (loss of appetite), nausea, weight loss, mental changes, and abdominal discomfort. Jaundice may last for six weeks, and a fatal outcome is possible.

Hepatitis B has a more insidious onset and a higher mortality rate since it tends to affect older patients who are in poorer health. With outbreaks of hepatitis B in nursing homes, it is important to remember that decubitis ulcers and materials contaminated with blood are infectious.

Treatment consists of adequate nutrition, relief of symptoms, and avoidance of further liver damage by the use of the appropriate drugs.

See HEPATITIS, DRUG-INDUCED.

Brocklehurst, J. C. *Textbook of Geriatric Medicine and Gerontology*, 3rd ed. New York: Churchill Livingstone, 1985.

Calkins E., *et al. The Practice of Geriatrics*. Philadelphia: W. B. Saunders, 1986.

hepatitis, drug-induced The liver is particularly vulnerable to drug-induced injury. In orally administered drugs, the highest concentration of medication goes directly to the liver. Thus, the liver is exposed for long periods of time to potentially toxic metabolites.

The elderly are apt to experience hepatotoxic reactions (severe inflammation of liver cells) because of the large number of medications they ingest and also because the aging liver is more susceptible to the hepatotoxic effects of medication.

Some drugs known to produce hepatotoxic reactions are: carbon tetrachloride, acetaminophen, tetracycline, nicotinic acid, and vitamin A. Several drugs that are capable of producing effects that may be indistinguishable from acute viral hepatitis are: methyldopa, phenytoin, isoniazid, nitrofarantoin, and aspirin. The elderly are frequently exposed to such drugs. These same drugs are responsible for the development of chronic hepatitis. Although drug-induced chronic hepatitis is rare, the mortality rate ranges from 10 percent to 50 percent.

When medication is suspected of causing hepatic damage, it should be discontinued immediately. The use of corticosteroid therapy for drug-induced hepatotoxicity has met with only sporadic success and needs to be further investigated.

Covington, T., and Walker, J. *Current Geriatric Therapy*. Philadelphia: W. B. Saunders, 1984.

hernia (inguinal, femoral, or umbilical) Hernia is a protrusion of an organ or structure from its normal cavity through a congenital or acquired defect. When an inguinal, femoral, or umbilical hernia occurs, a lump or swelling appears on the abdomen underneath the skin. The swelling may be large or small depending on how much of the viscera has protruded.

Congenital defects account for a large portion of hernias. It may appear in infancy or adulthood due to increased intro-abdominal pressure, which can occur during heavy lifting, sneezing, coughing. Hernias that develop in mid-life and old age are due to obesity and the weakening of muscles.

Inguinal hernias are the type that occur most commonly. Men are more likely to develop inguinal hernias. Umbilical and femoral hernias are more frequent among women. In the elderly man an inguinal hernia commonly exists with an enlarged prostate.

Hernias may be asymptomatic other than the appearance of swelling on the abdomen.

The swelling may be painful but disappears when the hernia is reduced. Incarcerated hernias cause severe pain.

A reducible hernia can be returned by manipulation to its own cavity. If it cannot be returned to its own cavity, it is called an irreducible or incarcerated hernia. If the blood supply to the structure within the hernia becomes occluded it is called a strangulated hernia. This leads to gangrene of the trapped tissues, which is a surgical emergency.

When a hernia becomes progressively larger in the elderly patient, early surgical intervention is advised since mortality risks are far greater for emergency repair. Reports indicate mortality rates range between 7 percent and 22 percent for emergency surgeries while elective repair carries only a 1.2 percent to 2 percent mortality rate.

See also HERNIA, HIATAL.

Phipps, W. J. *Essentials of Medical-Surgical Nursing.* St. Louis: C. V. Mosby Co., 1985.
Steinberg, F. U. *Care of the Geriatric Patient,* 6th ed. St. Louis: C. V. Mosby Co., 1983.

hernia, femoral See HERNIA.

hernia, hiatal Hiatal hernia is the protrusion of the stomach through the diaphragm into the chest. The development of hiatal hernia is associated with old age, obesity, chronic illness, straining with bowel movements, and wearing of tight belts and garments.

Symptoms of hiatal hernia include difficulty swallowing, heartburn, acid vomiting, spitting up blood, and regurgitation when stooping, lying flat, or eating a large meal.

Treatment for hiatal hernia is frequently conservative and may include the use of antacids, sleeping with the head elevated with either pillows or by elevating the head of the bed, and avoiding stooping or bending over. In people who are obese, weight loss may give symptomatic relief.

Avoidance of tight garments, eating small bland meals, and not reclining immediately after eating may also be helpful.

Barium swallow and esophagoscopy are useful in confirming the presence of a hiatal hernia. Surgical correction is rarely required unless disabling symptoms or complications arise.

See also HERNIA.

Phipps, W. J. *Essentials of Medical-Surgical Nursing.* St. Louis: C. V. Mosby Co., 1985.
Scherer, J. C. *Introductory Medical-Surgical Nursing,* 3rd ed. Philadelphia: J. B. Lippincott Co., 1982.
Steinberg, F. U. *Care of the Geriatric Patient,* 6th ed. St. Louis: C. V. Mosby Co., 1983.

hernia, inguinal See HERNIA.

hernia, strangulated See HERNIA.

hernia, umbilical See HERNIA.

herpes zoster (shingles) Herpes zoster, or shingles, is a viral infection of the peripheral nerves. It occurs as a result of reactivation of latent varicella virus (the virus that causes chicken pox) from sensory ganglia. It is seen frequently in the elderly; in illnesses that alter cell-mediated immunity such as Hodgkin's disease; in other lymphomas; in corticosteroid therapy; and in immunosuppression and radiation therapy. Incidence of herpes zoster in the elderly is 6.5 per 1,000 in persons 60 to 79 years of age and 10 per 1,000 in persons over age 80.

The patient usually develops a rash characterized by clusters of vesicles on an erythematous base in a dermatomal distribution. The rash usually lasts one to two weeks with varying degrees of pain. Postherpetic neuralgia (pain along nerve pathway) may occur in 30 percent to 40 percent of the elderly and occurs more frequently after involvement of the trigeminal nerve.

Treatment consists of the administration of prednisone in rapidly tapering dosages over one to two weeks. Topical analgesia with lotions containing benzocain is frequently effective. Other drugs used in treating postherpetic neuralgia are phenytoin, the combination of amitriptyline and prolixin, or chlorprothixene. Because herpes zoster is frequently a recurrent problem, some people take lysine (dietary supplement-amino acid) on a regular basis as a preventive measure.

Covington, T., and Walker, J. *Current Geriatric Therapy*. Philadelphia: W. B. Saunders, 1984.

hiring age   Many safety-related jobs have a maximum hiring age. Firefighters are not hired after age 35 and are forced to retire at age 55. The federal government will not allow anyone over the age of 60 to fly a commercial airplane. Police departments often consider a 29-year-old applicant too old. This type of age discrimination has caused a lot of bitterness in the United States. Many people are suing companies for age discrimination.

The Age Discrimination in Employment Act enacted by Congress, as well as other amendments, seeks to protect most workers between the ages of 40 and 70 years old from age discrimination.

See also GOLD-COLLAR WORKER.

Gilgoff, H. "How Old Is Too Old?" in *Aging*, Goldstein, E. C., ed. Vol. 3, Art. 5. Boca Raton, Fl.: Social Issues Resource Series, Inc., 1981.

hirsutism   See HAIR, EXCESSIVE.

hobbies (crafts)   People who sew, crochet, embroider, knit, paint, write poems, or play musical instruments generally want to continue when they grow older. It is relatively easy to renew interest in these activities even if it has been a few years since the older individual has been active in them. Sometimes it is necessary to make a few alterations if eyesight or manual dexterity have decreased.

Many projects can be made manageable by using simpler patterns, larger needles, or a magnifying glass. New materials and techniques are constantly coming along and an occasional visit to a craft or hobby shop can prove helpful for new ideas.

Some people do not develop their hobbies or crafts until they are older because they never felt they had time to devote to them. Leathercrafts, ceramics, needlework, painting, china painting, woodwork, stamp collecting, and playing musical instruments are some of the favorite activities of older people. Many cities offer programs for senior citizens that teach crafts and hobbies.

Fromme, A. *Life After Work*. Glenview, Ill.: AARP, 1984.
Gillies, J. *A Guide to Caring for Coping with Aging Parents*. Nashville: Thomas Nelson Publishers, 1981.

hospice   The development of the hospice is one of the great forward steps in human services in this century. Until this concept was established by Dr. Cicely Saunders at St. Christopher's Hospital (now Hospice) in London, England, in 1967, there was a tendency to ignore dying people simply because there was no therapeutic treatment that could turn away their oncoming deaths. Under the revolutionary idea of the hospice, however, the aim is to help dying people, often cancer victims, to retain as much control over their lives as possible, and to experience death with dignity.

When a patient has been diagnosed as terminally ill and is expected to live only a few weeks or months, a hospice program will provide a continuum of care consisting in the relief of pain, spiritual and psychological counseling, help with bodily care and functions as needed, and social services. Providers of hospice services not only include health professionals and staff specially trained to deal with the dying, but volunteers, clergy, and, of course, the individual's family. The aim is to help both patient and family come to terms and deal positively with the imminent death and to strengthen their capacity to meet death with dignity.

In home-based hospice programs, family members give most of the direct care to the dying individual, but they have the help of an interdisciplinary team (physician, nurse, clergy, social worker). In hospice residences care is supplied by professional staff, employees, and volunteers, with the family playing the supportive role. When a patient decides to follow the hospice approach, aggressive techniques (i.e., chemotherapy, radiotherapy, surgery, etc.) to preserve life are discontinued. The alleviation of pain and assurance of physical and psychological comfort—a personal rather more than a medical approach—become central.

A hospice was first established in the United States in 1971 in Branford, Connecticut, following the model established by Dr. Saunders in London. The concept has since spread across the United States, and today there are more than 1,900 hospice programs, which serve over 100,000 patients each year. About 65 percent of the people utilizing hospice programs are over 65, and 80 percent are dying of cancer.

A number of states (15 at last count) have passed laws or regulations dealing specifically with hospices. These laws provide for licensure and regulation, and promote the growth of hospice services.

Several states require health insurance policies to include home health care and provide optional coverage for hospice care to individuals and groups. Medicare has been modified to include hospice benefits, although the specific regulations have not been worked out.

Atchley, R. C. *Social Forces and Aging*, 4th ed. Belmont, Calif.: Wadsworth Publishing Co., 1985.
Millard, S. "Older Citizens Seek Independence," in *Aging*, Goldstein, E. C., ed. Vol. 2, Art. 64. Boca Raton, Fl.: Social Issues Resource Series, Inc., 1981.

Hottentot elderly   The Hottentots are a seminomadic African tribe who were one of the numerous social groups worldwide who engaged in a fairly common form of euthanasia directed at older people. The custom was to leave feeble or mentally incompetent elderly people in a remote place where they would either starve to death or be killed by wild animals. Like many other societies around the world (including some west coast American Indian tribes) the Hottentots could not support disabled people, and, with a migratory way of life, had to abandon those who could no longer perform work or move with the group. Extensive documentation of worldwide practices of this and other forms of euthanasia dates back at least to 1922, in the research reported by the distinguished American psychologist, G. Stanley Hall, in his book *Senescence*.

Pratty, J. "No Roles for the Elderly," in *Aging*, Goldstein, E. C., ed. Vol. 1, Art. 7. Boca Raton, Fl.: Social Issues Resource Series, Inc., 1981.
Russell, C. H. *Good News About Aging*. New York: John Wiley and Sons, 1989.

housing, age-segregated   Two million or about 6 percent of the U.S. elderly reside in communities and housing that have been designed especially for their occupancy.

Age-segregated housing holds many advantages for the elderly. One of the most obvious advantages is the things this age group have in common. Older people can relate to and sympathize with other older people's problems. Since the people are in the same age group they were born and raised at similar times and share a common history. The elderly can also decrease their involvement with a society that is preoccupied with the desirability of youth. Older people can "talk out" their fears of death and confront the frequent deaths of others. Most of the retirement villages are heavily secured. This offers the older person a sense of safety and protection. The older person is more likely to be noticed in an age-segregated community if he or she is in need of help. The elderly people living in such a community also receive lower rates because of the quantity of similar goods and services needed by their communities.

Some of the disadvantages of age-segregated housing are isolation from mainstream society, preventing older people from sharing wisdom and experiences with younger people and leading old people to have restricted sets of friendships and neighbors. In some elderly people age-segregated housing can contribute to low morale and feelings of uselessness and rejection.

See RESIDENTIAL CHOICE AND DESIGN FOR THE ELDERLY.

Golant, S. M. "Age-Segregated Housing," in Aging, Goldstein, E. C., ed. Vol. 2, Art. 86. Boca Raton, Fl.: Social Issues Resource Series, Inc., 1981.

hygiene, personal   As people grow older sometimes they feel that their appearance is not important anymore. For many people, a physical handicap, failing eyesight, or a loss of the sense of smell may restrict their personal grooming. Cleanliness is important not only for good health and comfort but for better self-esteem.

See also BATHING; FOOT CARE; HAIR CARE; INCONTINENCE; ORAL HYGIENE.

Gillies, J. A Guide to Caring for and Coping with Aging Parents. Nashville: Thomas Nelson Publishers, 1981.

hyperbaric oxygen   Tests have shown that senility is not due to a deterioration of the brain cells, which seem to be the strongest, longest-living cells in the body, but rather to a clogging of the arteries that cuts off the oxygen and nutrients the brain needs to function to full capacity.

Oxygen flow to the brain can be increased by using hyperbaric oxygen (HBO). This oxygen under pressure has been useful in many cases of presenility or in the first year of senility.

After treatment, these patients show excellent improvement. Their minds become sharper, memories are better, and their outlook and energy improve. The HBO treatment also frequently reverses the arthritis that accompanies aging.

See also AGING, BIOLOGICAL THEORY OF.

Martin, P. "Good News About Growing Older," in Aging, Goldstein, E. C., ed. Vol. 2, Art. 41. Boca Raton, Fl.: Social Issues Resource Series, Inc., 1981.

hypernephroma, malignant   See CANCER, KIDNEY.

hyperopia (far-sightedness)   The hyperopic eye is one that is deficient in refractive power so that rays of light from a distant object come to a focus at a point behind the retina with respect to the unaccommodated eye.

In most hyperopia, the chief cause is a shortening of the length of the eye. Such an eye is smaller than the normal eye and is called axial hyperopia. Another cause of hyperopia is found when the cornea or lens has less curvature than normal so that the image formed is focused at a point behind the normally placed retina. This is called curvature hyperopia. The third cause of hyperopia is a change of the refractive power of the lens, which can occur with age or in diabetes. This is called index hyperopia.

It is usually in older people that the symptoms of hyperopia become apparent, as educational demands and the time allotted for close work increase. Symptoms of hyperopia are the inability to see well closely at a young age. Other symptoms include headaches, burning of the eyes, a pulling sensation, and eyestrain. These symptoms are generally related to the constant excessive accommodation that is required for close work in a hyperope. In older people no symptoms may appear until the power of accomodation has diminished to the extent that the near point is beyond the range of comfortable reading distance.

The treatment of hyperopia involves the use of convex-lens, spectacles or contact lens. Older people, particularly those between 55 and 65 years of age, find it difficult to accommodate. This type of hyperopic patient usually needs convex lenses for both distance vision and close work.

See also ASTIGMATISM; MYOPIA; and PRESBYOPIA.

Newell, F. W. *Opthalmology Principles and Concepts,* 6th ed. St. Louis: C. V. Mosby Co., 1986.

Slatt, B. J., and Stein, H. A. *The Ophthalmic Assistant Fundamentals and Clinical Practice,* 4th ed. St. Louis: C. V. Mosby Co., 1983.

hypertension (high blood pressure)

Hypertension is increased vascular resistance, especially in the arterioles and small muscular arteries. Hypertension may be associated with Cushing syndrome (excessive secretion of adrenal cortical hormones), hyperthyroidism, coarctation of the aorta (constriction of the major channel of the arterial trunk), pheochromocytoma (encapsulated vascular tumor of the inner portion of the kidney), renal failure, increased intracranial pressure, and hyperaldosteronism (abnormality of electrolyte metabolism causing water retention). The most common type is essential hypertension in which the exact cause is unknown.

Hypertension occurs in 20 percent to 33 percent of the population over age 55, peaking at 55 to 64 years of age. The symptoms of hypertension may include headache and palpitation, but more likely the person is asymptomatic. Hypertension is characterized by a sustained elevation in arterial pressure, but the systolic, diastolic, and mean arterial pressure may all be elevated. Ventricle hypertrophy, congestive heart failure, and strokes may be consequences of undetected or poorly controlled hypertension. A diagnostic workup is important to determine the cause of the hypertension. Finding the exact cause allows more accurate treatment.

The treatment for hypertensive patients consists of four classes of drugs:

1. Diuretics—drugs that have a compensatory increased renin activity, presumably causing a depletion of intravascular fluid volume

2. Sympatholytics—drugs that decrease sympathetic nervous system activity often leading to an increase in intravascular fluid volume

3. Vasodilators—drugs that produce tachycardia, which can offset the blood pressure lowering effects of the other drugs

4. Beta blockers

With all the effects of these drugs, a combination of drug therapy permits the greatest therapeutic effects with lowered doses of any one drug, thus decreasing the chance or likelihood of dose-related side effects.

Placing the patient on a weight-reduction and low-sodium diet lowered the blood pressure in a number of patients. As little as a 10-pound weight loss can lower the pressure to a normal level in some cases.

Scherer, J. C. *Introductory Medical Surgical Nursing,* 3rd ed. Philadelphia: J. B. Lippincott Co., 1982.

Steinberg, F. U. *Care of the Geriatric Patient,* 6th ed. St. Louis: C. V. Mosby Co., 1983.

hyperthermia (fever, sunstroke, heat exhaustion, heatstroke, heat cramps)

Unusually high body temperature is known as hyperthermia. The causes of elevated temperature are exposure to excessive heat, impaired thermoregulatory reflexes, and infections.

Dangerous increases in body temperatures are more likely to occur in the elderly. During heat waves they may be unable to lose body heat adequately through sweating and peripheral vasodilatation, thus their temperature rises.

Mortality, from all causes, rises dramatically during heat waves in people over 50 and it progresses with increasing age. Many deaths are attributed to cardiovascular or cerebrovascular disease when, in fact, they can be directly related to a high body temperature. Deaths have occurred when air conditioning has failed or in residences where fans or air conditioning were not available. Older people traveling to unaccustomed hot climates have been susceptible to hyperthermia.

Those people with impaired thermoregulatory reflexes have difficulty controlling their body temperature even on exposure to moderate heat. The primary causes are lesions of the hypothalamus, lesions of the spinal cord, and extensive skin lesions. But even in the absence of lesions, the elderly show a higher threshold of elevated temperature and a decrease in sweating. Impaired temperature regulation, from diminished or absent sweating, is probably the main factor in increased mortality in the elderly during heat waves.

Infections cause fever, probably by raising the set point of the temperature-regulating mechanisms. In the elderly, fever gives rise to headache, dizziness, restlessness, and confusion. Delusions, hallucinations, and paranoia may also occur. Dehydration can occur rapidly since the elderly do not exhibit thirst as early as a younger person. Peripheral circulatory failure from sodium and water depletion can occur.

In moderate fever, the use of aspirin and correction of the underlying cause may be all that is necessary, with attention also given to early dehydration. In high fever, as in heatstroke (sunstroke), speed is essential to prevent brain damage. The skin becomes hot, dry, and flushed and body temperature rises to over 104 degrees. Without treatment most heatstroke victims will die. Treatment consists of sponging with cold water or immersion in ice water. Wet blankets and fans, to aid in evaporated cooling, are also effective.

The mortality from heatstroke is extremely high in the elderly. If the high temperature continues, serious and permanent brain damage results. Treatment should continue until body temperature is reduced to at least 102 degrees. If the person does not then respond, brain damage may have already occurred. Impairment of consciousness may lead to coma. Cardiac dysrhythmias, pneumonia, purpura, and gastrointestinal bleeding are common with sequelae hyperthermia.

See also HEAT INDEX.

Brocklehurst, J. C. *Textbook of Geriatric Medicine and Gerontology* 3rd ed. New York: Churchill Livingstone, 1985.

Phipps, W., *et al. Medical Surgical Nursing.* St. Louis: C. V. Mosby Co., 1983.

hyperthyroidism (Grave's disease, thyrotoxicosis, Basedow's disease, and exophthalmic goiter) Hyperthyroidism is a common chronic disorder that is caused by an excessive secretion of thyroid hormone. Twenty percent of hyperthyroid patients are over the age of 60.

Symptoms of hyperthyroidism include anxiety, insomnia, sweating, tremors, palpitations, tachycardia, heat intolerance, diarrhea, weight loss, muscular weakness, and angina. Some people with hyperthyroidism have exophthalmos (protrusion of the eyeball).

There are several types of medical and surgical treatment available for hyperthyroidism. Antithyroid drugs are used to block the production of thyroid hormone. This group is the initial therapy for all severely toxic patients and is preferred therapy for young adults. There is a 20 percent to 25 percent chance of remission after one to two years of treatment. This drug group includes propylthiouracil, methimazole, and radioactive iodine. The effects of these drugs will not be noticed until the excess thyroid hormone in the thyroid gland has been secreted into the blood stream. This will take several weeks. The complications of antithyroid drugs include rash, fever, hepatitis, and agranulocytosis.

Radioactive iodine (I-131) may be administered to a patient with hyperthyroidism to destroy the hyperplastic thyroid tissue by radiation. The dose of I-131 is based upon the weight of the person's thyroid gland, age, clinical symptoms, and the emanations from the gland as shown on a geiger counter. The side effects include nausea, vomiting, malaise, and fever. Radioactive iodine was thought to cause cancer; however, it has not been demonstrated in extensive studies. Hypothyroidism may be a possible delayed complication of I-131 treatment. Therefore a person should remain under medical supervision long after this treatment. Radioactive iodine is the preferred definitive therapy for people over 20, those who relapse after surgery, and those who cannot tolerate antithyroid drugs or refuse surgery. Within eight to nine weeks of the first dose of I-131, the person will begin to notice a remission of the symptoms.

Surgery (thyroidectomy) is another choice of treatment. It is the preferred treatment for children or adolescents who cannot tolerate antithyroid drugs or those who relapse after one or two years on antithyroid drugs. The possible side effects of a thyroidectomy include the immediate surgical and anesthetic risks, hypoparathyroidism, voice injury, and permanent hypothyroidism.

Since I-131 treatment is so effective, surgery is usually performed only on malignant thyroid disease, on people under 35, and on pregnant women.

Roger, C. S. and McCue, J. D. *Managing Chronic Disease.* Oradell, N. J.: Medical Economics Co. Inc., 1987.
Scherer, J. C. *Introductory Medical-Surgical Nursing.* Philadelphia: J. B. Lippincott Co., 1982.

hypochondriasis Hypochondriasis is a mental disorder characterized by constant preoccupation with health and one's own body. The essence of hypochondriasis is a clinical picture in which the predominant disturbance is an unrealistic interpretation of physical signs or sensations as abnormal. This leads to a preoccupation with the belief of having a serious illness. This disorder is not uncommon among the elderly, since physical changes and physical disabilities are frequently taking place.

Symptoms may include excessive worry about bowel movements, body temperature, aches, pains, coughs, sneezes, and cancer. A variety of physical conditions of disease, may simulate symptoms and it is often difficult to determine whether a person's complaints of pain or discomfort are physical, psychological, or both.

There is a high suicide risk for patients with persistent physical complaints whether hypochondriacal or due to an actual disease. Therefore, attempts should be made to resolve all such complaints. A medical check-up should be the first step to evaluate symptoms. If it is determined that the symptom is psychological, psychotherapy may be necessary. It is important to avoid complex diagnostic workups and the use of potentially addictive drugs. It is also important for those dealing with the hypochondriac to maintain a good relationship in order to lessen the distress of the individual.

Reichel, W. M. *Clinical Aspects of Aging.* Baltimore: The Williams & Wilkins Co., 1979.

hypotension, orthostatic Orthostatic hypotension is a fall in the arterial blood pressure when the person moves to a more upright position. Orthostatic blood pressure instability is common in the elderly. It should be suspected in people who become faint or experience dizziness when rising from a chair or bed. Many falls of the elderly can be traced to orthostatic hypotension.

Symptoms include light headedness, blurring of vision, and a sense of weakness and unsteadiness. The two major causes of this disorder are depletion of the total blood volume and impairment of autonomic cardiovascular reflex activity. Both of these causes may coexist.

Treatment of chronic orthostatic hypotension involves three basic methods: mechanical maneuvers, volume expanders, and pharmacologic agents. Mechanical measures include elevation of the head while resting, wearing a lower body compression garment, and exercises such as calf-muscle flexing. Patients should be taught to rise slowly and to remain as mobile as possible. Volume expanders include a high-salt diet and fluorocortisone acetate, which causes a uniform expansion of plasma volume. This expansion does not persist permanently in all patients. There are several pharmacologic agents used either alone or in sequence for the treatment of orthostatic hypotension. These drugs may include sympathomimetics, vasoconstrictors, Beta-receptor blockers, Alpha-receptor agonists, prostaglandin synthesis inhibitors, and antiserotonergics. These drugs mimic the actual effect of the body's natural vasopressors, although no single agent is uniformly successful.

Hurst, J. W. *The Heart*, 6th ed. St. Louis: McGraw-Hill Book Co., 1986.

Schatz, I. J. *Orthostatic Hypotension*. Philadelphia: F. A. Davis Co., 1986.

hypothermia   Exposure to cold can result in a low body temperature known as hypothermia. The most common victims are older people who have difficulty keeping themselves or their homes warm.

In order for the human body to function properly, body temperature should be around 98.6° F (37° C). When body temperature drops below 95° the heart begins to slow, the body becomes weak, and the mind becomes confused. Death could soon follow. Many older people die in their own homes because they become too confused and disoriented to sense the danger and seek help.

Many things such as living in a cold house, poor diet, stroke, diabetes, certain prescription drugs, or alcohol can increase the risk of becoming hypothermic. Outdoor temperatures do not have to be below freezing for hypothermia to develop. Indoors, room temperatures below 70 could be dangerous for some people if they are not dressed warmly enough.

Some of the danger signals of hypothermia are: confusion, difficulty speaking, forgetfulness, shivering, stiff muscles, stomach cold to touch, difficulty waking up, puffy face, trembling on one side of the body or in one arm or leg.

If hypothermia is suspected, call a doctor, ambulance, rescue squad, or local emergency room immediately. Handle the person very gently, covering him or her with blankets, quilts, or extra clothing. Make sure that the head and neck are covered. Do not give hot drinks or food or any medication. Do not massage the arms or legs or raise the legs. Wait for medical help before attempting to treat the patient in any way.

Dressing warmly is the best defense against hypothermia. Wear several layers of loose clothing, keeping the clothing dry. When outdoors, wear a wind-proof outer garment and mittens rather than gloves. Wearing a hat will enable the body to send warm blood to the hands and feet. Use a scarf around the neck. At night, hot water bottles, heating pads, and electric blankets will help to keep the bed warm. Utility companies provide programs for home insulation and other tips for home heating. State agencies can be contacted for assistance in paying fuel bills or providing services for the elderly.

Published by Center for Environment Physiology. *Hypothermia Bulletin*. Washington, D.C.: 1985.

hypothyroidism (myxedema)   Hypothyroidism is a chronic disorder that is caused by an underactive thyroid gland. The thyroid does not secrete enough thyroid hormone, therefore the rate of all metabolic processes is decreased. Hypothyroidism may occur after thyroidectomy. Hypothyroidism is the most common thyroid disease in the elderly. Moderately advanced and severe hypothyroidism is found almost exclusively in the elderly. Early hypothyroidism is easily confused with the progression of normal aging. Gait disorders are common and can easily be misdiagnosed.

The most common causes in the elderly may include high-dose radiation therapy for a laryngeal carcinoma or lymphoma, Graves' disease or colloid goiter; drugs that interfere with intrathyroidal iodide metabolism and surgical or I-131 ablation of the thyroid gland.

Symptoms of hypothyroidism include coarse hair and skin, deep voice, slow speech, cold intolerance, weight gain, constipation, depression, pseudodementia, hyponatremia (salt depletion), and hypothermia. Hypothyroidism may go untreated for years since many of the symptoms are nonspecific.

Hypothyroidism is treated by the replacement of the thyroid hormone. This may come in the form of thyroid extract or in a synthetic product. The prescription is taken orally once a day. The possible side effects of this treatment may include palpitations, hyperactivity, dyspnea (labored breathing), rapid pulse, insomnia, dizziness, and gastrointestinal disorders.

People who have had severe hypothyroidism should see a doctor regularly in order to check for the correct dosage of the thyroid extract.

Ham, R. J. *Geriatric Medicine Annual-1986.* Oradell, N.J.: Medical Economics Co., 1986.
Scherer, J. C. *Introductory Medical-Surgical Nursing.* Philadelphia: J. B. Lippincott Co., 1982.

I

ideas about aging in literature   observations about aging probably date back to the earliest human times, and written records of thoughts about age appear as early as the biblical *Book of Ecclesiastes* in the Old Testament. Recent writers on age have included Simone de Beauvoir and Betty Friedan. The latter is best known for *The Feminine Mystique* and is the author of *The Fountain of Age,* released in 1989.

Analysts have observed that a good deal of the literature about age contains three general approaches to aging, which have been labeled as the "antediluvian," "hyperborean," and "rejuvenation" themes. The first of these refers to the time before Noah in the Bible, and means literally "before the flood." It reaches back to the time of Adam, who according to the Bible, lived to be 930 years old, and to other patriarchs like Noah, who reached 950, and Methuseleh, who attained 969.

The underlying idea in this theme is that people long ago lived much longer than they do now—a mistaken notion, according to modern research, because studies in the ruins of ancient Egypt and Rome and elsewhere show that the average length of life in ancient times was about 25 years. Although some people did live to advanced years, no evidence of exceptional length of life has appeared in archeological studies in these or other locations. Today the average life expectancy, about 75 years in the United States, is much greater than it ever was in the past.

The hyperborean theme refers to the notion that somewhere in far away places people live to an exceptionally old age. This theme is still very much alive in the Soviet Union, where gerontologists insistently claim that an individual, Mezhid Agayev, residing in a remote region of Azerbaijan in the Caucasus mountains, lived to be 139. They have also claimed that a woman in Bolivia had reached 205, while two other persons in the USSR, a woman named Ashura Omarova and a man, lived to 195 and 165 respectively.

The hyperborean idea originated with the Greeks before the time of Christ. It surfaced again in modern times in one of the best-sellers of 1930s, the book *Lost Horizon.* In this tale a group of Europeans and Americans crash-land a plane on a flight west from China and accidentally happen on the city of Shangri-La, an earthly paradise of peace in remote Tibet where residents live virtually forever.

A film by the same name featured matinee idol Ronald Colman as the hero. After enjoying the peaceful enchantments of Shangri-La for a time, Colman leaves with a Tibetan woman, played by the actress Margo, who manages to convince him that the place is fraud. Once outside this earthly paradise, Margo, who had actually lived in Shangri-La long beyond the human life span, goes through a transformation of aging before Colman's horror-stricken eyes and dies in the midst of a howling blizzard.

Colman is rescued and makes his way back to Europe, but there he finds his memories of Shangri-La too strong to resist. He struggles once again to return to that happy place, and after a harrowing search in the mountains of Tibet he manages to rediscover his paradise. In real life, of course, there is no such place as Shangri-La; and, because they live with better sanitation and receive better health care and nutrition, the residents of industrialized western nations have a longer average life expectancy than those of remote places no matter how peaceful the latter may appear.

The rejuvenation theme is familiar to most Americans because they have heard the story of Ponce de León (the second largest city in Puerto Rico—Ponce—is named after him) and his discovery of Florida made while in search of the Fountain of Youth. The idea of rejuvenation has great appeal because of its promise to restore youthful vitality, beauty, and strength. It stands behind the success of nostrums like Queen Bee jelly, a popular ingredient in face creams and other emollients a few years ago, which sweep the American consumer market from time to time. It also fuels the thriving plastic surgery industry, which generates millions of dollars annually in face lifts, forehead lifts, chin lifts, breast lifts, fat tissue removal, and what-not. Retin-A, or resorsinal, a drug that removes some wrinkles by restoring collagen in the skin (but can also cause serious allergic reactions for some people), is one of the well-publicized promises of eternally youthful appearance.

Besides expressing these themes, many literary treatments of aging have gravitated to one of two poles—age is the best of times or it is the worst of times. Proponents of the pessimistic view—age is the worst of times—included the Greek philosopher, Aristotle, tutor to Alexander the Great. Aristotle saw the elderly as filled with faults—he believed that they were rigid, small minded, suspicious, cynical, ungenerous, cowardly, and shameless. They survive by shrewdness and calculation rather than through decency and moral values. They may seem self-controlled, but this is only because they do not have the physical power to generate emotional feelings.

On the other hand Plato, who once was Aristotle's teacher and who some consider the greatest philosopher of all time, took the opposite view. He thought that only the old had the necessary wisdom to be the governors of society, the politicians. Aristotle disagreed—he felt that old people had such grave defects of character that they should be disqualified from holding any political office.

The biblical book of Ecclesiastes, which was probably written about two hundred years after Aristotle's time, shared a pessimistic view of age. This was expressed in a haunting and enormously powerful passage of poetry known as the "Allegory of Age":

> Remember your Creator . . . before the sun and the light of day give place to darkness, before the moon and the stars grow dim, and the clouds return with the rain—when the guardians of the house tremble, and strong men stoop, when the women grinding the meal cease work because they are few, and those who look through the windows look no longer, when the street-doors are shut, when the voice of the mill is low, when the chirping of the sparrow grows faint and the song-birds fall silent.

Other spokespeople for the negative view of age have included Shakespeare and the modern writer Simone de Beauvoir, who published her highly negative ideas in 1973 in a book called *La Vieilliesse* (Age). Best known for her work *The Second Sex,* which helped to launch the women's liberation movement worldwide, de Beauvoir's book on age concentrates on illness and decline. Even more, de Beauvoir attacks society in general for the maltreatment of elder people—blaming the social milieu for what she describes as the poverty, uselessness, loneliness, and depression of the elderly.

Young people, she says, dismiss age with an indifferent shrug, and this has intensified the plight of the elderly and increased the stigma attached to age. At one point in her book she describes age as a "natural curse" because human societies treat the old so poorly that apes treat their own elderly comparatively better.

Her views can be summed up with a few dramatic quotations like this one:

> . . . the vast majority of mankind look upon the coming of old age with sorrow and rebellion. It fills them with more aversion than death itself. . . . When memory decays . . . former happenings . . . sink and vanish in a mocking darkness; life unravels stitch by stitch, leaving nothing but meaningless strands of wool in an old person's hands. . . . Those (elderly) who escape utter poverty and pinching want are forced to take care of a body that has grown frail, easily fatigued, often infirm, and racked with pain. Immediate pleasures are forbidden or parsimoniously measured out: love, eating, drinking, smoking, sport, walking.

While many gerontologists were much impressed by de Beauvoir's description of age, her account was probably heavily influenced by the illness and decline of her beloved friend and lover, Jean-Paul Sartre, a leader in the French school of existentialist writing, who went blind in his later years. De Beauvoir's study of age did not take into account ongoing gerontological research; which was beginning to show that most people take their senior years in stride, and that the old are actually happier and more self-composed than people usually have thought.

In fact, proponents of the positive view of aging have easily held their own against the pessimists. The earliest of these, the Roman statesman Cicero, who lived about 60 years before the birth of Christ, wrote a highly spirited defense of age. Active in Roman politics at the time of Julius Caesar and Mark Antony, Cicero exercised his famous oratorical powers in a treatise entitled *de Senectute (about Aging)*. In this defense Cicero answered four charges against aging—that it: weakens the body; withholds enjoyment of life; stands near death; and, prohibits great accomplishments.

His principle defense against such views was that age is really superior to youth because it is a time of spiritual growth. Age, he argued, is greater than youth because it stands above the trivial pursuit of pleasure typical of the early years of life.

Cicero's essay includes innumerable passages that deserve to be quoted, but two stand out especially for their appeal to modern minds. One is a forerunner of the idea that life is a series of passages, a concept which author Gail Sheehy was to adopt when she wrote her best-selling book *Passages* in the early 1980s. In Cicero's words:

> There is a fixed course for life's span and a simple path . . . for Nature. A fitting timeliness has been allotted for each part of the journey, so that the helpless dependency of infancy and the fiery intensity of youth, the dignity of the established years, and the maturity of old age have each a certain natural endowment, which must be perceived and fulfilled in its own season.

Cicero here not only identified the broad passages of life but observed that each age has its own unique qualities and excellent features, and therefore that late life is in no way inferior to early life.

At another point Cicero expressed a view about life and death that offers useful guidance to anyone who happens to consider these subjects:

> I have no regret at having lived, for I have so conducted my life that I do not feel that I was born to no purpose, and I cheerfully depart

from life as though I were leaving a guest chamber, not my own house. Nature has granted us an inn for a moment . . . not a permanent dwelling.

Living at a time before the rise of Christianity, Cicero held that there were philosophical reasons to believe in the immortality of the soul. Still, he felt that even if his belief in immortality was mistaken, he had no fear of death. Should there be no such thing as immortality, then he would happily go forward into the future, for when life simply ends there can be no sense of hardship or pain. Cicero's treatise is probably one of the world's great writings on age.

Daniel Defoe, author of the famous adventure book *Robinson Crusoe*, in the mid-1700s wrote a less-known work titled *Moll Fanders*. Quite scandalous for its time, the book develops an unexpectedly positive outlook on the virtues of old age. Moll's lifestyle was lurid, one of involvement with a variety of lovers and husbands, which led her at one point to describe herself as a whore. On two occasions she traveled form her home in England to America, but underlying her flamboyantly adventuresome life lay a moral theme: She was independent, courageous, self-reliant, resourceful, and made her way against all hardships.

Her second journey to America came in her fifties and sixties as a result of a criminal sentence for stealing (Australia later became the prison colony for England, but at Moll's time England's American territories served as its main prison colony). Once in America Moll managed to retrieve the one husband whom she really loved, a man separated from her years before because he was caught and convicted as a highwayman, a life he undertook due to abject poverty. Together they achieved success by running a plantation in Virginia, and in due time they returned to England.

There they lived an old age that redeemed them from their sin-filled youth. Now comfortable and wealthy, Moll's closing words are that she and her husband had determined

"to spend the rest of our lives in sincere penitence for the wicked lives we have lived." For Moll, age was a time of cheer and good humor where one can make up for the failings of a lifetime.

Robert Browning, a major poet of the Victorian England now celebrated with a spot in Poet's Corner in Westminster Abbey in London, was another writer who expressed a favorable view of old age. This he set forth in a memorable poem about the reflections of the thoughtful Rabbi Ben Ezra. A man with a philosophical turn of mind, the rabbi praised long life because it gave one a chance to witness the unfolding of God's plan for humankind.

> Grow old along with me,
> The best is yet to be,
> The last of life,
> For which the first is made.

According to the poem the years of youth are merely an introduction to seniority, the time when the really important events of life happen. In our present era, when most people attribute the best only to youth, the rabbi's ideas come like a breath of fresh air, stating a truth that ought to spread wide to the growing millions who are reaching their advanced maturity.

Russell, C. H. *Good News About Aging.* New York: John Wiley and Sons, 1989.

immune system rejuvenation One theory of aging proposes that the immune system declines with age, failing to protect the body from disease. The immune system may also play an important role in many aging processes as well. Many methods of bolstering the immune system are currently being researched. Two methods that have been studied are dietary restriction and transplanting immune cells from a young animal to an old animal. Another method that has been studied is the administration of hormones from the thymus gland. These methods lengthen life in some rodents with immune deficiencies but they have no life-extending effects on normal animals.

A drug called CoQ has also been investigated because of the theory that the immune system decline is caused partly by a deficiency of these quinone compounds. When the drug is administered to mice it prevents tumors. The drug may have damaging effects, which are currently being studied.

Interleuken-2, a substance that stimulates the growth of immune cells, restores certain immune functions in old mice.

See also AGING, BIOLOGICAL THEORY OF; COQ.

Kurz, M. A. "Theories of Aging and Popular Claims for Extending Life," in *Aging*, Goldstein, E. C., ed. Vol. 2, Art. 88. Boca Raton, Fl.: Social Issues Resource Series, Inc., 1981.

immunization in the elderly (tetanus immunization, diptheria immunization, influenza immunization, pneumonia immunization) *Tetanus and Diptheria:* Every adult should be immunized against tetanus and diptheria. For those who are certain of having been immunized, boosters should be given every 10 years. The mortality from tetanus in those over age 70 is greater than 60 percent—three to four times greater than in younger adults and children.

Influenza: Current recommendations for influenza vaccination include all people over age 65 and high-risk patients of all ages with chronic illnesses such as heart disease, diabetes, renal failure, chronic obstructive pulmonary disease, immunosuppression therapy, and malignancy. The only contraindications to use of the vaccine is patients with an allergy to eggs, and patients on chemotherapy. The vaccine should be administered yearly, two to three months prior to the expected epidemic seasons.

Pneumonia: The elderly in the high-risk group and asplenic patients should receive polyvalent pneumococcal polysaccharide vaccine. Immunity generally lasts five years. The vaccine should not be given more fre-

quently than every three years because more severe local reactions may occur. Major side effects of the vaccine are local tenderness and swelling.

Covington, T., and Walker, J. *Current Geriatric Therapy*. Philadelphia: W. B. Saunders, 1984.

impotence See SEXUALITY.

incontinence (see Table 27) There are two types of incontinence—urinary and fecal.

Urinary incontinence is the inability to control urinary function. This is a distressing symptom for many older people. There are many causes for incontinence. Mental impairment, brain damage associated with dementia, urinary tract infection, irritable bladder, prostate hyperatrophy (enlargement), and pelvic relaxation all can be responsible for incontinence.

Treatment for incontinence is varied. If the incontinence is intermittent the contributing cause should be treated. If there is a significant degree of pelvic relaxation, as in stress-related incontinence, when a person's urination is associated with coughing, sneezing, or running, a trial of Kegel exercises may be tried. These are relatively simple and involve contracting muscles to the point of stopping the urine stream up to 100 times a day. If this is not effective, surgery may be necessary.

Drug therapy may be useful, especially if bladder spasms are a problem. Anticholingeric drugs are used for this purpose. There are frequent side effects to these drugs including dry mouth, blurred vision, and constipation. These drugs should not be used in people with congestive heart failure, urinary obstruction, and narrow-angle glaucoma.

Often, a program of bladder retraining can be useful. People who are unable to feel the need to urinate may benefit from this program. The program includes regularly scheduled toileting and limiting the amount of fluid intake after the evening hours. It is important not to limit overall fluid intake, however. Adequate hydration alone may correct incontinence, by preventing fecal impaction, constipation, and urinary tract infection.

The Brantley Scott artificial urinary sphincter is a sophisticated device to control incontinence. This does, however, require a rather extensive surgical procedure but is about 90 percent successful in carefully selected candidates.

If none of these treatments are successful, a catheter may be necessary. This is regarded as a last resort because of the serious risks of urinary infection. Those with an indwelling Foley catheter must be careful to maintain proper drainage, remove encrustation, and apply antibiotic ointment in the urethral area daily. Periodic replacement of the catheter, irrigation of the catheter, maintaining good fluid intake, and sometimes antibiotic therapy are necessary to prevent infection. External catheters may be the best choice for males with at least partial emptying function.

Intermittent catheterization may be suitable, especially if the older person or a family member can be taught this relatively simple procedure.

Fecal incontinence is the inability to control bowel function. There are several causes for fecal incontinence. The external anal sphincter may be relaxed, the voluntary control of defecation may be interrupted in the central nervous system or messages may not be transmitted to the brain because of a lesion within the spinal cord or external pressure on the cord. The most common cause in the elderly is relaxation caused by general loss of muscle tone.

Treatment for fecal incontinence should involve a bowel training program. Ordinarily, the bowel is trained to empty at regular intervals. Once a day or every other day after breakfast is common. Foods and fluids increase peristalsis. Glycerin suppositories help stimulate evacuation of the bowel;

they should be inserted about two hours before the usual time of defecation. Occasionally, it is necessary to use a laxative suppository, such as Dulcolax, to provide additional stimulus. Routine enemas and laxatives should be avoided because they can caused dependence.

If incontinence cannot be managed, it can be made easier to live with by using plastic incontinence pants, penile clamps, condom drainage systems, and incontinence pads. Generally, these are available at medical equipment stores or large drug stores.

The psychological factors of incontinence are very important. Incontinence contributes to physical and social isolation and frequently leads to admission to extended-care facilities. It is important to maintain the older person's quality of life by managing incontinence with all available methods.

Brocklehurst, J. C. *Geriatric Medicine and Gerontology*, 3rd ed. New York: Churchill Livingstone, 1985.
Calkins, E. *et al. The Practice of Geriatrics.* Philadelphia: W. B. Saunders Co., 1986.

incontinence care   When living with incontinence, accept the fact that accidents will happen. Since incontinence is a major cause of bad odor in elderly people, every effort should be made to prevent this. The incontinent person should try to use the bathroom just before departing. Furniture and beds can be protected with water resistant pads. The incontinent person should change underwear and clothing as often as necessary, take frequent sponge baths, and use a lot of powders and deodorants.

If incontinency is constant, protective liners, disposable adult pants, or a catheter may be considered. Catherization is more easily accomplished with males, since it can be worn externally.

It should be remembered incontinence is not planned or deliberate and there is never a reason for scolding. Although it is often embarrassing, if handled with discretion and patience, discomfort can be kept to a minimum.

See also INCONTINENCE.

Gillies, J. *A Guide to Caring for and Coping with Aging Parents.* Nashville: Thomas Nelson Publishers, 1981.

Individual Retirement Account See IRA.

inflation See PERSONAL FINANCIAL PLANNING FOR RETIREMENT.

influenza Influenza is an acute respiratory tract infection accompanied by fever, cough, and myalgias. It is usually epidemic, occurring during the winter months with peaks from January through March. Respiratory mortality is increased, particularly in the elderly and those with underlying cardiac and pulmonary diseases.

The incidence of influenza may be decreased by immunization. All individuals over age 65 and those with cardiorespiratory illnesses or other risk factors should be vaccinated every year, two to three months before the expected flu season. A 70 percent to 80 percent success rate can be anticipated.

Those high-risk patients who remain unvaccinated may be partially protected by the use of amantidine, 100 mg twice daily. Since amantidine appears to prevent the entry of virus into cells and cell-to-cell transmission of virus, it may also be of some benefit in the treatment of active cases of influenza.

See also IMMUNIZATION IN THE ELDERLY.

Covington, T., and Walker T. *Current Geriatric Therapy.* Philadelphia: W. B. Saunders, 1984.

influenza immunization See IMMUNIZATION IN THE ELDERLY.

insomnia Insomnia is the inability to sleep during the period when sleep should normally occur. It may vary in degree from restlessness or disturbed sleep to curtailment of the normal length of sleep or absolute wakefulness. The causes of insomnia are varied but some of the most common are anxiety, renal failure, drug-induced insomnia, physical discomfort, and physical inactivity.

If insomnia is a result of anxiety, short-acting minor tranquilizers are usually very effective. They are used only for a relatively short period of time.

Urinary tract disturbances play a significant role in insomnia in the older person. Reduction of high levels of urea nitrogen and creatinine through lower intake of protein or dialysis bring sleep patterns more toward normal. Coffee, tea, and caffeinated soft drinks should be avoided after late afternoon and consumption of all liquids should be reduced in the evening.

Some patients may suffer insomnia as a result of being overmedicated. A review of the medications is indicated to be sure the dosages are within tolerance.

Physical discomforts such as back or neck pain or being too hot or too cold will interrupt sleep. These patients could be given mild analgesics and attention should be directed to regulating temperature control in their rooms.

The elderly frequently take naps during the day. These should be limited so that sleeping at night is not affected. Physical activities may help eliminate insomnia.

Scherer, J. C. *Introductory Medical-Surgical Nursing,* 3rd ed. Philadelphia: J. B. Lippincott Co., 1982.
Steinberg, F. U. *Care of the Geriatric Patient,* 6th ed. St. Louis: C. V. Mosby Co., 1983.

insurance, supplemental Many insurance companies offer supplemental insurance policies designed to help cover the cost uninsured by Medicare. Known as "Medigap" insurance, these policies will frequently cover the deductible and some of the shared costs.

Supplemental insurance usually does not require a physical examination. Most insurance companies may offer one such a plan and some companies may offer several with different ranges and types of health costs covered. Generally, the more a plan covers, the more it will cost the individual. Blue Cross/Blue Shield, the AMERICAN ASSOCIATION OF RETIRED PERSONS (AARP) and many other groups have plans that can be explored to help cushion the financial impact of health problems, especially during extended illnesses of the older individual.

Older people should be wary of mail-order or newspaper-supplement insurance offers and be sure to read the fine print. Many of these plans do not pay for the first week of hospital care or provide nursing home or psychiatric care benefits. Buying insurance policies that duplicate one another is unnecessary and can lead to payment of excessive premiums.

See also MEDICAID; MEDICARE.

Deedy, J. *Your Aging Parents*. Chicago: The Thomas More Press, 1984.

Gillies, J. *A Guide to Caring for and Coping with Aging Parents*. Nashville: Thomas Nelson Publishers, 1981.

intelligence, elderly The notion that everyone becomes senile with age is as widespread as it is false. Research on the intellectual abilities of older people does show some evidence of slowing of mental powers over the years (for example in ability to assimilate new information, speed of learning, solving of problems, and retention of short-term memory), yet the question is not how much mental power one loses, but rather how much mental power one retains. On that score the research is quite unequivocal—the overwhelming majority of older people retain the mental ability necessary to get along satisfactorily even in very old age. Of all the body organs, the brain normally deteriorates least, and only about 5 percent of the total population over 65, and about

20 percent of the population over 85, suffer senile dementia.

Actually, the peak of intelligence as measured by IQ tests—most of which stress speed in performance of mental tasks—comes in the teen years. By comparison with their teen years even people in their twenties are not as swift at mental tasks. According to research done by a leading gerontological psychologist, K. Warner Schaie of Pennsylvania State University, there is no uniformly reliable evidence of any notable decline in performance on mental tests until age 74, and even then the decline depends on the specific abilities being measured.

Schaie has conducted more than 30 years of research with hundreds of individuals who fairly well represent the U.S. population. His subjects have been residents of Seattle, Washington, from all walks of life, whose common characteristic was membership in a large health maintenance organization (HMO). He gave mental tests to this group in 1956, and over the years has tested and retested their mental abilities.

Through this research Schaie has identified the factors that promote favorable cognitive aging (ability to understand, to learn, to process information—other types of aging that involve the mind relate to the emotions, the senses, motor skills, etc.). These factors include: freedom from cardiovascular disease and other severe chronic illnesses; a good environment supported by a good education and a comfortable job and income; a complex and mentally stimulating environment; a flexible personality style in midlife; a spouse with a high cognitive status; and maintaining a level of perceptual processing speed (i.e., ability to take in information, understand it, and use it).

Further, Schaie has shown that *disuse* of the mind may account for much of the decline in mental power in late life; and, training in mental tasks can reverse decline of mental power for many people. In general, the research done by Schaie and others suggests that although mental abilities decline just as physical abilities do, individuals who keep active and use their minds remain mentally keen and competent as long as their health permits.

Schaie, K. Warner. "The Hazards of Cognitive Aging." *The Gerontologist.* 29:4, 484–493 (August 1989).

IRA (Individual Retirement Account)
IRAs were established under federal tax law to encourage the average wage earner to prepare for old age income by sheltering savings from taxes. Up to $2,000 of annual earnings ($2,250 for couples with one wage earner) can be invested in IRA accounts at this time. The interest income that is invested in IRA accounts does not have to be included in taxable income. Participants must pay a 10 percent penalty if they draw on their accounts before age 59½. The invested funds collect tax protected interest over the years. Investors are required to begin withdrawal in the year they reach 70½. Retirees are taxed on the withdrawals, but usually at a lower rate since their tax bracket is probably lower than during their working years.

People who wish to take deductions from their federal income taxes for IRA contributions should obtain the appropriate Internal Revenue Service publicaton and follow the instructions, however the basic rules can be summarized briefly. The deduction limit is $2000, and this amount may be reduced or eliminated depending on two factors: whether the individual or the individual's spouse is covered by an employer retirement plan; whether the individual's income exceeds specified limits.

Various rules apply to income limits depending on the individual's filing status as a single head of a household, married and filing joint return, or married filing separate returns. For the single person the allowable deduction is reduced beginning with a modified Adjusted Gross Income of $25,000, and it is eliminated for incomes above $35,000. For married couples filing jointly the reduction begins at $40,000 and is eliminated at $50,000 and for those filing separately the reduction range is 0 to $10,000.

Proposals have been made for restoring the full deductibility of IRA contributions for all income levels, and, in any case, tax rules change nearly annually. Taxpayers, therefore, need to contact the Internal Revenue Service or work with a qualified tax accountant to learn about changes.

The source on the above IRA information is: Internal Revenue Service, "Individual Retirement Arrangements (IRAs) for use in preparing 1990 Returns," Washington, D.C.: Internal Revenue Service, 1990. Publication 590, Catalog Number 15160X. p. 5.

Crichton, J. *The Age Care Sourcebook.* New York: Simon and Schuster, Inc. 1987.

iron   See VITAMINS.

itching   See PRURITIS.

J

Japanese Americans   See also STRESS OF LIFE.

Japanese elderly   Japan now has one of the fastest-growing aging populations in any world society, with a projected increase of its 65+ age group from 10 percent of its population in 1985 to 16.5 percent in the year 2005 (the comparable change during these years for the United States is from about 12 percent to about 14 percent). The life expectancy for Japanese men is about 75 years, and the average woman lives to about 80 (for the United States the comparable figures are about 73 years for men and 78 years for women). The relative longevity of the Japanese is attributed to their low-cholesterol diets rather than to heredity or lifestyle factors.

Though no one has yet attributed the longevity of the Japanese to their lifetime work patterns, these also differ from those of Americans and Europeans. In 1980 (the last date when worldwide statistics were compiled by the United Nations), Japanese women were somewhat more likely than European and American women to remain at work after age 65—about 20 percent of Japanese females were still working after that age compared to less than 10 percent in Europe and the United States. For Japanese men, 46 percent remained at work past 65 compared to 18 percent of American men and less than 10 percent of the Europeans. Today these figures remain approximately the same for Europe; however, the overall percentage of both sexes in American working past age 65 has dropped to about 10 percent compared to the 40 percent who remain at work in Japan.

Some people have attributed the unusually long work life of the Japanese to their national customs that stress intense commitment to their jobs. A more likely explanation is that pensions available to many Japanese are insufficient at age 65 to support retirement. Japan is one of the few industrialized nations that does not have a government sponsored retirement pension program. Instead, Japanese individuals and companies are obliged by law to create pension savings plans, but this apparently does not lead to lifelong saving rates that provide sufficient retirement income for many Japanese workers.

A new proposal made by Japan's Bureau of Planning in the Science and Technology Agency calls for a multilevel scheme for assisting Japan's burgeoning older population. It involves guaranteed incomes, the formation of special health and medical services, creation of "lifelong" study programs, and guaranteed housing for Japan's seniors.

By tradition the elderly in Japan live with their children, but this practice has started to decline in recent years. Some might think that this change reflects a decline of filial devotion or a growing generation gap in Japan, but the major cause is the improvement of pensions, which now provide enough income to allow more older people to maintain their own separate residences.

U.S. Bureau of the Census. *An Aging World.* International Population Reports Series P-95. No. 78. Washington, D.C.: U.S. Government Printing Office, 1987.
Yates, R. E. "Japan Has No Room to Be Old," in *Aging,* Goldstein, E. C., ed. Vol. 3, Art. 16. Boca Raton, Fl.: Social Issues Resource Series, Inc., 1981.

jaundice   Jaundice is yellowness of skin and eyes caused by an excess of bile pigment.

The assessment and management of jaundice is no different in the elderly and young adults. The types of jaundice are classified by whether the predominant pigment is unconjugated or conjugated.

- *Unconjugated*—The most common cause in the elderly person is the breakdown of hemoglobin from a pulmonary infarct in a person with cardiac failure. If cardiac failure is absent, some impairment of function of the congested liver presumably contributes.
- *Conjugated*—Usually subdivided into hepatic and posthepatic. In the hepatic classification, hepatocellular damage may be associated with cardiac failure, hepatitis, macronodular or primary biliary cirrhosis, or associated with other diseases. In the posthepatic classification there is often extrahepatic cholestasis due to gallstones or carcinoma in the ampullary region. Obstructive jaundice was much more common than hepatocellular jaundice in a study of elderly jaundiced people. Malignant causes of obstruction outnumber gallstone jaundice.

See also CANCER, LIVER; HEPATITIS.

Brocklehurst, J. C. *Textbook of Geriatric Medicine and Gerontology.* New York: Churchill Livingstone, 1985.

K

keratoconjunctivitis sicca (dry eyes)
Decreased tear production occurs as a part of the aging process. This diminished tear secretion is caused by an atrophy of the lacrimal gland. Absence of tears can cause keratinization (loss of moisture and thickening) of the corneal and conjunctival epithelium and can result in blindness. Decreased tear secretion occurs predominantly in keratoconjunctivitis sicca, and may occur in amyotrophic sclerosis (disease affecting nerve impulses in the connective tissue), Sjogren syndrome (connective tissue disease characterized by dry eyes, dry mouth, and arthritis), and some bulbar palsies.

Symptoms of dry eyes include a foreign body sensation, burning, itching, and excessive tearing. Each of these symptoms are worsened by a hot dry atmosphere and tobacco smoke. These symptoms may be aggravated by reading or infrequent or incomplete blinking. A propensity for dry eyes may be aggravated by keratitis, dellen, and pterygium.

Treatment for dry eye is often unsatisfactory. People experiment until they find a method of relief. Artificial tears and long-acting lacrimal inserts are commercially available. Hot soaks applied to the eyelids several times a day may be useful. Avoidance of dry atmospheres and direct wind, which may encourage tear evaporation, is helpful. People with dry eyes should avoid riding with the car windows down and having air-conditioner vents and fans directed on them. Humidifiers may also be helpful, especially in the winter when the humidity is low. If all of these fail, punctal occlusion, either temporary or permanent, can be used to diminish the symptoms.

It is important that dry eyes not be overlooked because untreated dry eyes may develop into irreversible corneal changes. The treatment for more extensive corneal changes may include surgery.

Newell, F. W. *Ophthalmology Principles and Concepts,* 6th ed. St. Louis: C. V. Mosby Co., 1986.

kidney cancer   See CANCER, KIDNEY.

Kuhn, Maggie
Maggie Kuhn founded the Gray Panthers when she reached age 65, and has served as National Convener of that Organization since 1970. Her motive in taking this leadership role grew out of her sense of injustice about America's treatment of the elderly, a sense that took strength from her own forced retirement from a post with the Presbyterian Church after 25 years of service. Quoted in *Parade* magazine, Kuhn insists that:

> old people should not be treated as wrinkled babies. . . . Old Folks have plenty to offer this country if only they are given half the chance. . . . America is caught up in the Detroit Syndrome, and we scrap-pile our old people like worn out car hulks. . . .

In an another interview with *Parade,* Kuhn remarked, ''Our society is Ageist . . . ageism goes both ways—hurting both the young and the old—depriving both groups of the right to control their lives.''

Quoted in Harris, D. K., and Cole, W. E. *Sociology of Aging.* Boston: Houghton Mifflin Company, 1980.

Kuhnt Junius disease   See MACULAR DEGENERATION.

L

larynx cancer   See CANCER, MOUTH, THROAT, AND LARYNX.

late great achievers   Elderly people can still make a contribution later in life. Continuing progress is being made in fighting cancer, heart disease, stroke, and other killers. A person watching his or her diet and exercise may live to the biological limit of 120 years.

Herein proof that life begins—or at least continues after 70:

1. Konrad Adenauer (1876–1967)—Seventy-three when he became the first chancellor of the Federal Republic of Germany. Resigned 14 years later.
2. Pope John XXIII (1881–1963)—Chosen Pope at 77, brought the Catholic Church into the 20th century.
3. Jomo Kenyatta (1894–1978)—Elected Kenya's first president at age 77. Led the country for 14 years.
4. Henri Matisse (1869–1954)—In his seventies did a series of paper cutouts that are exhibited at New York's Museum of Modern Art.
5. Golda Meir (1898–1978)—Named prime minister of Israel at 71; held the job for five years.
6. Pablo Picasso (1881–1973)—Completed his portraits of "Sylvette" at 73, married for the second time at 77, then executed three series of drawings between 85 and 90.
7. Anna Mary Robertson Moses (1860–1961)—Seventy-six when she took up painting as a hobby; as Grandma Moses she won international fame and staged 15 one-woman shows throughout Europe.
8. Arthur Rubinstein (1887–1982)—At age eighty-nine gave one of his greatest performances at New York's Carnegie Hall.
9. Sophocles (496–406 B.C.)—After the age of 70 wrote *Electra* and *Oedipus at Colonus;* held office in Athens at age 83.
10. Guiseppi Verdi (1813–1901)—At age 74 wrote *Otello* and at age 78 wrote *Falstaff.*
11. Frank Lloyd Wright, (1869–1959)—Completed New York's Guggenheim Museum at age 89; continued teaching until his death.
12. Adolph Zukon (1873–1976)—At age 91, chairman of Paramount Pictures.

See also ACHIEVEMENTS AT AN ADVANCED AGE.

Coniff, R. "Living Longer," in *Aging,* Goldstein, E. C., ed. Vol. 2, Art. 8. Boca Raton, FL.: Social Issues Resource Series, Inc., 1981.

later life expectancy   People who reach the advanced years of life have good news ahead, according to several sources. These include, perhaps surprisingly, the Internal Revenue Service, which has developed a longevity table as part of payout schedule for annuities to guide individuals in their income tax calculations.

Whether they rely on the IRS or someone else, individuals should be pleased to learn that they can disregard average life expectancy figures (now age 75) when they reach age 50 because new life expectancies take over as the years go on. For example, anyone born in 1925 had a life expectancy of 59 years at the time of birth, but if they beat the averages and survive to age 65 they will fall into a new life expectancy table because people at that age have a known life expectancy of about another 20 years. Recent figures on later life expectancy are as follows:

Age	Years of Life Expectancy Remaining
50	33.1
60	24.2
70	16
80	9.5
90	5
99	2.8

These Internal Revenue Service figures appeared in Table V, p. 47, of IRS publication #575, in 1988. They provide a useful guide for planning pay-outs from annuities, pension options, IRA, and Keogh plans because the chances are even that one will reach the average for one's age group (men should subtract about three years from and women add three years to the foregoing life expectancy tables).

Although age 65—the year of retirement with full benefits under Social Security—does not show on the table, the average 65-year-old can expect to live about another 20 years, and can set up withdrawals or pension payments to reflect that fact. If a male age 65 has a spouse aged 60, then he might set up a withdrawal plan that reflects her life expectancy—24.2 years—rather than his own.

Tucker, E. "How Long Must You Plan For?" *United Retirement Bulletin,* 14:5 (May 1988, Issue 157).

laxatives   (see Tables 19, 20) Laxatives are mild cathartics that loosen the bowels without pain. They are classified in several different categories including bulk-forming, stimulant, saline, emollient (stool softner), hyperosmotic (increased osmosis), and surfactant laxatives.

Laxative use is prevalent in the elderly, but only in a few cases must laxatives be taken chronically. Between 15 percent and 30 percent of the population older than 60 years of age take at least one dose of laxative per week.

Most constipation should be relieved with diet. A good intake of fruit (prunes, apples), high-fiber foods (bran, vegetables), and fluids help most elderly regulate bowel function. An acute episode of fecal impaction or constipation can usually be treated safely with a saline enema. Once acute constipation has been relieved, dietary manipulation, suppositories, and even weekly enemas may be used.

Bulk-forming laxatives are effective through absorption and retention of large amounts of water and are also useful in treating diarrhea. Effects are normally seen within 12 to 24 hours but could take up to three days for a full effect. These laxatives must be taken with water. Special care should be taken with diabetics and those on a salt restricted diet, although side effects are infrequent. An example of a bulk-forming laxative is Metamucil.

Stimulant laxatives are the type most abused by the public. They can induce a mild laxative action or, in high doses, produce severe cramping and fluid and electrolyte imbalance. With chronic abuse enteric loss of protein and malabsorption can occur. When used correctly, stimulants are useful for acute constipation secondary to other medication, due to prolonged bed rest or hospitalization, and as preparation for abdominal X-rays. Caster oil is in this group of laxatives. Chronic use of caster oil can cause erosion of the intestinal villi, leading to malabsorption of nutrients.

Saline laxatives include sulfate and magnesium salts. People are advised to drink at least eight ounces of water with the laxative to avoid dehydration. Effects are usually produced in three to six hours. In an elderly person, especially one with renal failure, toxic serum levels of magnesium can result. This is characterized by central nervous system depression, hypotension, muscle weakness, and electrocardiographic changes. An example is magnesium sulfate (milk of magnesium).

Mineral oil is an emollient laxative and should not be used in elderly patients. Most problems occur from chronic mineral oil aspiration. Aspiration can produce acute and chronic pneumonitis (inflammation of the lungs), localized granuloma, and pulmonary fibrosis. Patients taking oral anticoagulants and mineral oil will find the anticoagulants (agents preventing clotting) absorbed poorly.

Hyperosmotic laxatives include glycerin and lactulose. Glycerin in suppository form is usually effective within a half hour. Because it is rapidly absorbed and broken down systemically it is ineffective when taken orally. Lactulose is especially useful in treating the elderly. Glycerin suppositories are ineffective if fecal impaction with hard dry stools is present.

Surfactant laxatives work by a detergent activity and are especially effective for conditions where straining should be avoided, such as after abdominal surgery. Surfactants appear to be of little value in preventing constipation, however.

See also FECAL IMPACTIONS.

Covington, T., and Walker, J. *Current Geriatric Therapy.* Philadelphia: W. B. Saunders, 1984.

legal representative (trust, guardianship, conservatorship, power-of-attorney, representative payee) Sometimes older individuals become unable to handle their financial obligations because of either a physical or mental handicap. There are several ways to provide for this type of sitution, including a trust, guardianship, power-of-attorney, or representative payee.

A simple trust can be drawn, naming a family member, friend, or bank as trustee. The older individual must be mentally competent for a trust to be drawn up, which means that trusts are suitable for individuals who have solely physical disabilities. Legal consultation is necessary to draw up a trust. Property transferred to the trustee is to be used for the care and protection of the individual. Upon the death of the individual, property is distributed as the trust instructs.

A guardianship (conservatorship) may be appointed by the court if the individual is mentally incompetent and unable to designate a trustee. Generally, this is someone the family recommends or someone the court feels can serve best in this capacity. In many states, recent legislation has been passed to help protect the incompetent person. Efforts have been focused on requiring an annual accounting of financial worth, itemizing ex-penditures, and notification of hearings on guardianship petitions. Guardianship is a drastic legal step in which the incompetent person losses control of his or her property and income, the right to determine where to live, and what medical treatment he or she will receive. A guardian must obtain court approval, however, to remove the incompetent's voting privilege, to authorize experimental surgery, or terminate lifesaving medical treatment.

Power-of-attorney is authorization for someone to act on another's behalf. This can be issued for general or specific authority. Some lawyers advise against power-of-attorney because it is valid only as long as the individual is competent and alive. These states make provisions for guardianship. Other states recognize the power of attorney even if the individual becomes incompetent.

Finally, a representative payee can be appointed. This is a person who serves as an agent in receiving and depositing Social Security checks. The representative payee must keep adequate records of transactions. The representative must apply for payee status at the local Social Security office.

Deedy, J. *Your Aging Parents.* Chicago: The Thomas More Press, 1984.
Gillies, J. *A Guide to Caring for and Coping with Aging Parents.* Nashville: Thomas Nelson Publishers, 1981.

leisure Over 2,000 years ago the Greek philosopher Aristotle celebrated the importance of leisure in human life with the statement, "We are busy that we may have leisure." Modern leisure researchers Gene and Lei Burrus-Bammel, writing in the *Handbook of the Psychology of Aging,* have observed that, "In leisure occur the most important events of one's life: insights, personal relationships, choice of careers, and delights in ourselves, our friends, and the natural world." Gerontologist Russell Ward notes that leisure is essential to old people as they go about defining new goals and directing their energies into new channels.

Because people live longer than they did in the past the old have more time for leisure than ever before—in previous times most people died by age 50, and they never stopped working until death put them to permanent rest. Modern researchers say that everyone, including the old, need to take leisure seriously to get the most out of it. Leisure can include idle whiling away of time, but at its best it reaches beyond idleness by becoming an activity in itself, a career of later life.

The notion that leisure and idleness are the same thing may reflect on the element of freedom in leisure activities—one engages in leisure activities out of one's own choice and free will. Work, by comparison, is something that one *must* do, like it or not; and one often works under unwanted direction and supervision. In leisure, one is not told what to do, or how to do things; one is free and accountable only to one's self. There is no paycheck issued for most leisure activities. The only pay-off from leisure activities is one's own pleasure and satisfaction—one performs leisure activities simply because one likes them. They have a therapeutic value and help to recreate one's energies.

Contrary to what many people think, most older people use their leisure time in constructive ways, not just to sit and watch TV all day. National surveys have shown that most older people spend about as much time watching TV as everyone else, and they usually watch fewer hours than children, teenagers, and even young adults. About 60 percent of all Americans (including the old) spend two to four hours a day in front of TV, according to the General Social Survey, an annual poll of the American people carried out by the National Opinion Research Center at the University of Chicago.

When people reach later life they commonly use their leisure time to build on activities and hobbies, like fishing, reading, gardening, crafts, knitting or meeting and chatting with friends—activities that they have enjoyed for many years. Some take adult education courses to learn new information or to develop new activities, while others invest more time in doing things they have never had enough time to do before— odd jobs, painting and repairing their homes, shopping for bargains, and so forth.

A Harris poll has shown that 25 percent of the older population also engages in volunteer services, spending anywhere from a few hours per week to almost full-time work. The same survey recorded a long list of volunteer activities that includes time donated to hospitals and mental health clinics, transportation of the handicapped, political activity, psychological support of shut-in people through telephone call networks, foster grandparent and day care for children and youth, staffing of thrift shops, supplying home delivered meals—to name only a few.

When it comes to exercise, experts agree that older people are like other Americans— they need to abandon their sedentary lifestyles and take part in more exercise activities. In age there is time for an hour or two of pleasant leisure recreation daily; it appears that physical activity is not only essential in age but that it may be one of the keys to good health and long life.

Still, experts on exercise physiology warn against sudden leaps into strenuous and vigorous aerobic fitness programs that may be suitable for early life but that can cause injury to anyone who has not maintained a high energy level over the years. Lowered lung capacity, weaker heart action, narrow and less responsive arteries and veins, less flexibility in muscles and tendons—all these and other physical changes typical of age recommend moderate exercise programs that emphasize low-impact activities like walking, swimming, gentle stretching and bending, and smooth, rythmic movements. Consulting with a physician about exercise from time to time makes good sense in late life.

Deedy, J. *Your Aging Parents.* Chicago: The Thomas More Press, 1984.

Fromme, A. *Life After Work*. Glenview, Ill.: AARP, 1984.

Gillies, J. *A Guide to Caring for Coping with Aging Parents*. Nashville: Thomas Nelson Publishers, 1981.

Russell, C. H. *Good News About Aging*. New York: John Wiley and Sons, 1989.

leukemia, chronic lymphocytic Chronic lymphocytic leukemia is a disease of the tissues in the bone marrow, spleen, and lymph nodes that interferes with the white blood cells' ability to combat infection. This type generally is seen in people over 50 years of age. The white blood cell count may be only modestly increased with chronic lymphocytic leukemia but the bone marrow will reveal lymphocytic infiltration.

Chronic lymphocytic leukemia may be asymptomatic such that the initial diagnosis is made during a routine exam or for an evaluation of another disorder.

If symptoms do occur, they are vague and include weight loss, loss of energy, weakness, anemia, joint pain, susceptibility to infections, lymphadenopathy (disease affecting lymph nodes), splenomegaly (enlargement of spleen), and purpuric disorders (hemorrhage into the skin).

If the leukemia is asymptomatic, no treatment is necessary.

If symptoms are present, with anemia or a high white blood count, steroids and antileukemic agents may be prescribed. Radiation therapy may be necessary and occasionally surgical removal of the spleen is required.

Generally leukemia in older people progresses very slowly and may continue as long as 15 years on a benign course. A complicating infection may be the first sign of the disease. Therefore, avoiding contact with infectious diseases is recommended.

Phipps, W. J., *et al. Medical Surgical Nursing*. St. Louis: C. V. Mosby Co., 1983.

Reichel, W. *Clinical Aspects of Aging*. Baltimore: Williams & Wilkins Co., 1979.

lifecare (continuing care, life-care centers)   "Lifecare" is a rapidly growing living arrangement for older people, increasing more than 50 percent in the past 15 years, from about 200 to over 700 residences nationwide. Enrollment in a lifecare facility requires a substantial one-time downpayment and subsequent monthly payments, similar to rent, to the facility operator (many centers are church-related or run by fraternal organizations like the Masons). In return for these payments, residents are assured of a lifetime of housing and service in a small house or apartment, with grounds and building maintenance provided, along with the possibility of moving to a hotellike facility, for an intermediate level of personal care or to a full-scale nursing home residence if required. Some centers do not guarantee all of these services, but provide for variations under differing contractual arrangements.

Residents who contract for these life-long services often begin by living independently in a small house, apartment, or condominiumlike structure, on the life-care facility grounds. Here they do their own shopping, cooking, cleaning, and continue all the usual routines of life except building and grounds maintenance. In the event that they become somewhat disabled and need moderate levels of assistance—as with meal preparation or help with bathing—they can move to the hotel-like area of the facility where intermediate levels of personal service are provided. Should they later need nursing home care, they can move to a skilled nursing unit that is often a part of property run by the center, or that may be an independently operated nursing home.

Some life-care centers are small multibuilding facilities arranged in various configurations around landscaped grounds. Others are high-rise apartment buildings located in cities, suburbs, or small towns, which include all levels of service in different floors of the structure. Whatever the type of facility, the environment and surrounding grounds are usually well designed and very attractive.

Although the initial admission fee to many life-care facilities is high (ranging from a low of about $40,000 to well over $200,000), and the monthly maintenance rates may run from $400 to $1500 or more, it is estimated that over half of today's elderly population could afford a life-care facility if they chose. Because there are many variations to contractual arrangements and services provided under life-care contracts, applicants should examine these in detail, with professional advice if possible, and assure themselves of the financial solvency of the operator before concluding any agreement. Studies have shown people who live in well-run life-care facilities enjoy better health and are hospitalized less frequently than older people of comparable age.

Residents of life-care facilities acquire no equity interest in these facilities, which has created an unfortunate climate for fraud and mismanagement in some cases. Eleven states have enacted laws aimed specifically at these institutions. These laws cover certification and financial regulation, including escrow and reserve fund projections and provisions for monitoring facilities and administering the statutes. A community-based life-care system, known as a social health maintenance organization, is being tested in four areas around the nation. Developed by Brandeis University under a federal grant, social health maintenance organizations seek to integrate services and funding sources for people who live in the community and as an alternative to institutionalization. Elderly participants would receive services such as case management, home health, chore services, drugs, congregate or delivered meals, and transportation from a single provider.

A prepaid fee covered by Medicare, Medicaid, and Title XX social service funds would fund much of these services; enrollees would pay premiums of $25 to $40 per month. The social health maintenance organization would be at risk financially for excess costs, with an annual dollar limit between $6,000 and $12,000 for services. These organizations would save Medicaid dollars without increasing Medicare costs.

For a list of accredited life-care facilities, contact:
American Association of Homes for the Aging
1129 20th Street N.W. Suite 400
Washington, DC 20036

Carlin, V. F., and Mansberg, R. *If I Live to Be 100: Congregate Housing for Later Life*. West Nyock, N.Y.: Parker Publishing Co., 1984.
Millard, S. "Lifecare," in *Aging*, Goldstein, E. C., ed. Vol. 2, Art. 64. Boca Raton, Fl.: Social Issues Resource Series, Inc., 1981.

life expectancy The terms *life expectancy* and *life span* need to be distinguished from one another because the first refers to the average number of years people actually live, whereas the second applies to the biological limit of human life—120 years. Although a few people do live past 110 years, and one Japanese man was even recorded as reaching 120, the average person dies at a much younger age—in fact, half the U.S. population dies by age 75.

The dictionary defines life expectancy as "an expected number of years of life based on statistical probability"—a probability that is calculated by examining the survival rate for a specific population (for example, everyone born in 1925 or everyone born in 1990), and then using that as the probability that people in that population will live to a particular year. In the United States the present overall life expectancy for women and men at birth is about 75 years.

Because women live longer than men, however, the rates for the sexes differ—the average is 71.5 years for men and 78.3 for women. White people have a longer life expectancy than black people—the latter average only 69.7 years.

Life expectancy is widely used as a standard for comparing the health and welfare of nations; a comparison that rests on the idea that countries with longer average lifetimes have better nutrition, health care, and so on. In this respect the United States, the wealthiest nation in the world, measures up less well than one might expect when compared to other industrialized nations. Japan, with 77 years, has the highest life expectancy in the world; Sweden ranks second at 76.6 years; and Norway is third at 76.2. Other nations that exceed the United States include Denmark, France, Italy, Canada, Australia, Hong Kong, and Israel—in that order. Other European nations (United Kingdom, West Germany, etc.) match the U.S. closely.

The relatively unfavorable showing of the U.S. is due in part to the high infant mortality that occurs in American minority groups, where many people are afflicted with poverty, disease, lack of education, inadequate prenatal care, and the social and family disorganization that typically accompanies such conditions. It is also true that the nations that lead the world in life expectancy are those with relatively little cultural or ethnic diversity—nations that can be described as having homogeneous populations.

Over the centuries average life expectancy has increased from about age 20 in ancient Rome some 2,000 years ago (death in childhood and youth were common there owing to the lack of sanitation and medical knowhow) to about age 40 at the time that the pilgrims came to America. Between the time of the pilgrims and 1900, life expectancy in America grew slowly to about age 47. After the turn of this century it exploded with an increase to 75 years, an unprecedented jump of almost 30 years between 1900 and 1975.

The most recent increases—those that occurred after 1960—have been due in part to better medical control of cancer, heart disease, and stroke. This advance, together with earlier progress, has brought the proportion of Americans over age 65 from 4 percent of the population and three million people in 1900 to about 12 percent of the total and 30 million people at the present time. The U.S. Bureau of the Census projects an even more rapid expansion of the 65+ population until the middle of the next

century, when growth will level off at 67.5 million and at 21.8 percent of the population.

The most explosive period of growth for people aged 65+ will occur after 2010, as shown by the following proportions and numbers of people over that age at various intervals: year 1990—about 12.7 percent and 31½ million; year 2000—13 percent and nearly 35 million; year 2010—13.8 percent and 39 million; year 2020—17.3 percent and 51.5 million; year 2030—21.2 percent and 64.5 million; year 2040—21.7 percent and 67 million.

See also LATER LIFE EXPECTANCY; LIFE SPAN.

Schick, F. L. *Statistical Handbook on Aging Americans*. Phoenix: Oryx Press, 1986.

U.S. Bureau of the Census. *An Aging World*. International Population Reports Series P-95. No. 78. Washington, D.C.: U.S. Government Printing Office, 1987.

life extension   Humanity has been searching in vain for the well-spring of eternal life since the beginning of recorded history, sometimes in ways so bizarre as to defy common sense. Ponce de León, well known to Americans for his explorations of Florida in the early 1500s while seeking to find the spring of the waters of eternal youth, could perhaps be excused because of the lack of scientific knowledge in his time.

Novelist Aldous Huxley wrote a fictional account of the strange results of an 18th-century search for eternal life that mocked modern fantasies about survival in present life held by some contemporary seekers after a biological rather than spiritual eternity. In this tale, titled *After Many a Summer Dies the Swan*, Huxley included a harshly satirical subplot involving a French nobleman of the late 1700s and his wife, who together eagerly sought to prolong their lives by consuming a secret formula made of bacteria extracted from the entrails of fish. Huxley's use of this fantastic idea was premised on his knowledge of the theories like those of Russian scientist Elie Metchnikoff, who hypothesized that the putrefying poisons, which develop within our bodies during digestion when intestinal flora break down food, cause aging and death. According to Huxley's tale, the nobleman and his wife did succeed in prolonging their lives by destroying the toxins caused by the process of digestion going on in their aristocratic bellies, but at a considerable cost—their bodies went into reverse evolution as they aged, and they eventually turned into barely human, apelike creatures who had to live in a cage.

In the real world of everyday life, the most powerful force in extending life has been the improvement of sanitation—the unexciting but profoundly important construction of modern sewage and water systems that dispose of disease-carrying human wastes, eliminate stagnant pools of water that breed malaria mosquitoes and other maladies, and supply us with fresh, clean water free of cholera, salmonella, and other infections. These have eliminated from most developed nations the plagues and epidemics that, until this century, destroyed people throughout infancy and youth and kept human life expectancy below age 40.

Better nutrition, with greater quantity and higher quality of food, has also been a factor in extending human life, as has the now prosaic but still revolutionary development of medical immunization against childhood diseases. We take such factors for granted these days, but they alone probably account for most of the increase in life expectancy since 1900, a year when the average length of life was about 30 years shorter than it is today.

More recent increases in length of life have been wrung from nature with greater difficulty, resting on the spectacular victories of scientific research and medical know-how that produced antibiotics, immunization against polio, artery bypasses, angioplasty, pacemakers, organ transplants, joint replace-

ments, blood pressure medications, chemical and surgical therapies for cancer, cataract excisions and corneal transplants, and all the many other scientific and medical breakthroughs that have made late life more healthful and hopeful than ever in human history. Sometimes called "life-extension technologies," these most recent advances in human health sciences not only lengthen life but substantially improve the quality of daily human experience by reducing ill health and overcoming, or at least mitigating, the effects of acute and chronic illness in old age.

A number of researchers studying the biological causes of aging at the cellular level predict even more remarkable progress if we can successfully attack the causes of aging within human cells themselves. No major researcher, however, has yet forecast the total elimination of death—only the prolongation of the average length of life.

Widespread lifestyle change on the part of the American public can also contribute to increased longevity in the future. Dr. Roy Walford of UCLA, for example, is personally experimenting with a reduced calorie intake following experiments that enabled researchers to prolong the lives of minimally fed laboratory mice. This research, he believes, suggests that people who control and reduce their food intake will bring their years closer to the maximum life span of the human species—about 120 years.

Further, research on exercise has shown a relationship between even moderate levels of physical activity and increased age. Still more, it has proven that exercise can forestall, and actually even *reverse,* the process of aging at the same time as it contributes to the greater enjoyment of life.

It is also known that major lifestyle changes in the use of tobacco will increase average longevity. To cite just one example, the well-known association between smoking, cancer, lung disease, and, ultimately, death, was strikingly documented in The General

Social Survey, which showed that the vast majority—nearly 83 percent—of men over 85 report being nonsmokers. Women generally outlive men, and GSS showed that none of the women over 85 were smokers.

Consideration of past advances and the possibility of future lifestyle changes has led some gerontologists to predict that we may expect more people in the future to live to the biological limit of the human life span. The term used to describe this possible development is known as *curve rectangularization,* which simply means that the curve of human survival, which now begins to slide downward like a ski slope in the late fifties, will continue on as a straight line past 110 years of age as more people reach toward the full potential for human years. After age 110 the curve of survival will drop off sharply, and it will look like the side of a square rather than a sloping hillside.

Even now thousands of people live beyond age 90 and 100, but the George Burnses and centenarians (a centenarian is 100 years old or more) are so few that they represent only very small numbers in the last decades of life. If we do succeed in extending life—or rectangularizing the curve of life—then everyone will reach close to the limit of the human life span—120 years.

See also AGING, BIOLOGICAL THEORY OF.

Kinney, T.: "Living Longer," in *Aging,* Goldstein, E. C., ed. Vol. 3, Art. 10. Boca Raton, Fl.: Social Issues Resource Series, Inc., 1981.
Russell, C. H. *Good News About Aging.* New York: John Wiley and Sons, 1989.
Russell, C. H., and Megaard, I. J. *The General Social Survey, 1972–1986: the State of the American People.* New York: Springer-Verlag, 1988.
Walford, R. L. *The 120 Year Diet.* New York: Simon and Schuster, 1986.

life insurance: locating policies of deceased persons Most experts feel that older people have lesser need for life insurance than younger people. Life insurance is important to midlife breadwinners who need to provide for their families if they die suddenly. But older people, whose children have left home and are independent, do not need high coverage. The older person should carry only enough life insurance to provide for their spouse, pay off their mortgage and other debts, pay federal estate and state inheritance taxes, and provide for burial costs and the costs of administering their estate.

When trying to locate the life insurance policy of a deceased person, check the deceased's personal papers. Look for canceled checks, premium or dividend notices, or other correspondence to or from an insurance company.

If any of the individual's friends are insurance agents check with them. Also, check with former employers, both for any company insurance and for a possible allotment from wages to an insurance company for the payment of premiums.

If you cannot uncover anything, write to the American Council of Life Insurance at the address below. Tell them that you are trying to track down a life insurance policy and they will send you a form to complete. They will circulate the form free of charge to most of the major insurance companies.

For more information write or call:
American Council of Life Insurance
Information Services
1850 K St. N.W.
Washington, DC 20006
(202) 624-2000

Avery, A. C. *Successful Aging.* New York: Ballantine Books, 1987.

life span The term *life span* refers to the biological limit of life for a species, which, in the case of humans, is about 115 to 120 years. Contrary to what many people think, animals like parrots, elephants, and tortoises do not have longer life spans than humans. On the contrary, human beings seem to have the longest life span of any vertebrate, (any creature with a spine, whether mammal, reptile, fish, amphibian, or bird). Interesting examples of the life spans of some vertebrates appear in an article found in *Hand-* *book of the Biology of Aging,* a major reference source in the field of gerontology. A sampling of these is as follows:

Maximum Life Spans of Selected Vertebrates

Species	Common Name	Scientific Name	Maximum Life Span in Years
Primates	Human	Homo sapiens	115–120
	Chimpanzee	Pan troglodytes	44
Carnivores	Domestic cat	Felis catus	28
	Dog	Canis familiares	20
Ungulates	Elephant	Elephas maximus	70
	Horse	Equus caballus	46
Rodents	House mouse	Mus musculus	3
	Black rat	Rattus rattus	5
Bat	Vampire bat	Desmodus rotundus	13
Birds	Eagle owl (longest-lived bird)	Bubo bubo	68
Reptiles	Snapping turtle	Macroclemys temmincki	58 +
	Galapagos turtle	Testudo elephantopus	100 +
Amphibians	Common toad	Bufo bufo	36
	African clawed toad	Xenopus laevis	15

Kirkwood, T. B. L. "Comparative and Evolutionary Aspects of Anatomy," in *Handbook of the Biology of Aging,* 2nd ed, Finch, C. E., and Schneider, E. L., eds. New York: Van Nostrand Reinhold Co., 1985.

Lifeline   Lifeline is a personal emergency response system that is attached to the participant's telephone. It is activated whenever help is needed by a small button worn on a chain around the participant's neck or wrist. Lifeline allows the older individual to be more independent and can prolong the ability to live alone.

When an emergency arises and the unit is activated, a call is automatically received at the Emergency Response Center (usually a designated hospital or health-care facility). Trained personnel are available at the center 24 hours a day. When the signal is received at the center, a call is placed to the home of the Lifeline participant to see what help is needed. If no answer is obtained a "responder" is called to go to the home and check on the caller. The responder is a predesignated friend or relative with access to the home of the participant. When the responder arrives contact is again made with the Emergency Response Center to implement whatever help is needed.

The Lifeline unit can still be activated during a power failure or if the phone to which the Lifeline unit is attached is off the hook. A timer button on the unit is pushed to reset it once every 24 hours. If the timer is not reset Lifeline automatically calls and starts the emergency procedure.

There is an installation fee and monthly charges, which vary from area to area. Lifeline was begun in 1970 and is available throughout the country.

For additional information write or call:
Lifeline Systems, Inc.
#1 Arsenal Marketplace
Watertown, MA 02172
(617) 923-4141

lip cancer   See CANCER, LIP.

lipectomy, submental   See COSMETIC SURGERY.

lipofuscin and glucose   Some scientists believe that certain chemicals are disruptive to cell production in the body, hastening the aging process. Two of those chemicals under suspicion are lipofuscin, a fatty brown pigment, and glucose, a sugar.

Lipofuscin, created when the body breaks down fats, is found within cells and collects with age. While scientists agree that cells choked with pigment cannot work correctly, some believe that lipofuscin does not cause aging; it merely indicates that aging is occurring.

Glucose, however, may actually be a prime cause of aging. Researchers have found that glucose damages proteins, including collagen, the main component of the connective tissues that supports the cells. In a test tube, glucose binds collagen fibers together. Such linking has been found in the tissues of elderly people as well.

Maranto, G. "Aging—Can We Slow the Inevitable?" in *Aging,* Goldstein, E. C., ed. Vol. 2, Art. 78. Boca Raton, Fl: Social Issues Resource Series, Inc., 1981.

liposuction   See COSMETIC SURGERY.

live, where to   Preretirement counselors advise prospective retirees to assess their current housing situation and consider where they should live in retirement. For some, this may mean selling their family home and purchasing a smaller one. Others may choose

to rent or move to an apartment complex so the burden of maintenance is on someone else. Some may want to hold onto the house that has been a home full of memories for so many years.

Most people want to retire in the same general area in which they live. But others look for that elusive paradise and seek a totally new environment. If a new locale is selected several basic needs should be fulfilled to ensure a smooth transition:

- health—a climate and housing suited to one's physical condition
- economic security—a price that is affordable
- status—a position or voice in the community
- friendship—a place where the retiree already has friends or where the opportunity exists to make new friends

If a location is selected on the basis of climate it is a good idea to research the area by spending an extended vacation there. Every area has both agreeable and disagreeable weather at times. Subscribe to the daily or weekly newspaper in the area and read it carefully for items on food prices, business activity, real estate prices, and taxes. Look for items that give a "feel" for the community such as social, recreational, and church activities.

Most experts would advise against moving just to be near one's children. Too often the retiree finds that children are caught up in the demands of their own daily lives and they are left living in a city they otherwise would not have chosen, with few friends and interests outside of their children and grandchildren.

As the retiree grows older, he or she may pass through three stages of activity—active, slowdown, and dependent. Most people think only of their current, active stage when selecting housing. It is important, however, to think ahead to the slowdown and dependent stages. The importance of medical facilities looms larger and should be nearby or within easy access. As eyesight deteriorates and driving becomes more difficult, public transportation may be needed. One-level living areas greatly facilitate the use of wheelchairs and walkers. It need not be depressing to consider these possibilities when changing housing and it will certainly ease the transition if it has been planned for in advance.

As the older person becomes more dependent due to deteriorating health, the choices of where to live become more complex and may be settled only with family consultations or professional guidance. Nursing homes, retirement centers, live-in care, or living with one's children are all options that need careful evaluation, so that not only are the needs of the older person met but those of the family as well. It is important, whenever possible, for the elderly to make their own decision about where to live. Generally, acceptance and contentment are more easily achieved.

See also LIVING WITH ONE'S CHILDREN; NURSING HOME, HOW TO SELECT, MONITOR, AND EVALUATE; RETIREMENT RESIDENCE CENTERS.

Fromme, A. *Life After Work*. Glenview, Ill.: AARP, 1985.
Gillies, J. *A Guide to Caring for and Coping with Aging Parents*. Nashville: Thomas Nelson Publishers, 1981.
Lester, A. D. and Lester, J. L. *Understanding Aging Parents*. Philadelphia: The Westminster Press, 1980.

liver cancer   See CANCER, LIVER.

living alone   Research shows that independence is vital to most older people and crucial to their self-esteem. The vast majority of elderly are eager to maintain their own homes to maintain their independence and the freedom to control their own lives—in short, their autonomy.

Maintaining a home provides mental and physical stimulation because it requires responsibility. Decisions must be made about what to clean, when to do the laundry, whether to paint the house this year or cut down that old tree. These decisions and their resulting activities keep the elderly physically active and mentally alert. Having one's own home also provides privacy, another factor contributing to self-esteem.

If the elderly become ill or incapacitated in some way, it may still be possible for them to remain in their homes. Friends, neighbors, and church are usually nearby, offering them support and reassurance. Many public and private services are available to provide assistance. Meals on Wheels will bring one hot meal a day, guaranteeing not only a balanced meal but personal contact to evaluate the aged person's needs. Telephone programs are available whereby a volunteer calls daily, usually at a predetermined time, and if no one answers, the caller immediately telephones the responsible parties (family members, neighbors, social worker) so that a visual check can be made.

Visiting nurses can provide medical care if needed and see that the elderly are taking medication as prescribed.

Sometimes it may be necessary to hire a live-in companion to assist the elderly with bathing, cooking meals, and daily maintenance of the home.

It is necessary to remember the emotional investment the elderly have in their home. Memories are attached to every room and are constant reminders of children playing, family gatherings, and happy holidays. Being forced to move from their home can have a negative impact on some older people. Many become confused, disoriented, angry, and depressed. With the resources available it is possible to help the elderly to remain in their own home. This usually results in a more comfortable, secure, and happy individual.

See also FOSTER CARE; LIVING WITH ONE'S CHILDREN; NURSING HOME, HOW TO SELECT, MONITOR, AND EVALUATE; RETIREMENT CENTERS.

Lester, A. D., and Lester, J. L. *Understanding Aging Parents*. Philadelphia: The Westminster Press, 1980.

living space   As people grow older a sweeping simplification in their lives may be beneficial. Moving usually makes such a simplification easy but if the person decides to stay in the same house deliberate action may be needed.

Giving unneeded things away to friends, family, or charities may be useful. Alterations may need to be made in the home as people grow older. As vision changes, more concentrated light may become necessary for reading, and higher-wattage light bulbs may be helpful. Rugs should be secured to avoid tripping. Doors or drawers that stick may make too great a demand on the person's strength and should be repaired. If the older person has a garage, an electric door opener may be considered. Older people often need a warmer environment. Changing the thermostat may make it unbearably warm for younger people and increase the cost for energy. One solution is heavier clothing. Thermal underwear, a sweater, shawl, or a lap robe may be useful. An electric blanket may solve the problem at night and an electric heating pad to warm cold feet during the day may be helpful. If circulation is poor or sensation diminished in the feet, care should be taken not to unknowingly burn the feet with the heating pad or electric blanket.

Deedy, J. *Your Aging Parents.* Chicago: The Thomas More Press, 1984.

living wills (right-to-die laws)   A living will is a directive made by competent adults to ensure that if they become terminally ill "heroic" means will not be employed to prolong their life. At press time, thirty-eight states and the District of Columbia have passed statutes known as "right-to-die" laws or natural death acts.

These laws place some limitations on binding advance directives. Under most statutes these directives only become operative if a consulting physician agrees that the patient is terminally ill. Some states even require the patient to reconfirm his or her wishes after the onset of the terminal illness.

The interpretation of "heroic" and the real intentions of the terminally ill patient are often open to debate. Therefore, many patients choose to delegate to a particular person the legal authority to enact their health-care wishes if they should become incompetent. Several states even require such delegation. The remaining states have durable power of attorney statutes that are generally broad enough to authorize someone to make health-care decisions.

Advance directives are clearly the preferred choice rather than have the court appoint a guardian to speak for the patient, which is the customary practice if there is no advance directive. However, in recent years, five states have authorized families of adult patients to make decisions on their health care without going to court and 12 other states have similar statutes.

These new statutes vary in many respects but all address five areas of concern:

1. The type of patient eligible
2. The type of treatment that may be withdrawn or withheld
3. Which family members can exercise authority
4. Measures to prevent abuse of power by family members
5. Provisions for physicians to make decisions for the patient

Areen, J. *The Legal Status of Consent Obtained from Families of Adult Patients to Withhold or Withdraw Treatment. JAMA.* Vol. 258: 229–235 (1987).

living with one's children   It may become undesirable for older individuals to live by themselves. One option is living with one's children or other family members. Sometimes this is the only alternative that is financially feasible.

Though adult children and their parents may have an amicable relationship, living together again may present numerous difficulties and adjustments. One of the major problems is that some parents can never seem to acknowledge that their children are adults and they continue to try to exert control in the child's life. The older adult may have difficulty adjusting to the fact that their child is the one now responsible for their care and well-being.

Another problem may be caused by the simple increase in the number of people expected to share the same space. It is essential that all those involved in the new living arrangement discuss and plan in advance whatever changes may be needed in their day-to-day routine.

Criteria that must be considered include:

1. Space available for all family members
2. If family members are compatible
3. Changes necessary to make the house accessible, such as grab bars in the bathrooms or handrails on the stairs
4. Necessary care available
5. All family members agreeable
6. The elderly person's financial contribution
7. Discipline the older person will have over the younger children or teenagers

The most ideal situation is for the older person to have his or her own room or suite. If possible, a bedroom with an adjoining bathroom can allow privacy and some independent living.

It is important to establish clear ground rules in advance to lessen conflicts between family members, especially in the area of authority. A grandparent may not approve of the hours a grandchild keeps but he or she can not reprimand him or her. A television set in the elder parent's bedroom need not mean he or she is expected to do all TV viewing there. And what about meal preparation and household chores? Is everyone expected to help? Unless such matters are discussed honestly and at the time they first come up they can mushroom into major disagreements.

Modifications may have to be made in the physical layout of the home. For example, ramps may have to be built at the entrances.

Doorways may have to be widened to accommodate wheelchairs. If the older person can use a telephone one could be installed in the bedroom. Perhaps a hospital-type bed would be more practical. Various furniture and equipment is available for rental or purchase through hospital equipment firms.

Many times it becomes necessary for an occupational therapist or social worker to help assess the home and make suggestions on necessary modifications.

When providing health care in the home, accidents must be expected. No matter what preventive measure are taken older people still fall and break bones.

The older person may not make it to the bathroom in time. It is necessary to be prepared to deal with damp and stained rugs and upholstery. If a wheelchair is being used, expect nicks and scratches on furniture, walls, and door frames. Providing a loving and caring environment for loved ones is usually worth these minor inconveniences.

Day-care centers are now being offered for older people. Supervised activities, such as games, crafts, field trips shopping sprees, programs, music, conversation, and exercise are held throughout the day. A hot, well-balanced meal is served at noon and assistance with taking medications and going to the restroom are offered. The purpose of the day-care facilities is to provide a safe and stimulating place for the older person to spend the day. This may be an appropriate alternative for families who work but want the older person to live with them.

Try to complete as many of the preparations as possible prior to the arrival of the parent. Older people who need to move in with adult children often feel they are intruding and feel guilty about upsetting their children's lives. If they witness a lot of changes because of them they may feel as if they are a burden and become more depressed.

All involved must understand that they are beginning a new lifestyle. Life is going to be different for everyone and feelings of anxiety and apprehension are to be expected. But with mutual respect, understanding, and love it can be a pleasant and rewarding experience.

See also FOSTER CARE; NURSING HOME, HOW TO SELECT, MONITOR, AND EVALUATE; RETIREMENT RESIDENCE CENTERS.

Deedy, J. *Your Aging Parents*. Chicago: The Thomas More Press, 1984.

Gillies, J. *A Guide to Caring for and Coping with Aging Parents*. Nashville: Thomas Nelson Publishers, 1981.

Horne, J. *Caregiving: Helping an Aged Loved One*. Glenview, Ill.: Scott Foresman, 1985.

loneliness   Loneliness has mistakenly become practically synonymous with old age. Although everyone is lonely at one time or another, studies show that as age increases, loneliness generally decreases. Elderly people are less lonely than other groups, such as college students, single people, and divorced people. Many factors, such as gender, health, former occupation, income, and living situation affect the levels of loneliness in the elderly. Elderly men, in general, are less lonely than elderly women. People who consider themselves to be in good or excellent health are less lonely than those who consider themselves to be in poor health. People whose former occupations were in the skilled labor category (carpenters, electricians, machinists) have lower levels of loneliness than other groups. Many people in this group develop their work interest into an enjoyable hobby in later life. The living situation is another important factor in the level of loneliness of an older person. Feelings of confinement, not the type of housing in which they live, cause increased loneliness among the elderly.

Hooks, G. "Poverty: Old Age's Unexpected Bequest," in *Aging*, Goldstein, E. C., ed. Vol. 1, Art. 6. Boca Raton, Fl.: Social Issues Resource Series, Inc., 1981.

long-term care   The designation *long-term care* has normally been associated with nurs-

ing homes, but today it applies equally to home health care, homemaker services, and even to hospice arrangements. People who require long-term care have chronic illnesses or disabilities that do not require the intensive supervision and levels of care typically provided in hospitals. Their health condition, however, makes them heavily dependent on others for supervision or assistance with activities of daily living. People who require long-term care might have become disabled as the result of a stroke, be victims of Alzheimer's disease, or have been crippled by arthritis. Not all people receiving long-term care are elderly, but the majority are.

Home care services have become an increasingly common part of long-term care because they are presumed to be less costly and they help to maintain independence on the part of the recipient. Skilled levels of nursing may be provided at home for a person who has experienced a bone fracture, a cardiac seizure, or who needs intravenous feeding.

A second level of long-term home care may be simple personal care, and could include such services as assistance with bathing, supervision of medications, physical therapy, or the like. A third level might involve homemaker help only—such as housekeeping, meal preparation, and laundry. Home care services may be found in country areas and small towns as well as cities, and may be provided either by public or private agencies or both. These services are subject to state and federal regulation when paid for by Medicare or Medicaid insurance.

Huttman, E. D. *Social Services for the Elderly*. New York: The Free Press, 1985.

longevity predictors and factors   Dr. Erdman Palmore of Duke University Center for the Study of Aging and Human Development has found that the best predictor of longevity for men over age 60 is satisfaction in their work or volunteer activities. For women of the same age, it is the ability to function physically.

Other predictors of longevity are: being happy, avoiding tobacco, and enjoying sex. Less active people and those in poor mental and physical condition tend to be older than their years. Studies at the Normative Aging Study in Boston support the belief that people who appear to be biologically older than their years, actually are and, in fact, may stand a greater chance of dying sooner.

Although American gerontologists have questioned the findings, one region where people of great age are said to live is in the Caucasus in the Soviet Union. While only 7 percent of the Soviet population lives in this area, 16 percent of the country's elderly and 35 percent of those of 100 years of age are found here.

Research shows that group longevity is determined by a combination of factors:

1. Ecological factors—a subtropical climate to which the population has biologically adapted in the course of many generations.
2. Genetic factors—some aspects of this adaptation have been reinforced genetically and transmitted to their descendants.
3. Morphological characteristics—small stature and muscular constitution.
4. Diet—little meat and hardly any animal fats, salt or sugar; they consume lots of milk products (especially cheese), fruits and vegetables.
5. Environment—generally live all their lives in the place where they were born.
6. Work—have always done the same kind of work, in farming or in the home, and continue to work as long as their strength permits.
7. Social factors—still see circle of friends and participate in various social activities.

While little evidence supports the idea, many person believe that the environment of city life may affect the elderly more negatively. One main reason is thought to be that city residents are unable to continue the type of work in retirement that they performed all their lives, and therefore experience a complete change in their daily routines. Those living in rural areas also seem to maintain closer ties with family and friends.

Kozlov, V. "The Fires of Winter," in *Aging,* Goldstean, E. C., ed. Vol. 2, Art. 35. Boca Raton, Fl.: Social Issues Resource Series, Inc., 1981.
"Your Body and Mind As the Years Go By," in *Aging,* Goldstein, E. C., ed. Vol. 2, Art. 23. Boca Raton, Fl.: Social Issues Resource Series, Inc., 1981.

longevity, rules of   Researchers at the University of California at Los Angeles, led by Dr. Lester Breslow, found that the healthiest people followed seven habits:

1. Never smoke cigarettes
2. Get regular physical activity
3. Use alcohol moderately or never
4. Sleep seven or eight hours each night
5. Maintain proper weight
6. Eat breakfast
7. Avoid eating between meals

Other physicians add to this basic list. Dr. Edward W. Campion, head of geriatrics at Massachusetts General Hospital in Boston, advises, "Avoid undue amounts of emotional stress, control blood pressure, and use reasonable caution in automobiles."

Hobbies and good reading habits may help. But Dr. Richard W. Besdine of Harvard maintains, "Work is best. It doesn't have to be the same work you did all your life. But it has to be something that keeps your mind busy and makes you feel useful."

Haney, D. Q. "Altering Habits Can Lengthen Life," in *Aging,* Goldstein, E. C. ed. Vol. 2, Art 11. Boca Raton, Fl.: Social Issues Resource Series, Inc., 1981.

lung cancer   See CANCER, LUNG.

lung disease, chronic obstructive (COPD)   *Chronic obstructive pulmonary disease* is a term used to describe a group of progressive respiratory disorders with diffuse abnormalities of gas transport and exchange.

The elderly are subject to COPD due not only to the biological process of aging, which includes decreased pulmonary tissue elasticity, but to prolonged exposure to pollutants or occupational environment.

Cigarette smoking is a major factor in the development of COPD. Environmental exposures to sulfur dioxide, asbestos, and cotton dust are causative factors that predispose the respiratory tract to chronic infection. Repeated pulmonary infections can result in the alteration of lung structure and destruction of pulmonary tissue. The disease is more prevalent in men than in women.

Corticosteroid therapy plays an important role in the treatment of COPD. Inhaled corticosteroids may reduce steroid side effects. Oral or parenteral corticosteroid therapy helps control inflammations and reduce secretions during acute exacerbations. The patient can be placed on a tapering regimen or alternate day steroid therapy. Patients even on short-term steroid therapy should be aware of the side effects of restlessness, mood changes, weight gain, and exacerbation of diabetes or hypertension. Cataracts, bone fragility, adrenal suppression, and immunosuppression are side-effects of long-term therapy.

See also BRONCHITIS, CHRONIC; EMPHYSEMA.

Rogers, S. C., and McCue, J. D. *Managing Chronic Disease—1987*. Oradell, N.J.: Medical Economics Co., 1987.

Scherer, J. C. *Introductory Medical–Surgical Nursing*. Philadelphia: J. B. Lippincott Co., 1982.

M

macular degeneration (senile macular degeneration, disciform degeneration of the macula, Kuhnt Junius disease)

Macular degeneration is a major cause of visual disability in the elderly. It is the second-ranking cause of blindness and responsible for 12 percent of all blindness in the United States. Macular degeneration is the leading cause of blindness for people age 75 and over and is the most common cause of new cases of blindness among those who are age 65 and over. It is characterized by a loss of central vision, with a retention of peripheral vision. Senile macular degeneration is generally caused by poor blood circulation to the macular area of the retina. Age, smoking, ultraviolet light, nutrition, stress, hereditary factors, illness, and certain drugs are all suspected factors in the decreased blood circulation.

There is no medical treatment effective for most macular degeneration. It is important that macular degeneration is properly diagnosed through a variety of eye tests including fluorscein retinal angiography (visualization of retinal vessel after the injection of fluorscein). In a small number of cases laser treatment may be beneficial. The cases benefited by laser treatment are those in which there is an overgrowth of blood vessels. Early detection is critical in this instance.

Treatments with vitamins, hormones, low-fat diets, regular exercise programs, and systemic vasodilators (agents that cause dilation of blood vessels) have been proposed but controlled studies have not confirmed their effectiveness. Although it is not felt it will be of much benefit for reversing macular degeneration, these methods may be useful as preventive measures. Several recent reports suggest that 25–200 mg of zinc may be of value to stabilize macular degeneration.

People with macular degeneration may be fitted with low-vision optical devices for reading. Stronger reading glasses, telescopic lenses, or high-intensity lights may also be helpful.

A person with macular degeneration will never go totally blind. Even if all central vision is lost the individual can continue many useful activities by relying on the side vision and the use of visual aids.

Another common misconception is that the use of the eyes for reading and sewing will hasten the deterioration. Patients need to be told that this is not so and that there is nothing gained by "saving their eyes," although reading may be difficult. They will not "strain" their eyes and should plan to use their eyes as much as their diminished vision will allow them to do.

Less common is disciform degeneration of the macula (Kuhnt-Junius disease), which occurs in people over 40 years of age. The lesion is an extravasation (escaping from vessel into tissue) of blood between Bruch's membrane (innermost layer of choroid) and the pigment epithelium. There is no treatment at the present time.

Newell, F. W. *Opthalmology, Principles and Concepts,* 7th ed. St. Louis: C. V. Mosby Co., 1986.

Scheie, H. G. and Albert, D. M. *Textbook of Opthalmology,* 10th ed. Philadelphia: W. B. Saunders, 1986.

macular degeneration, senile See MACULAR DEGENERATION.

mammoplasty see COSMETIC SURGERY.

mania Mania is a disordered mental state of extreme excitement. Mania is frequently associated with alternating periods of depression (manic depression).

Between six and 19 percent of all effectively ill hospital patients over 60 have a form of mania. Women are affected about three times more often than men. When it occurs in old age, the first attack is usually around the age of 60. The person's behavior may be seen as elation, overactivity, aggressiveness, sleeplessness, inattention to bodily needs, grandiose delusions of ability, wealth, and/or personal importance. In the elderly, a mood of anger, hostility, or impatience is the most common symptom.

Recognition may be difficult when the patient is highly disordered. The patient is often playful when answering test questions. These people may also experience perplexity, elated moods, speech disorders, incoherence, and depression.

See also DEPRESSION.

Brocklehurst, J. C. *Textbook of Geriartric Medicine and Gerontology.* New York: Churchill Livingstone, 1985.

marriage contract See PRENUPTIAL PROPERTY AGREEMENT.

Masai By studying other cultures scientists can find out how different aging cultures respond to various factors. Blood pressure, blood cholesterol, and body weight have been studied in the Masai.

The Masai, a group of nomadic herdsmen of east Africa, have a diet that averages 3,000 calories per day. Sixty-six percent of its caloric value is animal fat. Their estimated average daily cholesterol intake ranges from 600 to 2,000 mg a day per adult. Despite a heavy parasite load and high prevalence of infectious diseases, such as malaria and syphillis, the physical fitness of Masai is remarkable. Studies have shown that no increase in body weight occurs between 25 and 35 years, and blood pressure and blood cholesterol were very low and did not increase with age. These people even with their high cholesterol intake have low blood pressures and low cholesterol levels and therefore are not at risk for stroke, heart attack, and blocked arteries. These biological characteristics are probably genetically determined.

See also BUSHMAN OF KALAHARI DESERT; NEW GUINEAN HIGHLANDERS; POLYNESIANS; SOLOMON ISLAND TRIBES; SOMALI CAMEL HERDSMEN; TARAHUMARA INDIANS; YANOMANO INDIANS.

Brocklehurst, J. C. *Textbook of Geriatric Medicine and Gerontology.* New York: Churchill Livingstone, 1985.

Medicaid Medicaid is medical insurance for those who do not qualify for Medicare, or who cannot afford to pay costs that are only partially covered by Medicare insurance.

Medicaid is free to people of all ages who are recipients of Supplemental Security Incomes (SSI) and other public assistance programs generally grouped under the caption of welfare. Because the over-65-year-old population experiences more frequent and more severe illness than the young, the elderly have absorbed about 35 percent of the Medicaid funds in recent years even though they represent only about 15 percent of the population that receives Medicaid assistance.

The program is financed by federal and state governments, and is administered by state welfare agencies. Medicaid is also available to people who do not receive public assistance but who have incomes sufficiently low to meet the program's eligibility standards.

For individuals who qualify for both Medicare and Medicaid, the Medicaid segment covers costs that would not be covered under Medicare alone. Medicaid also pays for up to three drug prescriptions per month, and eyeglasses, hearing aids, and dental care. Most importantly, Medicaid covers long-term care costs in nursing homes or at home, whereas Medicare does so only in exceptional circumstances and for a limited number of days.

Individuals who exhaust their income and property resources while personally paying for long-term care become eligible for Medicaid. Under the Medicaid program they continue to receive long-term care, and, therefore, are not deprived of help because of impoverishment.

The law and regulations governing Medicaid eligibility change from time to time, but under present elibigility requirements a married couple with one member in a nursing home may transfer jointly owned property, such as a car or house, to the other member. The purpose of this arrangement is to allow the spouse remaining at home to be financially independent and to prevent that individual from becoming an impoverished charge of the public. Because single people are not assumed to have dependents, their assets must be liquidated to cover the costs of long-term care.

Medicaid eligibility criteria and benefits vary from state to state. Each state sets and governs it own rules. The older individual should contact the local public assistance or welfare office for requirements in his state.

Deedy, J. *Your Aging Parents.* Chicago: The Thomas More Press, 1984.

Gillies, J. *A Guide to Caring for Coping with Aging Parents.* Nashville: Thomas Nelson Publishers, 1981.

Medicare   Medicare is the health-care coverage provided to anyone over 65 except for the few not covered by Social Security or Railroad Retirement and those who refuse it (the program is also avialable to disabled people under 65). Medicare is a shared-cost program with a monthly premium automatically deducted from the individual's Social Security check. Medicare has annual deductibles that may change from year to year. Medicare's part A provides coverage for hospital costs after the yearly deductible is met. For the first 60 days in the hospital Medicare covers the cost. From days 61 through 90, the individual is required to share part of the costs. Each individual is given 60 reserve days during his or her lifetime. If the individual must be hospitalized more than 90 days he or she will be required to share a larger part of the cost for these reserve days.

Medicare pays for some nursing home costs if the older individual's doctor decides the patient can continue therapy and convalese in a nursing facility rather than staying on in a hospital. Medicare will pay all the costs for the first 20 days. Thereafter, up to the 100th day, the individual must share the costs. Medicare does not pay for nursing home care after the 100th day, nor does it customarily pay for care not associated with a hospital stay (i.e., long-term care).

Medicare's part B provides medical coverage and pays for physicians and surgeons fees, medical services, outpatient hospital care, and some home health care. The individual must pay a yearly deductible for part B also. After this deductible is met, Medicare then pays 80 percent of the remaining "reasonable charges." Medicare determines what is reasonable. If the doctors' fees are higher than the Medicare standard then the individuals must pay the difference, plus their share (20 percent) of the "approved charge." If the physician "accepts assignment," however, that means he or she accepts what Medicare considers reasonable as payment in full and the individual will owe only the 20 percent not covered after the deductible is met.

Examples of Charges and Payments

	Unassigned	Assigned
Doctor bill	$150.00	$150.00
Medicare's reasonable or approved amount	$100.00	$100.00
80 percent of approved amount	$80.00	$80.00
Yearly deductible—1987	$75.00	$75.00
Amount individual responsible for (If deductible has not been met)	$145.00	$95.00
Amount individual responsible for (If deductible has been met)	$70.00	$20.00

Everyone who has Medicare should have a Medicare card that is issued by the Social Security office. This card will give the Medicare number, which may be the Social Security number plus a letter although this is not always the case.

Medicare's rules and regulations change from year to year. What has been described here is a basic, overall picture of Medicare. For exact amount of deductibles and other rules the older individual should contact his or her local Social Security office to obtain a current Medicare handbook.

See also INSURANCE, SUPPLEMENTAL; MEDICAID; MEDICAL BENEFITS; SOCIAL SECURITY.

Deedy, J. *Your Aging Parents*. Chicago: The Thomas More Press, 1984.
Gillies, J. *A Guide to Caring for and Coping with Aging Parents*. Nashville: Thomas Nelson Publishers, 1981.

medication, difficulties in prescribing
A number of factors make prescribing drugs for the elderly difficult.

They include:

1. Atrophy of Disuse—Many elderly people are forced into a sedentary, inactive lifestyle. Their functional ability is decreased by this disuse. Even though large tissue and organ losses do not always jeopardize life itself, they can greatly influence drug action.
2. Sex Difference—Females generally react to drugs differently than males.
3. Malnutrition—Poor eating habits and malnutrition are a common problem in the elderly, making drug therapy more complicated.
4. Chronic Drug Use—Little is known about the long-term effects of continued drug use. But it is established that chronic use of certain drugs may interfere with a patient's nutritional status.

5. Multimorbidity—Many elderly patients suffer from multiple physical problems and may be seen by several physicians. They also may patronize more than one pharmacy to have their prescriptions filled. Thus, one physician or pharmacist may not be aware if a drug is duplicated or if a potential negative interaction exists.

6. Diagnostic Difficulties—At times it is difficult to prescribe for the elderly because it is difficult to diagnose the problem. Some symptoms that are often ascribed to old age (confusion, falls, fatigue) can be indicators of serious illness. The elderly frequently do not give a reliable history, by attributing many symptoms to age and failing to mention them to the doctor.

Covington, T., and Walker, J. *Current Geriatric Therapy.* Philadelphia: W. B. Saunders, 1984.

medication, noncompliance   Over the past decade it has become increasingly evident that a significant percentage of patients fail to follow precisely advice on the use of their medication as well as other prescribed regimens such as diet, exercise, and the use of tobacco and alcohol. Noncompliance rates are estimated to be in the range of 25 percent to 50 percent. The elderly use more medications than the rest of population and are more likely to confuse or forget their medications.

Noncompliance with drug therapy generally consists of four problems:

1. Failure to have a prescription filled
2. Improper administration of the medication
3. Premature discontinuation of the medicine
4. Taking inappropriate medication

Prescriptions are not filled usually for one of two reasons—the patient does not have the money or the patient does not understand or believe in the benefits of the medication.

Errors can occur in both overdosing and underdosing. It is a common misconception that if one tablet is good, two will be better. Sometimes dosages are decreased to conserve on use because of the expense of the medication. Some medicines that should be taken with meals may be missed if the patient does not eat three meals a day as is presumed when prescribing such medicine.

When a patient begins to feel better medication may be discontinued too soon. This is a common occurrence with antibiotics, which need to be used for 10 full days.

The use of inappropriate medication occurs for a variety of reasons. A person may save old prescriptions and use at will at an incorrect time. If the physician is not aware of all the medications that a patient is taking, a noncompatible drug may be prescribed. Often, older people will share medicines of family members who develop similar illnesses.

To assist in encouraging proper compliance, medication calendars are available to record the names and times for taking each drug. Packaging devices have been developed to enable the patient to take the prescribed dosage. Though such packaging increases the cost of the medication, it may be well worth it since it promotes better compliance.

See also MEDICATION, SELF; POLYPHARMOCOTHERAPY.

Covington, T., and Walker, J. *Current Geriatric Therapy.* Philadelphia: W. B. Saunders, 1984.

medication, self   The availability of "safe and effective" nonprescription medicines leads many elderly people to self-medicate rather than consult a physician. They are especially susceptible to the influence of modern advertising techniques.

In the last two decades, television has had a tremendous impact on health-care attitudes with graphic ads extolling products to combat irregularity, diarrhea, hacking coughs, and tension headaches. The easy availability of these over-the-counter products masks the potential for abuse and dependency.

The most commonly used nonprescription medications include laxatives, antacids, analgesics, vitamins, sedatives, and cold preparations. Withdrawal symptoms from physical dependency on these products can present a significant medical problem as can cardiovascular effects from cold preparations.

The elderly are also prone to the use of "quack remedies." A person who fails to obtain relief or the promise of hope from a debilitating illness through prescription medication will be more likely to rely on quackery. Such therapies usually offer the promise of "cures" and "guaranteed" improvements tempting alternative to someone in pain. Dissatisfaction with impersonal attitudes and high costs of the established medical profession leads a patient to investigate unorthodox treatments. Cancer patients and those suffering from arthritis are particularly vulnerable to unproven remedies.

See also MEDICATION NONCOMPLIANCE; POLYPHARMOCOTHERAPY.

Covington, T., and Walker, J. *Current Geriatric Therapy.* Philadelphia: W. B. Saunders, 1984.

meditation   Meditation is recognized by health professionals and the general public as a good method for attaining physical and mental calm. Participants in meditation focus their attention on one particular object, image, or phrase, along with breathing exercises. One method of meditation that deepens physical and mental relaxation is visualization. In one type of visualization, for example, participants are asked to visualize spheres of light of specific color in specific centers of their body. Many elderly people participate in meditation and find its benefits very rewarding.

See also AUTOGENIC TRAINING; BIOFEEDBACK TRAINING; GESTALT DREAM ANALYSIS; HATHA YOGA; POSITIVE ATTITUDE; SELF-IMAGE EXERCISE; TAI CHI CHUAN.

Field, S. "Sage Can Be a Spice in Life," in *Aging,* Goldstein, E. C., ed. Vol. 1, Art. 26.

Boca Raton, Fl.: Social Issues Resource Series, Inc., 1981.

memory pill   Choline, a common vitamin found in eggs, fish, and lecithin, has often been called the "memory pill." Choline has been found to improve short-term memory loss and make its users "brighter." Researchers at the University of Massachusetts and Massachusetts Institute of Technology (MIT) are exploring uses of choline to improve memory and intellectual function in the senile.

Hanson, D. "Some Golden Years Have a Silver Lining," in *Aging,* Goldstein, E. C., ed. Vol. 2, Art. 5. Boca Raton, Fl.: Social Issues Resources Series, Inc., 1981.

memory, sensory   Sensory memory is the mental faculty that enables a person to retain and recall sensory perceptions. The capacity of visual sensory memory can be determined by the number of letters correctly identified in a briefly presented visual field. Studies have been done to determine whether or not the capacity of the sensory memory decreases with age. In the studies conducted, a six-letter display was shown to the subjects. The mean age of the subjects was 21. The older adults identified fewer letters than did the younger adults. The elderly subjects performed much more poorly than the younger adults. These studies suggested that sensory memory decreases as a person grows older, although confirmation with studies of the same people over long periods of their lives is also needed.

See also FORGETFULNESS.

Brocklehurst, J. C. *Textbook of Geriatric Medicine and Gerontology.* New York: Churchill Livingstone, 1985.

memory, tertiary   Tertiary memory, or long-term memory, does not seem to be affected by the aging process. Fozard gave four pieces of evidence to support the theory that long-term memory does not decline with age. The four lines of evidence are:

1. The rate of forgetting for pictorial learning does not vary with age over a two-year period.
2. Material of significance learned under natural conditions 10 to 30 years earlier is easily recalled by adults.
3. Older people remember colloquial expressions and names of well-known events as well as young people do.
4. Total knowledge increases with age but efficiency of memory remains constant.

These results supported the theory that long-term memory does not decrease with age.

See also FORGETFULNESS.

Brocklehurst, J. C. *Textbook of Geriatric Medicine and Gerontology*. New York: Churchill Livingstone, 1985.

Fozard, J. L. "The Time for Remembering," in L. D. Poon, ed., *Aging in the 1980's: Selected Contemporary Issues in the Psychology of Aging*. Washington, D. C.: American Psychological Association, 1980.

meningitis   Meningitis is an inflammation or infection of the lining of the brain and spinal cord. The three major categories of meningitis are bacterial, fungal, and viral. Rarely, infections are secondary to protozoa (e.g., amoeba, Toxoplasma) and other parasites. One of the most silent neurologic abnormalities of old age is meningitis. All elderly who show mental confusion, disorientation, or coma should be carefully evaluated for meningitis.

The most common bacteria that cause meningitis are *Pneumococcus* and *Meningococcus*. Fungal meningitis forms include crytococcal, coccidioidal, and histoplasmal. Viral meningitis is most frequently caused by enteroviruses (coxsackie, ECHO, polio), mumps, and lymphocytic choriomeningitis virus. Sporadic viral encephalitis is primarily caused by herpes simplex, whereas epidemics of encephalitis are frequently due to arboviruses (those borne by arthropods).

Infecting agents gain access to the central nervous system primarily through the circulatory system. Bacterial meningitis in the elderly is frequently associated with an underlying illness such as diabetes, decubitus ulcers (pressure sores), or following neurosurgery or trauma to the central nervous system.

The most common symptoms of meningitis are fever, headache, stiff neck, and alterations in the state of consciousness. In the elderly, it may be difficult to separate these symptoms from their underlying disorder. Confusion, stupor, and headache are usually present. Lumbar puncture usually confirms the suspicion of meningitis. Treatment of sporadic meningitis without associated illness is with penicillin or chloramphenicol in penicillin-sensitive people. Staphylococcal infections should be treated with nafcillin or an equivalent drug. Gram negative organisms should be treated with carbenicillin, chloramphenicol, maxalactam, or cefotaxime. Fungal meningitis is usually treated by the intravenous or intrathecal administration of amphotericin B. The only form of viral encephalitis that responds to therapy is herpes simplex–induced encephalitis. This is treated with adenine arabinoside for 10 days. Biopsy of brain tissue is usually required to make this diagnosis.

Covington, T., and Walker, J. *Current Geriatric Therapy*. Philadelphia: W. B. Saunders, 1984.

menopause (climacteric, "change of life")   Menopause, or climacteric, is the transitional phase between reproductive and nonreproductive ability. Menopause occurs when there has not been menstrual flow for one year. During menopause, which usually lasts 12 to 18 months, there is a gradual decline in ovarian function. Menopause usually occurs between ages 45–55, with 50 percent of women experiencing it between 45 and 55, 25 percent before 45, and 25 percent after.

Ovulation ceases gradually and with it menstruation and reproduction. This change usually occurs gradually, menstruation decreases or is very heavy and irregular for a time before the menses stops permanently. The uterus, the vagina, and vulva decrease in size. As ovarian function decreases so does the production of estrogen and progesterone. The endocrine imbalance may lead to fatigue, nervousness, sweating, palpitations, severe headaches, and hot flashes. These may be mild and infrequent or last as long as two minutes, occurring every 10 to 30 minutes around the clock. Sometimes they are severe enough to interfere with sleep.

Women have varying emotional reactions to menopause. The idea that menopause is inevitably accompanied by emotional and psychological problems has been rejected in recent years as the "menopause myth." Some view it as a loss of role, particularly women whose interests were focused entirely on children and the home. Some are concerned about changes in the marital relationship, continued sexual satisfaction, or the husband's response to aging. Feelings of depression are common among women experiencing menopause. These women require factual information and sometimes counseling to maintain a good attitude and productive life. Peer support groups can be helpful.

Women should be counseled about contraception because the menstrual cycle and ovulation are irregular. Oral contraceptives are reliable but there is an increase in the incidence of blood clots and cancer. Yearly physical examinations are recommended due to the higher incidence of uterine cancer. Bleeding after menopause, menstrual periods that become heavier, and bleeding after intercourse or douching require the attention of a physician.

Hot flashes and excessive perspiration that may occur are associated with lack of estrogen, increased luteinizing hormone, increased prostaglandins, and high levels of follicle-stimulating hormone. Estrogen deprivation may cause urinary frequency, painful urination, joint and muscle pain, cardiovascular disorders, and osteoporosis.

Estrogen is often the treatment of choice. Other methods that have proven effective are vitamin E, ginseng and B-complex vitamins. Good sources of vitamin E are vegetable oils, soybeans, spinach, peanuts, and wheat germ. Good dietary sources of B-complex vitamins are whole grains, Brewer's yeast, wheat germ, yogurt, liver, and milk.

The advantages and disadvantages of estrogen therapy have been debated for many years. Studies suggest an increased risk of endometrial cancer associated with the administration of estrogen. The benefits and the risks need to be discussed before therapy is started. It is desirable to use the lowest dose possible to relieve symptoms. During estrogen therapy women should be examined at least every six months. The examination should include breast exam, pap smear, and blood pressure check.

Menopause does not mean the end of an active sexual life. An active sexual life maintains pliability of the vaginal tissue. Sexual function does not depend on the release of ova or hormones, women can enjoy sexual activity during the climacteric and after menopause. The loss of estrogen causes the vagina to lose its elasticity and become shorter and narrower. Vulvar changes include flattening of the labia, thinning of pubic hair, and shrinking of the introitus. This may lead to dyspareunia (painful sexual relations).

Dyspareunia is treated by local applications of a vaginal cream. Vaginal infections are common because the lack of estrogen causes the vaginal secretions to become more alkaline. Vaginal infections are treated according to the causative organism but frequently respond to vinegar douching.

Menopause may be artificially induced in cases of specific diseases by irradiation of the ovaries, surgical removal of both ovaries, or hysterectomy. When the uterus is removed but the ovaries are left in place menstruation ceases, but the ovaries continue to function until the age of climacteric has been reached.

Many women view the "change of life" negatively. This negative image is reinforced by the media, books, health professionals, and the general public. Education preceding the onset of menopause can help dispel many myths and misconceptions. Women need to be informed about what menopause is, how it affects reproductive and sexual ability, and what can be done to make it more comfortable.

See also DYSPAREUNIA; OSTEOPOROSIS; VAGINITIS.

Calkins, E., *et al. The Practice of Geriatrics*. Philadelphia: W. B. Saunders Co., 1986.
Scherer, J. C. *Introductory Medical-Surgical Nursing*. Philadelphia: J. B. Lippincott Co., 1982.

metabolic rate theory The exact link between higher metabolic rates and aging is not known. Some researchers suggest that the higher metabolic theory connects with the oxygen radical theory of aging.

In the oxygen radical theory, it is suggested that the act of breathing contributes to aging. When oxygen is taken into the body to fuel its metabolic activity the chemistry of living creates a highly reactive form of oxygen, which is called a free radical of oxygen. These free radicals bounce around in cells and cause damage to the first molecule they contact. Radicals can inactivate enzymes, hormones, proteins, and fats, and even DNA. The oxygen radical model is used to explain degenerative disease linked to aging such as atherosclerosis, cancer, hypertension, and Alzheimer's disease.

See also AGING, BIOLOGICAL THEORY OF.

Thompson, L. "Old Age Doesn't Kill People, Disease Does," In *Aging*, Goldstein, E. C., ed. Vol. 3, Art. 17. Boca Raton, Fl: Social Issues Resource Series, Inc., 1981.

middle age People between 40 and 60 years of age are considered middle-aged. About 21 percent of the U.S. population is between 40 and 60. Research on the psychological and social characteristics of middle age is relatively new, so that generalizations about this period of life need to be made cautiously and tentatively. Long-standing folk wisdom, however, has it that "life begins at 40," and to some extent this idea appears to be confirmed by research studies that show that individuals in middle age re-evaluate their lives to determine anew the things they value, to re-examine their career choices, and to reconsider their goals. By this period of life, the natural, almost accidental, strength and beauty of youth have begun to decline, so that psychologists observe that individuals reaching midlife need to learn to emphasize their powers of mind because these will help them to withstand the forces of aging.

Perhaps the most famous characterization of middle age was made by psychiatrist Erik Erickson, who described the period as one where one either develops "generativity" or slides into "ego stagnation." In essence, generativity means creating things and doing things that will last beyond one's own lifetime. Most often individuals achieve creativity through their family relations and/or a successful career, but creativity in the arts and altruistic service to others also represent possible avenues.

Ego stagnation, on the other hand, is a state of boredom, psychological poverty, and sometimes excessive concern with physical and psychological decline. Erikson, a psychiatrist who developed his observations about middle age from therapy sessions with individuals and small groups of clients, is not alone in his view that midlife is a time of change; this view is also shared by other researchers who have made large-scale surveys of the American population.

Erikson, however, argues that all stages of life are times of change—each stage of life requires a struggle to achieve a positive psychological development (e.g., in midlife this is "generativity") in response to the unique challenges of that stage. Just as infants must struggle to become autonomous, independent beings (or else, according to Erikson, slip into shame and doubt) so the middle-aged adult must successfully grow into generativity or collapse into stagnation.

Studies by Paul Costa and Robert McCrae of the National Institute on Aging appear to contradict the popular notion that individuals go through a "midlife crisis." Although their research was restricted to men, they designed a questionnaire derived from extensive analysis of writings about "the midlife crisis," and administered it to two separate groups of men. In neither group was there any evidence of a crisis, leading the two scholars to observe that "The mid-life crisis, whatever it was, did not appear to be confined to mid-life." They concluded that most people maintain a vigorous and positive approach to life, and that they adapt readily to the changes brought by aging.

The General Social Survey supports the Costa and McCrae finding by showing that there is no decline in happiness in the American population in midlife, even though this is a period of considerable adult responsibility and pressure. At this age, for instance, the incidence of death in one's family reaches a lifetime peak—as much as 55 percent of the middle-aged population sees one or more family members die, according to the General Social Survey.

The middle aged have also been labeled "the sandwich generation," because people at this stage of life may find themselves responsible for helping their adult parents while their children still need assistance in getting through college or with starting family life. Research shows that the majority of individuals successfully navigate these and the other challenges of midlife.

Saline, C.: "Entering Middle Age: What To Do With The Rest Of Your Life." In *Aging*, ed. Goldstein, E. C., Vol. 2, Art. 61. Boca Raton, Fl. Social Issues Resource Series, Inc. 1981.

Schaie, K. W., and Willis, S. L. *Adult Development and Aging*, 2nd ed. Boston: Little, Brown and Company, 1986.
Ward, R. A. *The Aging Experience*, 2nd ed. New York: Harper and Row, 1984.
Russell, C. H. *Good News About Aging*. New York: John Wiley and Sons, 1989.
Russell, C. H., and Megaard, I. *The General Social Survey, 1972–1986: The State of the American People*. New York: Springer-Verlag, 1988.

midlife crisis   See MIDDLE AGE.

minerals   See VITAMINS.

mobility, home   The aged often have trouble moving around because of physical problems. Some improvements in the home can allow an older person more mobility.

Grab bars and nonslip surfaces in the bathroom can be helpful to older people. Grab bars for the bathtub can be bought in many local stores and are easy to install. Safety mats can be purchased at a hardware store.

Adjusting furniture heights can also be helpful for elderly people. You can adjust a regular bed to a height that will help the older person to get in and out easier. Elevated toilet seats and safety benches for the tub can also be bought.

Rearranging cupboards so that often-used foods, utensils, and cleaning supplies are at the front can also be helpful to an older person. Moving heavy dishes to lower and more convenient shelves can also be helpful.

Many common household items can be helpful in maximizing mobility. A child's wagon can be used to move heavy objects around the house. An office chair with wheels can help an older person move from room to room.

These are only a few of the home improvements that enable people to have more mobility.

Crichton, J. *The Age Care Source Book*. New York: Simon and Schuster, Inc., 1987.

mortality, disease-specific in the elderly   In all industrialized societies the major causes of death in the elderly are the cardiovascular diseases such as ischemic heart disease, cerebrovascular diseases, and strokes. In developed nations infectious diseases and cancer are not as deadly as they were 50 years ago. Death due to disease has steadily decreased over the years. This is probably due to better medical care.

Brocklehurst, J. C. *Textbook of Geriatric Medicine and Gerontology.* New York: Churchill Livingstone, 1985.

mortgages, reverse   A reverse mortgage, or home-equity conversion, is one way to increase income during retirement, but financial managers advise that such a plan should be adopted only after careful consideration of financial alternatives. Monthly payments are received by the homeowner for a negotiated period of time. When the home is sold, usually upon the death of the owner, principal and interest are deducted from the sale. Home-equity conversions are only practical for an older person who owns a home that is fully paid for or has only a small remaining mortgage. Three variations of home-equity conversions are: reverse annuity mortgages (RAMs), sale/leasebacks, and deferred payment loans.

Reverse annuity mortgages (RAMs) are usually limited to 60 percent to 80 percent of the appraised value of the property with a fixed interest rate for a set number of years, e.g., 10 years. The homeowner would receive a monthly income for the duration of the loan. At the end of that period of time, the loan must be renegotiated or repaid in full.

In a sale/leaseback agreement, an investor purchases the home and grants the seller life tenancy in the home or the right to tenancy for a fixed number of years at a specified rent. Payment is received in one of several ways: a lump sum, equal monthly payments, or monthly mortgage payments from which rent is deducted.

The deferred payment loan is another way homeowners can draw on the equity built up in their home for use to maintain and repair the structure. This type of loan allowed the homeowner to defer payment of both principal and interest, either for a specified period of time or until the home is sold.

It is extremely important to investigate these options by seeking legal advice or by talking to a reputable financial consultant. The Federal Council on Aging (FCA), an advisory panel to the president, recommends that all these loan arrangements should involve a lawyer and the homeowner's potential heirs, since a reverse mortgage agreement may drastically reduce or eliminate the estate the family may inherit.

Averyt, A. *Successful Aging.* New York: Ballantine Books, 1987.

mourning   It is useful to distinguish the word *mourning* form the word *bereavement.* The first usually applies to the socially defined period of time and set of activities that follow the death of an intimate person, whereas the second usually refers to the inward pain or sense of loss that accompanies such a death.

Mourning events include funerals, visiting hours with the bereaved person or family members, customs regarding dress and behavior following bereavement, and the like. Such practices differ widely from country to country and among ethnic groups—ranging from festive and joyful occasions celebrated with firecrackers and feasts (as carried out in parts of China and Indonesia) to periods of wailing and despair demanded from women in the near East.

In the United States mourning customs before World War I used to include wearing of black clothing by widows, black arm bands or diamond-shaped black sleeve patches worn by men (more so in Europe than in the United States), and a period of withdrawal from social activity. These kinds of customs have all but disappeared in the United States within the past 50 years, but some thanatologists (people who study death and its surrounding customs) hold that the decline of mourning customs deprives bereaved persons of due recognition of their grief, and of the social support needed to complete their grief work.

Ward, R. A. *The Aging Experience,* 2nd ed. New York: Harper and Row, 1984.

mouth cancer See CANCER, MOUTH, THROAT, AND LARYNX.

multiple myeloma Multiple myeloma is a series of malignancies composed of plasma cells scattered through the bone marrow, interrupting the antibody production. Multiple myeloma usually appears in people over 50 years of age.

Symptoms of multiple myeloma are traced to the proliferation of plasma-cell tumors from the bone marrow into the hard bone tissue causing an erosion of the bone. These symptoms include lack of energy, weight loss, recurrent infections, anemia, bone pain, chronic renal failure, and spontaneous pathologic fractures.

Treatment of multiple myeloma consists of systemic chemotherapy and radiation. The therapy helps to relieve symptoms and extend the useful life of the person. A balanced diet, physical activity, and sometimes steroids can be suggested to prevent symptoms.

Multiple myeloma may be asymptomatic for years and can be discovered by a routine blood test. Early detection is important and any older person with bone pain and anemia should be tested for multiple myeloma. Once the symptomatic stage is reached and renal failure occurs, the prognosis is poor. If the disease is detected and treated early, the person may experience a remission for years.

Ham,, R. J. *Geriatric Medicine Annual—1987.* Oradell, N.J.: Medical Economic Books, 1987.
Phipps, W. J., *et al. Medical Surgical Nursing.* St. Louis: C. V. Mosby Co., 1983.

muscle cramps See MUSCLE DYSFUNCTION.

muscle dysfunction (muscle wasting, muscle cramps, muscle strain) Wasting of skeletal muscles and a general decrease in muscular strength, endurance, and agility are common in the aged. Their posture tends to become one of general flexation. The head and neck are held forward, the dorsal spine becomes bent forward, the upper limbs are bent at the elbows and wrists, and the hips and knees are also slightly flexed. The aged person usually shows a decrease in movement and in reflexes.

Muscle cramps become more troublesome with advancing age. They are characterized by sustained involuntary and painful contractions of a muscle group, frequently following unusual muscular effort and especially at night. Various diseases can contribute to this problem but in most instances the cause is unknown. Their incidence may be diminished by a hot bath at bedtime or by the use of certain drugs such as quinine sulfate or Benadryl.

Muscle strain is a common problem with older people because of poor muscle tone and atrophy from lack of exercise. The most common location of muscle strain is the neck and lower back. It frequently occurs following an activity that may not have been attempted for some time or is performed for a longer period than usual.

Treatment for muscle strain consists of the use of muscle relaxants, aspirin, or other anti-inflammatory drugs. Muscle spasms may be relieved with hot packs, ultrasound, whirlpool, and ice applications. The best treatment, however, is prevention. This can be accomplished through education related to proper back usage and the need for proper exercise. Prolonged inactivity causes a stiffening of the joints and atrophy of the muscles, leading to an increased chance of muscle strain.

Reichel, W. M. *Clinical Aspects of Aging.* Baltimore: The Williams & Wilkins Co., 1979.

muscles strain   See MUSCLE DYSFUNC-
TION.

muscles wasting   See MUSCLE DYSFUNC-
TION.

myocardial infarction (heart attack)

Myocardial infarction is the rapid death of
part of the heart muscle as a result of the
sudden blockage of one of the branches of
a coronary artery. This blockage may be
caused by the formation of a blood clot in
the coronary artery, progression of atherosclerotic changes, or prolonged constriction
of the arteries. A myocardial infarction may
be extensive enough to cause immediate death
or it may cause necrosis of a portion of the
myocardium (heart muscle) with subsequent
healing by scar formation or fibrosis. Heart
attack is the major cause of death in people
over age 65. Over 2,000 per 100,000 population in the United States suffer heart attacks.

Symptoms include chest pain, sweating,
nausea, vomiting, cyanosis, shock, decreasing blood pressure, confusion, weakness,
and a rapid weak pulse. The pain is described as sudden, severe, crushing, or vise-
like in the substernal region that may radiate
to the neck, jaw, arms, back, or abdomen
and lasts longer than 10 minutes. This pain
occurs at random and is not associated with
effort as angina is. Although pain is the
most common symptom, it is not necessarily
present. The incidence of painless myocardial infarcts increase with age and in the
elderly the chief complaint may be a sudden
shortness of breath.

Treatment usually involves hospitalization
to resuscitate and stabilize the person. During the acute phase of the myocardial infarction the goal of treatment is to reduce
the workload of the heart. Generally, an
intravenous route is established and the patient is given morphine sulfate to relieve
pain and apprehension, and to produce dilation of the blood vessels. The person is
placed on bed rest for 24 to 48 hours in
order to limit the size of the infarction. Rest
and reassurance are essential. Sometimes,
sedation with Valium or an equivalent is
necessary to achieve this. Ventricular fibrillation is one of the most serious threats
during an myocardial infarction. Because of
this, the person should be constantly monitored with EKG and frequent vital signs. If
premature ventricular beats (PVBs) are documented, intravenous lidocaine is usually
administered. Oxygen therapy is administered for 24 hours or until symptoms resolve
to correct a decrease in arterial oxygen pressure caused by ventilation-perfusion abnormalities. Anticoagulation therapy may or may
not be administered. Some physicians feel it
might be beneficial to give intravenous heparin until the patient is ambulating well.

A soft, low-salt diet is recommended for
the first few days following a myocardial
infarction. A stool softener should be given
since the intense straining may trigger arrhythmias, cardiac arrest, or pulmonary embolus.

The clot may be dissolved, in some cases,
with streptokinase (an enzyme). Some people may benefit from balloon dilation of the
coronary blockage. If these methods are not
useful, coronary bypass surgery may be necessary. Coronary bypass surgery involves
bypassing an obstructed area of the coronary
vessels with a graft or artificial substitute.
During hospitalization a rehabilitation program will begin. Progressive activity is closely
monitored. If cyanosis (blueness of the skin),
arrhythmias, resting heart rate greater than
100, or resting blood pressure greater than
160/95 during an exercise session are present, the session should be terminated.

After discharge from the hospital the person is usually put on a gradually increasing
walking program. Education is an important
part of the treatment for myocardial infarction patient. The education program should
include an individualized presentation of risk
factors, medications, diet, and it should stress
the importance of gradual progressive activity. Contrary to a common myth, a person

can resume sexual intercourse following a myocardial infarction. In general, the person should abstain from intercourse for four to six weeks. If the person can walk two flights of stairs without cardiac difficulties he or she is generally able to perform sexual intercourse safely.

Myocardial infarction is a serious event and one of the major causes of death among the elderly. Many people, however, live an active and comfortable life for years following a myocardial infarction.

Phipps, W. J., et al. Medical Surgical Nursing. St. Louis: C. V. Mosby Co., 1983.
Scherer, J. C. Introductory Medical-Surgical Nursing. Philadelphia: J. B. Lippincott Co., 1982.

myopia (near-sightedness) Myopia is a condition in which parallel rays of light come to focus at a point in front of the retina. The myopic eye has basically too much plus power for its size. Elderly patients with cataracts will become more near-sighted as their cataracts develop. Frequently, they will discover they can read without glasses. This is sometimes referred to as "second sight."

In axial myopia the eyeball is too long for the normal refractive power of the lens and the cornea. In curvature myopia the eye is of normal size but the curvature of the cornea and the lens is increased. In index myopia a change in the index of refraction of the lens is present. This is witnessed in two pathologic states, diabetes mellitus and cataract. In diabetes the lens loses water because of the high level of blood sugar in the anterior chamber and therefore its index of refraction increases. In the cataract patient the center of the lens becomes increasingly hard. This hard inner core increases the index of refraction of the entire lens structure, thereby increasing the converging power. The chief symptom of myopia is an inability to see at a distance. Treatment of myopia usually involves the use of glasses or contact lenses to correct the refractive error. Radial kera-

totomy is a procedure in which multiple radial cuts are made in the cornea to help correct the near-sightedness. An older adult also may need to wear reading glasses if he or she does not wear glasses for distance following this procedure.

In spite of extensive research and clinical investigations the cause of myopia is poorly understood. Myopia is familial in nature and is passed from one generation to another as a dominant trait.

See also ASTIGMATISM; HYPEROPIA; PRESBYOPIA.

Newell, F. W. Ophthalmology Principles and Concepts, 6th ed. St. Louis; C. V. Mosby Co., 1986
Slatt, B. J., and Stein, H. A. The Ophthalmic Assistant Fundamentals and Clinical Practice, 4th ed. St. Louis: C. V. Mosby Co., 1983.

myxedema See HYPOTHROIDISM.

N

near-death experiences Pollster and American public opinion analyst and statistician, George Gallup surveyed a sample of physicians to determine whether or not they felt that the growing reports of near-death experiences gave any confirmation to the commonly held view that life continues after death. Most physicians thought that near-death experiences provided no support whatever for a belief in life after death, and some compared these experiences to hallucinations caused by drugs or simply to recovery effects from anesthetics. In terms of this survey, life after death remains a matter of faith and hope, not a scientifically proven fact.

Russell, C. H., Good News About Aging. New York: John Wiley and Sons, 1989.

near-sightedness See MYOPIA.

Nepalese Sherpas The stamina that an older individual exhibits is dependent on his or her physical activities according to the findings of a study of Nepalese Sherpas. Residents of the (Himalayas, the Sherpas are justly famous for their service as guides on mountain climbing, and it was Sherpa Tensing Norgay who shared the honors with Sir Edmund Hilary in the first human conquest of Mt. Everest. As a result the Nepalese Sherpas have often been studied by scientists in order to determine the benefits of exercise. One particular study divided the Sherpas into two groups—the "high-activity" group and the "low-activity" group. The high-activity group was made up of males who were farmers, herders, and who worked occasionally as porters and guides. The low-activity group consisted of traders who moved from village to village. Both of the groups were examined at high altitudes (3,400 m). The study found higher levels of performance among the highly active at all ages. This suggests that at every age, overfed, affluent societies, such as the United States, probably develop and use only a fraction of their physical capacity and fail to achieve their full mental and physical potential.

See also PRIMITIVE TRIBE NATURAL SELECTION.

Brocklehurst, J. C. *Textbook of Geriatric Medicine and Gerontology.* New York: Churchill Livingstone, 1985.

New Guinean Highlanders The New Guinean Highlanders subsist on low-caloric diets consisting mostly of sweet potatoes. These supply about 90 percent of the Highlanders total caloric intake. Adult Highlanders do not consume more than 25 grams of protein a day. Therefore, their lean body mass decreases noticeably with age. The muscles in the arms and the calves become measurably smaller after age 30. The one advantage of a low-calorie diet is the low intake of fats. A diet lacking fats keeps blood pressure low and serum cholesterol levels

low. People who are concerned about excess weight in their upper arms, thighs, and buttocks may wish to consult their physicians about the possible value of a similar diet.

See also MASAI; POLYNESIANS; SOLOMON ISLAND TRIBES; SOMALI CAMEL HERDSMEN; TARAHUMARA INDIANS; YANOMANO INDIANS.

Brocklehurst, J. C. *Textbook of Geriatric Medicine and Gerontology.* New York: Churchill Livingstone, 1985.

NIA See U.S. NATIONAL INSTITUTE ON AGING.

nosebleeds See EPISTAXIS.

nose cancer See CANCER, NOSE.

nursing homes, adjustment to Residence in a nursing home is the exception rather than the rule for the vast majority of older Americans—only about 5 percent of the population over age 65 and 22 percent of the population over 85 reside in nursing homes. When entry into a nursing home does occur, it is practically always associated with a disabling chronic condition or impairment, such as organic brain syndrome or paralysis resulting from a stroke, that obliges the affected individual to depend on others for help with personal activities (bathing, dressing, toileting, and consuming meals).

Though nursing homes do discharge about 20 percent of their patients, they serve as the last homes for most people who enter them. Largely because of the growing size of the elderly population, the United States now has 22,000 nursing homes with over 1.5 million residents. This rate of growth is expected to continue after the year 2000, when the nursing home population is expected to increase to about 2.25 million and then to more than three million.

Accounts of nursing home placements generally allege that moving to a nursing home is traumatic for both the client and family members. Such accounts disregard the obvious fact that transfer to a nursing home may come as a considerable relief to all concerned, not excepting the client— especially so when one considers that the average nursing home resident has at least four times as many chronic disabilities and impairments as elderly community residents, and faces severe problems when attempting to reside in a conventional home.

Once in a nursing home, individuals no longer need to struggle with the tasks of daily living that are routinely managed by the rest of the population but impossible for nursing home residents. Needs for personal hygiene and good nutrition are met, medications are taken under supervision, and increased social contact frequently occurs. Research shows that relocation stress following a move into a nursing is usually quite temporary, and the client comfortably adjusts to the new situation.

Some years ago nursing homes perhaps did suffer from low regulatory standards and did resemble dreary hideaways for the helpless, but industry self-regulation along with rising state standards for licensure have greatly improved the quality and character of nursing home life. When an individual or elderly couple is reluctant to move into a nursing home even in the face of obvious need, professional counsel from physicians, nurses, and social workers, as well as agencies that serve the elderly and the homes themselves, can be helpful.

The success of these sources in advising with moves to a nursing home grows out of their customary sympathetic understanding and their extensive experience with problems of relocation. Most professionals who offer services for the elderly can offer advice on how to make a move seem like a desirable solution to the individual's problem of coping with daily living.

Professionals recommend that plans for a move into a nursing home be discussed honestly with the person(s) who need to move, and advise candor when stress of caregiving becomes excessive. When a person does move to a nursing home, family members need to develop a routine of regular visits and supportive help. A number of valuable and well-written guidebooks are now available to assist individuals with arrangements and follow up of a move of an older family member to a nursing home.

Atchley, R. C. *Social Forces and Aging,* 4th ed. Belmont, Calif.: Wadsworth Publishing Company, 1985.

Deedy, J. *Your Aging Parents.* Chicago: The Thomas More Press, 1984.

Gillies, J. *A Guide to Caring for and Coping with Aging Parents.* Nashville: Thomas Nelson Publishers, 1981.

Hooyman, N. R., and Lustbader, W. *Taking Care.* New York: The Free Press, 1986.

Lester, A. D. and Lester, J. L. *Understanding Aging Parents.* Philadelphia: The Westminster Press, 1980.

Ward, R. A. *The Aging Experience,* 2nd ed. New York: Harper and Row, 1984.

nursing homes, how to select, monitor, and evaluate   Generally, there are four main reasons for residing in a nursing home. These are: disturbances in thinking; illness that requires special medical attention not available at home; harmful behavior to one's self or others; and environmental factors that include not having people who can adequately care for the older person or non-accessibility of special equipment, such as wheelchairs, lifts, and special tubs.

Several factors should be considered when selecting a nursing home. The older person and/or family should understand how finances determine the options. They should know the amounts Medicare and Medicaid will pay for accredited facilities and then find out which facilities are accredited in the area. (At present, Medicare coverage is generally not available for nursing home stays unless they follow a hospitalization episode.)

There are several types of nursing-home care available and these should be matched to the individual's needs. If intensive care is needed, a 24-hour skilled nursing facility is necessary. This means that there are qualified nurses on duty 24 hours a day. If constant medical care is not necessary an intermediate-care facility will be quite satisfactory at about half the cost. In an intermediate-care facility, care will be administered by unskilled staff under the supervision of at least one registered nurse. The older individual's doctor can be helpful in determining the type of care necessary. Frequently, the doctor can recommend a facility since he or she visits nursing homes with some regularity and knows how well his or her orders are followed. Another source of referral may be family clergy who can probably recommend church-owned facilities in the area.

Once the list of nursing homes that are available has been narrowed down by the type of care and cost, it is probably a good idea to check with the Better Business Bureau to determine whether all are reputable facilities.

At this point it is advisable for the older person and family to visit some of the prospective homes. If the older person is able, allow him or her as much input in the decision as possible.

Official statements of overall nursing home policy issued by operators and organizations have value because they define broad goals of nursing home care. The best of these include the following principles. The resident comes first; individual feelings, emotions, and wants are considered of utmost importance; the comfort and happiness of the resident is paramount.

Residents' rights desirably include:

1. Being fully informed of their medical condition
2. Participating in planning of medical treatment
3. Being transferred or discharged only for medical reasons
4. Being free from mental and physical abuse

5. Being free from drug and nonemergency physical restraints, except as ordered by a physician for a specified period of time, or to protect from self-induced injury
6. Being treated with consideration, respect, and dignity
7. If married, being assured of privacy for visits by spouse and if both spouses are residents, being permitted to share a room.

Three broad areas to assess when visiting prospective homes are medical, nursing, and therapeutic services; food and housekeeping services; and the social and pyschological atmosphere.

When evaluating a specific nursing home, individuals should pay attention to the rapport between staff and residents, how clean the residents are, if there are enough bathrooms, if there is proper lighting and ventilation, whether there is sufficient storage space, and general appearance of the rooms.

Nursing homes that are most readily accepted by both family and resident are those with pleasant environments. Some things that help to provide these types of environment include providing residents with safe patio areas so that they can enjoy the fresh air and sunshine and not feel "penned in," varying the colors of rooms and hallways, allowing residents to decorate their own areas, and having wall hangings, plants, and aquariums to give the facility a more homelike appearance. Other factors include providing enough living space to allow for group exercise, programs, crafts, and group interaction, and promoting opportunities for spiritual involvement by having a retired pastor or pastoral student in attendance regularly or having choirs or a hymn sing-a-long.

It is important for the nursing home to provide enough opportunities and activities to enrich the residents' lives, instead of simply providing a place to exist.

It may be helpful for the family to carry a checklist on the nursing home visit so as not to overlook anything. The U.S. Department of Health and Human Services (HHS) has a prepared list, which may be helpful. This list is as follows:

1. Does the home have a current license from the state?
2. Does the administrator have a current license from the state?
3. If you need and are eligible for financial assistance, is the home certified to participate in government or other programs that provide it?
4. Does the home provide special services such as a specific diet or therapy that the patient needs?
5. Location:
  A. Pleasing to the patient?
  B. Convenient for patient's personal doctor?
  C. Convenient for frequent visitor?
  D. Near a hospital?
6. Accident prevention
  A. Well-lighted inside?
  B. Free of hazards underfoot?
  C. Chairs sturdy and not easily tipped?
  D. Warning signs posted around freshly waxed floors?
  E. Handrails in hallways and grab bars in bathrooms?
7. Fire safety
  A. Meets federal and state codes?
  B. Exits clearly marked and unobstructed?
  C. Written emergency evacuation plan?
  D. Frequent fire drills?
  E. Exit doors not locked on the inside?
  F. Stairways enclosed and doors to stairways kept closed?
8. Bedrooms
  A. Open into hall?
  B. Windows?
  C. No more than four beds per room?
  D. Easy access to each bed?
  E. Fresh drinking water at each bed?
  F. Drapery for each bed?
  G. Nurse call bell by each bed?
  H. At least one comfortable chair for each patient?

  I. Reading lights?
  J. Clothes closet and drawers?
  K. Room for a wheelchair to maneuver?
  L. Care in selecting roommates?
9. Cleanliness
  A. Generally clean, even though it may have a lived-in look?
  B. Free of unpleasant odors?
  C. Incontinent patients given prompt attention?
10. Lobby
  A. Is the atmosphere welcoming?
  B. If also a lounge, is it being used by residents?
  C. Furniture attractive and comfortable?
  D. Plants and flowers?
  E. Certificates and licenses on display?
11. Hallways
  A. Large enough for two wheelchairs to pass with ease?
  B. Hand-grip railings on the sides?
12. Dining room
  A. Attractive and inviting?
  B. Comfortable chairs and tables?
  C. Easy to move around in?
  D. Tables convenient for those in wheelchairs?
  E. Food tasty and attractively served?
  F. Meals match posted menu?
  G. Those needing help receiving it?
13. Kitchen
  A. Food preparation, dishwashing, and garbage area separated?
  B. Food needing refrigeration not standing on counters?
  C. Kitchen help observe sanitation rules?
14. Activity rooms
  A. Rooms available for patients' activities?
  B. Equipment (such as games, easels, yarn, kiln) available?
  C. Patients using equipment?
15. Special-purpose rooms
  A. Rooms set aside for physical examinations or therapy?
  B. Rooms being used for stated purpose?
16. Isolation room
  A. At least one bed and bathroom avail-

able for patients with contagious illness?

17. Toilet facilities
    A. Convenient to bedrooms?
    B. Easy for a wheelchair patient to use?
    C. Sink?
    D. Nurse call bell?
    E. Hand grips on or near toilets?
    F. Bathtubs and showers with nonslip surfaces?

18. Grounds
    A. Residents can get fresh air?
    B. Ramps to help handicapped?

19. Medical
    A. Physician available in emergency?
    B. Private physician allowed?
    C. Regular medical attention assured?
    D. Thorough physical immediately before or upon admission?
    E. Medical records and plan of care kept?
    F. Patient involved in developing plans for treatments?
    G. Other medical services (dentists, optometrists, etc.) available regularly?
    H. Freedom to purchase medicines outside home?

20. Hospitalization
    A. Arrangement with nearby hospital for transfer when necessary?

21. Nursing service
    A. R.N. responsible for nursing staff in a skilled nursing home?
    B. L.P.N. on duty day and night in a skilled nursing home?
    C. Trained nurses' aides and orderlies on duty in homes providing some nursing care?

22. Rehabilitation
    A. Specialists in various therapies available when needed?

23. Activities program
    A. Individual patient preferences?
    B. Group and individual activities?
    C. Residents encouraged but not forced to participate?
    D. Outside trips for those who can go?
    E. Volunteers from the community work with the patients?

24. Religious observances
    A. Arrangements made for patient to worship as he or she pleases?
    B. Religious observances a matter of choice?

25. Social Services
    A. Social worker available to help residents and families?

26. Food
    A. Dietitian plans menus for patients on special diets?
    B. Variety from meal to meal?
    C. Meals served at normal times?
    D. Plenty of time for each meal?
    E. Snacks?
    F. Food delivered to patients' rooms?
    G. Help with eating given when needed?

27. Grooming
    A. Barbers and beauticians available?

28. General atmosphere friendly and supportive?

29. Residents retain human rights?
    A. May participate in planning treatment?
    B. Medical records kept confidential?
    C. Can veto experimental research?
    D. Have freedom and privacy to attend to personal needs?
    E. Married couples may share room?
    F. All have opportunities to socialize?
    G. May manage own finances if capable, or obtain accountant if not?
    H. May decorate own bedrooms?
    I. May wear own clothes?
    J. May communicate with anyone without censorship?
    K. Are not transferred or discharged arbitrarily?

30. Administrator and staff available to discuss problems?
    A. Patients and relatives can discuss complaints without fear of reprisal?
    B. Staff responds to calls quickly and courteously?

31. Residents appear alert unless very ill?

32. Visiting hours accommodate residents and relatives?

33. Civil rights regulations observed?

34. Visitors and volunteers pleased with home?

Once a home has been chosen and the family member moved in, personal observation and visits are the best means of monitoring care. Visit the facility at different times of the day and week in order to observe different shifts.

If the resident is mentally competent he or she can frequently help to monitor the quality of care. If, however, the resident is unable to reason, it will be necessary to identify a responsible staff member to help monitor care and resolve problems. Remember to speak with the staff when pleased with the care as well as when displeased. Positive comments go a long way and will help when trying to work out problems in the future.

Some facilities plan regular "family meetings," which are held several times a year, at which senior staff, relatives, and the resident meet to share concerns, questions, and suggestions for new programs or care.

A few facilities have organized "resident councils" in which residents participate in some of the decision-making that affects their lives.

Deedy, J. *Your Aging Parents*. Chicago: The Thomas More Press, 1984.
Gillies, J. *A Guide to Caring for and Coping with Aging Parents*. Nashville: Thomas Nelson Publishers, 1981.
Lester, A. D. and Lester, J. L. *Understanding Aging Parents*. Philadelphia: The Westminster Press, 1980.

nutrition   Eating habits are established early in life and by the time a person reaches old age, likes and dislikes are deeply entrenched. Foods are often chosen for their appetite-filling value rather than for their nourishment. Because of this, malnutrition is a problem of the elderly.

Eating is basically a social activity. Appetites improve when meals are shared. A person living alone soon loses interest in preparing and eating nutritious meals. Apathy and loneliness are a big deterrent to an appetite even if cooking facilities are available.

Other factors in inadequate nutrition of the elderly include digestive changes, loss of appetite due to decreased sensitivity in smell and taste, and chewing problems due to ill-fitting dentures or the absence of teeth.

See also FLUID INTAKE; FOOD GROUPS, BASIC; VITAMINS.

Deedy, J. *Your Aging Parents*. Chicago: The Thomas More Press, 1984.

O

obesity   Obesity is a condition resulting from an abnormal increase of fat in the subcutaneous connective tissues. It results when caloric intake greatly exceeds energy expenditure. Obesity contributes to increased mortality from various diseases. Although the elderly are less affected than those at younger ages, obesity is a common problem in older individuals.

Diseases closely affected by obesity include HYPERTENSION, coronary artery disease, pulmonary abnormalities, DIABETES MELLITUS, and OSTEOARTHRITIS.

Treatment of obesity is generally unsatisfactory and discouraging to the patient but attempts at control should be continued because of its known positive effects on health and longevity. The various types of therapy include dietary manipulation, behavior modification, exercise therapy, surgical procedures, medication, and drugs used to inhibit starch absorption or to simulate the taste of fat without caloric content.

Attempting to change a lifetime of habits in the elderly is extremely difficult and may, in part, account for the poor results. An understanding, sympathetic approach by the physician is important in helping the patient deal with this frustrating disorder.

Covington, T., and Walker, J. *Current Geriatric Therapy*. Philadelphia: W. B. Saunders, 1984.

oldest old   The term *oldest old* refers to people over 85 years of age—the fastest growing segment of the American population. As the most recent indicator of the progress of the aging population in America, the 85 + age group will have nearly doubled between 1980 and the year 2000, growing to nearly five million persons from only 2.6 million during that time period. Estimates for future years project a continued growth of the oldest old to nearly 13 million persons by 2040.

Altman, L. K. "Science Takes Heed: 'Oldest Old' Post Significant Challenge," in *Aging*, Goldstein, E. C., ed. Vol. 2, Art. 98. Boca Raton, Fl.: Social Issues Resource Series, Inc., 1981.
Rosenwaike, I. "A Demographic Portrait of the Oldest Old," *Milbank Memorial Fund Quarterly: Health and Society*. Vol. 63:2 (Spring, 1985).

oral hygiene (dental care)   The condition of teeth affects the total health of an older individual. Poor oral hygiene can result in loss of appetite and weight and cause mouth infection. Regular dental checkups should be continued, even if all teeth have been removed and dentures fitted. Electric toothbrushes and Waterpiks may be useful in older people whose eyesight and manual dexterity is diminished. Regular flossing is also important to prevent gum disease and cavities. Unfortunately, neglect of teeth in the early years of life leaves a large percentage of older people faced with the prospect of wearing dentures. Dentures must be cleaned daily with running water and a brush. Then they should be soaked each night in some kind of cleaning agent. Dentures should be stored in a safe container to prevent chance of breakage and warpage. A mouthwash or gargle may be refreshing to use regularly. Many older individuals take medications that tend to dry the mouth and lips. Lips should be coated with a light coat of cream or petroleum jelly to protect against cracking.

Gillies, J. *A Guide to Caring for and Coping with Aging Parents*. Nashville: Thomas Nelson Publishers, 1981.

organic brain syndrome (acute reversible dementia)   Organic brain syndrome is the deterioration of the mental or intellectual ability of a person. Generally, organic brain syndrome is preceded by physical problems such as cerebral arteriosclerotic disease, degeneration of nerve tissue, head injuries, reduced blood flow to the brain, a minor stroke, fever, intoxication of alcohol and drugs, nutritional deficiency, metabolic disturbances, pneumonia, myocardial infarction, diabetes, syphilis, renal failure, or fluid and electrolyte imbalances. Organic brain syndrome is usually reversible, which differentiates it from Alzheimer's disease.

Symptoms or organic brain syndrome include impaired judgment, loss of memory, emotional instability, deterioration of the thought process, disorientation, and incoherence. Symptoms may come and go, which is probably related to the amount of blood flow to the brain at any given time.

Treatment involves determining the cause of the condition. Many times the condition is reversible when the underlying medical problem is discovered and treated.

See also ALZHEIMER'S DISEASE.

Rossman, I. *Clinical Geriatrics*, 3rd ed. Philadelphia: J. B. Lippincott Co., 1986.
Scherer, J. C. *Introductory Medical-Surgical Nursing*. Philadelphia: J. B. Lippincott Co., 1986.

orthodontia (braces)   Until recent years, orthodontists believed that anyone past adolescence was not a good candidate for braces. It was believed that teeth could only move within developing bone. Today, adults make up 20 percent to 30 percent of all orthodontic patients. Some are even as old as 70 years of age.

The most common problem of adults is overcrowding complicated by loss of teeth. People who cannot floss between their teeth are prime candidates for cavities, periodontal disease, and loss of teeth. A few years ago, this loss of teeth and resultant need for dentures was considered the price of a long life. But today, following the loss of a tooth, orthodonic treatment may enable the person to save their remaining teeth for the rest of their life.

Technological advances have eliminated the heavy metal wires and brackets of the past except in the most difficult cases. Research in space age metallurgy has developed ultrathin wires that move teeth more efficiently. These wires are lighter and more resilient and patients experience less discomfort when they are tightened during treatment. But even more appealing is the cosmetic effect. Today's appliances are nearly invisible.

Although age itself is no deterrent to orthodontic success, the teeth, gums, and bone structure must be reasonably healthy before treatment can begin. Orthodontia cannot help anyone who has suffered major bone loss of the jaw.

With so much emphasis placed on appearances in today's lifestyles more and more adults are turning to orthodontia.

Peake, J. "Braces—At My Age!" *Modern Maturity*. Aug.–Sept., 1987.

osteitis deformans See PAGET'S DISEASE.

osteoarthritis (arthritis) Osteoarthritis is a noninflammatory degenerative joint disease occurring chiefly in older people. Five percent of individuals over the age of 50 have clinical symptoms of arthritis. By age 60, 15 percent of men and 25 percent of women have clinical symptoms. Causes are not always known but injury to joints, no matter how minor, may predispose to osteoarthritis. This is perhaps due to irregular pressure. Excessive use of a joint for occupation or sport accelerates local changes. Obesity and familial occurence are also factors.

Initial changes occur in the cartilage, which first loses its elasticity and later becomes softened and frayed, losing its ability to cushion the joint. The main symptom is joint pain, which occurs on motion and weight bearing. The pain is characterized as aching and is rarely intense. Decreased range of motion, localized tenderness, and enlargement of the joint are other symptoms. The knees and hips are most commonly affected.

Rest is the primary treatment for osteoarthritis. The use of canes and crutches is helpful when weight-bearing joints are affected. Heat, massage, and isometric exercises are helpful in improving muscle strength around the joint and in preventing atrophy. Analgesics are the usual drug used since agents with greater risks of toxicity are seldom justified because of the need for long-term usage.

Traction and surgery are indicated when severe symptoms are not relieved by other measures. Total joint replacements are usually quite successful and should be considered once a joint has become sufficiently painful or disabling enough to limit the quality of life.

See also ARTHRITIS, RHEUMATOID.
For additional information write or call:
National Arthritis Foundation
1314 Spring Street N.W. #103
Atlanta, GA 30309
1-800-282-7032

Reichel, W. M. *Clinical Aspects of Aging.* Baltimore: The Williams & Wilkins Co., 1979.

osteoporosis (brittle bones) The most prevalent metabolic disease of bone is osteoporosis, a disorder characterized by a decreased volume of bone from reduced calcium levels, resulting in a thinning of the skeleton. Bones are easily fractured with little or no trauma.

Osteoporosis is found in increasing frequency in women over 45 and in men over 55 years of age and affects almost 11 million aged in the United States. It is four times more prevalent in women and very common among Caucasians and northern Europeans.

Lack of estrogen and reduced intake of calcium are thought to be primary factors leading to osteoporosis. Reduced physical activity is now thought to be an equally important reason for bone loss. Drugs and toxins such as heparin, dilantin, corticosteroids, and alcohol may contribute also to the loss of bone. Osteoporosis is also found in certain diseases such as hyperthyroidism, hyperparathyroidism, diabetes, sickle-cell disease, and multiple myeloma.

Osteoporosis is often asymptomatic and is frequently discovered accidentally. Fractures and the collapse of vertebrae can occur insidiously. The patient only becomes aware with the realization that his or her stature has shortened or perhaps when found on an unrelated X-ray. The most frequent symptom is a dull aching in the lower thoracic or lumbar region. The pain is exacerbated by sitting or standing for some time and is usually relieved by lying down.

The loss of height is due to vertebral compression with the resultant "dowager's hump." This progressive deforming process leads to downward angulation of the ribs and a narrowing of the normal gap between the lower ribs and the iliac crest. Measurable reduction in height ceases when the coastal margins come to rest on the iliac crests.

By the time osteoporosis has become symptomatic, it is not possible to restore normal bone mass. Treatment of osteoporosis, therefore, centers around preventing further fractures and deformities and helping the person to continue daily activities. Calcium supplements, estrogen therapy, and fluoride therapy are used with varying degrees of success.

Loss of strength and muscle tone enhances osteoporosis. One of the best preventive and rehabilitative exercises is walking. If a patient is bed-ridden, isometric exercises should be employed until the patient is able to get out of bed and start walking again. Since many fractures occur as the result of a fall, the use of a cane or walker for support should be encouraged. If surgery is necessary, prolonged immobilization should be avoided, since osteoporosis invariable increases with the vicious cycle of pain, rest, and fractures. Intense remedial treatment is suggested utilizing heat applications, range of motion exercises, and whirlpool therapy.

Reichel, W. M. *Clinical Aspects of Aging.* Baltimore: The Williams & Wilkins Co., 1979.
Steinberg, F. U. *Care of the Geriatric Patient,* 6th ed. St. Louis: C. V. Mosby Co., 1983.

otitis media   Otitis media, infection of the middle ear, occurs primarily in childhood but can extend into adulthood, becoming chronic. Incidence of otitis media increase with the occurence of upper respiratory infections. Respiratory infections occur most frequently in those with the least resistance (the very young and very old) and therefore the incidence of otitis media tends to increase as individuals age.

The onset of chronic ear disease is insidious. The patient usually presents with fully developed symptomatic disease with pain and decreased hearing.

Chronic disease of the middle ear has two aspects. The primary disability is due to continuing or recurrent infection of the ear with the symptoms of drainage from the ear. The second area of disability is the attendant loss of hearing due to damage to the sound conduction mechanism and to cochlear damage from toxicity or direct extension of the infectious process.

Culture and sensitivity tests may be indicated, especially if antibiotics have been used for prolonged periods. Corticosteroids may be added to antibiotics to control local allergic manifestations. The addition of heparin is of value to control local histamine response in the tissues. Systemic antibiotics are indicated in acute infections superimposed on the chronic infection. Alcohol should not be used in strengths greater than 70 percent since it is both irritating and painful.

Surgical intervention is indicated in cases with: presence of threatened or an actual complication; presence of irreversible pathologic conditions in the mastoid of middle ear, such as osteomyelitis (bone inflammation), cholesteatoma (cystlike mass), or sequestration (formation of dead bone); lack of response to an adequate medical regimen.

Surgical reconstruction, eradication of irreversible disease, and adequate drainage result in the possibility of aural rehabilitation for many individuals suffering from chronic ear diseases.

See also EXTERNAL OTITIS.

Ballenger, J. J. *Diseases of the Nose, Throat, Ear, Head and Neck,* 13th ed. Philadelphia: Lea & Febiger, 1985.

ovary cancer   See CANCER, OVARIAN.

overweight   See OBESITY.

P

PABA   (para-aminobenzoic   acid)
PABA is an anti-aging remedy that is suppose to reverse graying hair if taken in large doses. Side-effects include nausea, vomiting, and blood disorders.

PABA is usually found in health food stores next to the B vitamins. PABA does not really belong there because it is not a vitamin for people. Some bacteria need it in their diets, but people do not.

Sulfa drugs act by interfering with a bacterium's use of PABA, because of this the use of PABA may inhibit action of antibacterial drugs.

See also AGING, BIOLOGICAL THEORY OF.

Meister, K. A. "The 80's Search for the Fountain of Youth Comes Up Very Dry," In *Aging,* Goldstein, E. C., ed. Vol. 2, Art. 76. Boca Raton, Fl.: Social Issues Resources Series, Inc., 1981.

Paget's Disease (osteitis deformans)
Osteitis deformans (Paget's disease) is a common bone disorder in the elderly. It is characterized by a combination of excessive bone resorption and deposition, which can result in enlargement of the bones and in severe deformity of the skeleton.

Paget's disease can occur at any site but is most commonly found in the tibia (shin bone), the bones of the pelvic girdle, and the skull. Bone enlargements can lead to pressure on other structures, producing deafness, back pain, and paraplegia (paralysis of lower extremities) due to spinal cord compression. Cardiac failure can occur and is usually due to associated ischemic heart disease. Osteogenic sarcoma (cancer of bone) is the most serious complication of Paget's disease but it is rare.

Calcitonin administered in daily doses is used in the treatment of those patients with bone pain, neurological complications, and high-output cardiac failure. Most patients with Paget's disease do not require treatment.

Brocklehurst, J. C. *Textbook of Geriatric Medicine and Gerontology.* New York: Churchill Livingstone, 1985.

pain management   The sensory experience of pain can be categorized as acute pain or chronic pain. Acute pain accompanies an active illness or injury and disappears when the individual recovers from the primary condition. It serves as a warning signal and alerts the patient and physician that something is wrong. All attempts are made to render the patient as comfortable as possible while the primary disorder is diagnosed and treated.

Chronic, or protracted, pain presents a different situation. Many patients with chronic pain have no discernible lesion or illness. More commonly, the severity of the pain is not explained by the disease that is detected. This is commonly found in geriatric patients who face many loses in their life, which force them to constantly adapt to new situations. It becomes easier for them to focus on physical symptoms rather than on the feelings of their loss.

However, it is unquestioned that the elderly must deal more often with chronic pain as a direct result of specific painful physical disorders such as intractable (uncurable) cancer.

Proper therapeutic management is of prime importance with administration of medication on a regularly prescribed schedule rather than sporadically when pain is at its worst.

The patient needs to accept the reality of the effects of chronic pain and the adjustments necessary to cope with daily life. The ability to sleep, the working quality of family life, the degree of independence, and the quality of interpersonal relationships all indicate the degree of adaptability. To achieve this level it may be necessary for some patients to seek psychotherapy either on an individual basis, in group therapy or family counseling.

For many patients with chronic pain, the regular visit to the family physician can be helpful. A sympathetic, caring doctor who can understand what they are suffering and empathize with them can have great meaning to the elderly patient. Family, recreational and church activities are other ways that maintain a patient's involvement with life. The more involved a patient is with other people and activities the less involved will he or she be with matters of pain and illness.

Covington, T., and Walker, J. *Current Geriatric Therapy*. Philadelphia: W. B. Saunders, 1984.

pancreas cancer See CANCER, PANCREATIC.

pantothenic acid Pantothenic acid is a vitamin that is promoted as an anti-aging remedy. Pantothenic acid is considered an anti-aging agent because it is a component of Royal Jelly, the substance that turns female bees into long-lived, fertile queens instead of short-lived, sterile workers. The Life Extention Foundation in Florida has found that large doses of pantothenic acid "extends the life of a black mouse by 20 percent." Though pantothenic acid is found in practically all foods and though it is almost impossible to develop a deficiency of it, it is sold as a vitamin supplement and can be expensive.

See AGING, BIOLOGICAL THEORY OF.

Lardner, J. "The People Who Want to Live Much, Much Longer," in *Aging,* Goldstein, E. C., ed. Vol. 2, Art. 48. Boca Raton, Fl.: Social Issues Resource Series, Inc., 1981.
Meister, K. "The 80's Search For the Fountain of Youth Comes Up Very Dry," In *Aging,* Goldstein, E. C., ed. Vol. 2, Art. 76, Boca Raton, Fl.: Social Issues Resource Series, Inc., 1981.

para-aminobenzoic acid See PABA.

paralysis agitans See PARKINSONISM.

paranoia Paranoia is a psychotic reaction that frequently involves delusions. In the older person, paranoid reactions may result from social isolation or from reduced sensory capabilities. For example, the person with a hearing impairment may not be able to determine what is actually being said and will impart hostile motivations to those who are present. This type of paranoid behavior is fairly common among older people.

Some people will have mild symptoms consisting of, for example, suspecting thievery while searching for articles that have been misplaced or lost. Such thoughts often respond to explanations and reassurance.

Other people are highly delusional and may have visual or auditory hallucinations, hearing or seeing things that do not exist. They frequently think people are playing tricks on them or conspiring against them.

In each case, treatment of the paranoia requires dealing with the underlying cause. This involves correcting visual or hearing defects and use of psychotherapy, tranquilizing drugs, and occasionally, in severe cases, shock therapy.

Elderly paranoid people are rarely dangerous but are often frightened and anxious. A devoted family who encourages the person to pursue treatment can be of invaluable assistance in the management of such cases.

See also ANXIETY.

Steinberg, F. U. *Care of the Geriatric Patient,* 6th ed. St. Louis: C. V. Mosby Co., 1983.

Parkinson's disease   See PARKINSONISM.

Parkinsonism (paralysis agitans, Parkinson's disease)   Parkinsonism is the third most common neurologic problem in the elderly. This disease affects one in 100 persons over the age of 55 of both sexes and of all races.

The cause of Parkinsonism is unknown, although some cases are induced by the use of drugs and encephalitis (inflammation of the brain).

Symptoms of Parkinsonism include tremors that disappear with sleep, rigidity of muscles, slowness of voluntary movement, dizziness, infrequent blinking, expressionless face, distorted posture, drooling, dermatitis, depression, constipation, urinary incontinence, shuffling gait, small cramped handwriting, and hoarse low voice.

Treatment of Parkinsonism is palliative (reducing severity) and symptomatic and depends on the pharmocologic manipulation of the pathophysiologic state. The drug treatment to be used is determined by the severity of the symptoms and the presence of associated diseases. The preferred anticholi-

nergic agents are Artane, Cogentin, Kemadrin, and Akineton. These drugs act selectively on the central anticholinergic activity. The side-effects that may occur include blurring of vision, dryness of mouth and throat, constipation, urinary urgency or retention, ataxia (loss of muscle coordination), and mental disturbances.

Levodopa therapy has dramatically changed the management of Parkinsonism. The side-effects associated with Levodopa include nausea, vomiting, orthostatic hypotension, insomnia, and mental confusion. Frequently an enzyme inhibitor will diminish the side-effects of Levodopa, and that too, may be prescribed. Usually a neurologist or internist, familiar with Levodopa, can properly adjust the dosage of Levodopa and enzyme inhibitors so that the disease is controlled with few side effects.

Surgery is another alternative in the treatment of Parkinson's disease. This experimental surgery consists of adrenal cortex transplantation to the basal ganglion. Many people, however, cannot be surgically treated. The results are best when the person is younger and has unilateral involvement.

The progress of Parkinson's disease may be slowed by improving the general health of the patient. The cure for Parkinson's disease has not been found but several treatments are available that help to decrease the degree of symptoms.

Scherer, J. C. *Introductory Medical-Surgical Nursing,* 3rd ed. Philadelphia: J. B. Lippincott Co., 1982.
Steinberg, F. U. *Care of the Geriatric Patient,* 6th ed. St. Louis: C. V. Mosby Co., 1983.

patient rights   The American Hospital Association has published a booklet of patients' rights. The patients' "bill of rights" is uniform in content at health-care institutions around the country.

1. The patient has the right to considerate and respectful care.

2. The patient has the right to obtain from his or her physician complete current information concerning diagnosis, treatment, and prognosis in terms the patient can be reasonably expected to understand.
3. The patient has the right to receive from his or her physician information necessary to give informed consent prior to the start of any procedure and/or treatment.
4. The patient has the right to refuse treatment to the extent permitted by law, and to be informed of the medical consequences of his or her action.
5. The patient has the right to every consideration of his or her privacy concerning his or her own medical care program. Case discussion, consultation, examination, and treatment are confidential and should be conducted discreetly.
6. The patient has the right to expect that all communications and records pertaining to his or her care should be treated as confidential.
7. The patient has the right to expect that within its capacity a hospital must make reasonable response to the request of a patient for services.
8. The patient has the right to obtain information as to any relationship of his or her hospital to other health-care and educational institutions insofar as his or her care is concerned.
9. The patient has the right to be advised if the hospital proposes to engage in or perform human experimentation affecting his or her care or treatment.
10. The patient has the right to expect reasonable continuity of care.
11. The patient has the right to examine and receive an explanation of his or her bill regardless of source of payment.
12. The patient has the right to know what hospital rules and regulations apply to his or her conduct as a patient.

Seskin, J. *Alone Not Lonely*. Glenview, Il.: Scott, Foresman and Co., 1986.

pensions, public and private plans
Today over 7.1 million federal, state, and local government employees are receiving government pension benefits, and another 13.9 million currently employed by government participate in public employee pension plans. Estimates place 75 percent of nongovernment private company employees as working for companies that offer pension plans, but only 62 percent of men in their fifties and sixties take advantage of such plans, and only 43 percent of both males and females in younger age groups make any use of these opportunities. As recently as 1979, 50 million working persons did not take part in private pension plan coverages.

Failure to participate in private company pension plans can be extremely short-sighted. The vast majority of people who do not participate in such plans are forced to rely on Social Security as their principal, or even exclusive, source of income. As the article on PERSONAL FINANCIAL PLANNING FOR RETIREMENT in the present volume makes clear, SOCIAL SECURITY was never intended, and is not now intended, to supply a total retirement income—rather, it serves as a secure, government-backed foundation upon which individuals may build private savings, annuities, and company pensions to achieve a financially comfortable retirement.

Short-sightedness in individual pension planning can come about in other ways than overreliance on Social Security. People who are self-employed or work for small companies often may not have pension plan coverage. Because many plans require continuous participation for a considerable period of years (10 years is not uncommon), individuals who change jobs frequently, are laid off, or take leaves of absence may not be covered.

In addition, some company pension plans provide a choice between Social Security or the company plan; or, the company plan is combined with Social Security so that the amount of the monthly Social Security check is subtracted from the company pension check. While many people enter retirement expecting a company pension check, until now only about one third of all workers have received them. Good judgment about planning for retirement recommends participating in pension and savings plans for old age.

See also PERSONAL FINANCIAL PLANNING FOR RETIREMENT.

Averyt, A. C. *Successful Aging*. New York: Ballantine Books, 1987.

U.S. Bureau of the Census, *Statistical Abstract of the United States: 1989*, 109th ed. Washington, D.C.: U.S. Government Printing Office.

pension rights for women   A relatively new law protects women; the REA (Retirement Equity Act) went into effect in 1985. In the past, many women lost a share of the husband's pension through widowhood when the husband had failed to provide for the wife as a survivor. Often a widow received nothing from her husband's pension if he died before the date of early retirement. Under the new REA, survivors' benefits continue if a worker dies and a spouse survives. The husband must have the spouse's written consent notarized and witnessed—to eliminate her from survivors' benefits. Also, if a worker leaves employment and returns within five years, the pension credits earned before the break are not lost. This is helpful to people who must take off a few years to care for young children or aging parents.

Averyt, A. C. *Successful Aging*. New York: Ballantine Books, 1987.

periodontal disease (pyorrhea, gum disease)   Periodontal disease (pyorrhea) is inflammation of the gum tissue caused by the presence of plaque and calculus. This results in gingival (gum) inflammation, re-

cession of the gums, pocket formations, and loss of bony support of the teeth. If the infection continues untreated it will spread to the bone in which the teeth are rooted, causing the teeth to detach from their supporting tissue.

Estimates of the incidence of periodontal disease in the over 65 age group range as high as 90 percent. This disease often starts in middle age and is accelerated by systemic disorders such as diabetes, osteoporosis, and metabolic deficiencies.

Symptoms of periodontal disease include gum inflammation, recession of the gum, and loosening of the teeth.

The prevention and treatment of pyorrhea is the key to the preservation of teeth in the elderly. Removal of food plaque and calculus is the initial step in treatment, but good oral hygiene and proper nutrition remain the primary preventive measures. For the person limited by physical disabilities the dentist may suggest modification in tooth brushes and other methods of oral hygiene such as Waterpiks and mouthwashes.

See also CARIES, SENILE.

Steinberg, F. U. *Care of the Geriatric Patient*, 6th ed. St. Louis: C. V. Mosby Co., 1983.

peritonitis   Peritonitis is an inflammation of the peritoneum, the serous sac lining of the abdominal cavity. The intestines normally filled with bacteria are enclosed in the peritoneum. A break in the continuity of the intestines that causes a leakage of the intestinal contents can lead to inflammation and infection of the peritoneum. Peritonitis can be caused by perforation of the appendix or a duodenal ulcer. The infection may be a generalized peritonitis or it may be localized and lead to formation of an abscess.

Severe pain and tenderness usually occurs over the area of the greatest peritoneal inflammation. The location of the pain helps the physician to determine whether the peritonitis is due to a perforation of the appendix or of the duodenum.

A white blood count and differential and an X-ray examination of the abdomen aid in the diagnosis.

Symptoms include severe abdominal pain and tenderness, nausea, and vomiting. The patient may be afebrile (without fever) initially but the temperature rises as the infection becomes established. The pulse becomes rapid and weak and respirations are shallow. Paralytic ileus (lack of intestinal activity) typically accompanies peritonitis with the person's abdomen becoming rigid and boardlike. As the condition progresses the abdomen becomes somewhat softer and very distended with the gas and the intestinal contents that cannot pass normally through the tract. Marked leukocytosis (increase in circulating white blood cells) commonly occurs in peritonitis.

Early diagnosis of conditions such as appendicitis have decreased the incidence of peritonitis. Strict surgical asepsis and use of antibiotics before performing surgery on the intestines have further reduced the number of patients who develop peritonitis as a complication of surgery.

Preventing further leakage of intestinal contents from a duodenal ulcer into the peritoneal cavity can be achieved by surgically closing the duodenum. If intestinal contents are leaking from a ruptured appendix the appendix is removed. Gastrointestinal decompression is used to drain the accumulated gas and intestinal contents.

Replacing fluids and electrolytes is important. Water and electrolytes are lost in vomitus and drainage from the gastrointestinal intubation and the person cannot take anything by mouth. Large quantities of body fluids and electrolytes collect in the peritoneal cavity instead of circulating normally throughout the body, increasing the problems of water and electrolyte imbalance.

Large doses of antibiotics are given to combat infection. Analgesics such as meperidine are often necessary to relieve pain and promote rest.

Scherer, J. C. *Introductory Medical-Surgical Nursing,* 3rd ed. Philadelphia: J. B. Lippincott Co., 1982.

Steinberg, F. J. *Care of the Geriatric Patient,* 6th ed. St. Louis: C. V. Mosby Co., 1983.

personal financial planning for retirement   The first step in sound financial planning for retirement is to recognize early in life that a systematic buildup of funds is essential, and that Social Security alone is not sufficient to support a comfortable retirement. While it is never too late to begin saving for retirement—whether through a company pension plan, buying an annuity, IRA, or Keogh, or other means—ideally retirement saving should start no later than the late thirties or early forties, or sooner if possible. The average person who retires at 65 can expect to live another 20 years (about three years more for women and three years less for men), so funds set aside to provide income during the retirement years must be substantial.

Too many Americans have made the mistake of assuming that Social Security should provide their entire retirement income when in fact it was always intended that individuals should supplement Social Security with their own retirement saving plans. (People who wish to know their probable monthly Social Security income can obtain this information by contacting regional Social Security offices). Social Security makes an excellent financial foundation for retirement because it is government guaranteed and comprehensive in its coverage, but it should be realized that it replaces well below half of the preretirement earnings of the majority of individuals. The table on page 181 shows the percentage of a single person's preretirement income replaced by Social Security.

Financial advisers point out that Social Security makes a good starting point for planning retirement income because it is usually unnecessary to replace 100 percent of the income that one had prior to retire-

Percentage of Income Replaced by Social Security Payments

Preretirement Income	Percentage Replaced
$ 6,500	57%
$10,000	49%
$15,000	42%
$20,000	34%
$30,000	23%
$50,000	14%

ment. Among the reasons for this are the following:

• Social Security itself, which represents anywhere from about 7.5 percent of every paycheck for employees up to about 15 percent for the self-employed, is no longer deducted from one's income. Instead of being withheld, Social Security is now paid over to the retiree.
• Other pensions contributions, either in the form of employer pension plans, personal savings, or both, which may constitute 5 percent or more of income, are no longer deducted, and, like Social Security, now become sources of income.
• Expenses related to holding a job, such as commuting and automobile costs, meals, clothing, etc., are no longer required.
• Standard deductions from income taxes may increase.
• Residential mortgages and household expenses (buying a refrigerator, washing machine, etc.), along with childrearing expenses (school and college, family health insurance, food and clothing for dependents) are often unnecessary.

Financial experts note that living expenses, which are often at their peak during one's forties and fifties when mortgages are not yet paid off and children are in college, tend to decline in the sixties and after. They estimate that these reduced costs all together can easily mount up to 25 percent to 30 percent of the income one received during one's forties and fifties. Consequently, many

retired individuals manage successfully on about 70 percent of the funds they received earlier in life.

Individuals who have maintained private savings need to estimate how much to withdraw from these annually so that their nest egg will last as long as they believe necessary—typically, this might be the 20 to 30 years that they and their spouse can expect to live. For example, if one had $50,000 in certificates of deposit at retirement, one would spend down the entire amount in little more than five years if one thoughtlessly drew out 20 percent, or $10,000, per year. Consequently, some lower withdrawal rate would normally be desirable.

But, if one has savings designed to stretch out for 10 or more years, one also needs to take into account the effect of inflation, now running at from four to five percent per year. As Peter Weaver and Annette Buchanan point out in *What to Do with What You've Got,* a book written under AARP auspices, the dreaded inflation monster can destroy a lifetime of careful planning for financial security in old age because the "Rule of 72" takes effect. This rule is that one divides the inflation rate into 72 to find out how soon one will have to double one's income in order to stay abreast of inflation—if one assumes an inflation rate of 4 percent per year, then one would have to double one's income in 18 years ($72 \div 4 = 18$) in order to offset inflation.

While Social Security offsets inflation through annual cost-of-living adjustments, inflation can be beaten in other ways. It is possible to take an inflation rate into account when estimating how long one wants one's savings to last if one assumes an inflation rate and a specific growth rate for one's savings under a definite withdrawal plan. The chart below shows how many years one's money will last at specified withdrawal rates.

In order to get a general idea of the effect of inflation, add an assumed inflation rate to the withdrawal rate. For example, someone who plans to withdraw 6 percent per year at a 4 percent inflation rate, and projects an annual growth rate of 9 percent, could probably expect to have their nest egg last some-what more than 20 years. (This estimate is only an approximation, and individuals who need more precise figures should consult a qualified accountant or financial planner).

Years Your Money Will Last

Withdrawal Rate	Annual Growth Rate of Funds									
	5%	6%	7%	8%	9%	10%	11%	12%	13%	14%
6%	36									
7%	25	33								
8%	20	23	30							
9%	16	18	22	24						
10%	14	15	17	20	26					
11%	12	13	14	16	19	25				
12%	11	11	12	14	15	18	23			
13%	9	10	11	12	13	15	17	21		
14%	9	9	10	11	11	13	14	17	21	
15%	8	8	9	9	10	11	12	14	16	20

Besides this, annuities and certain employee pension plans provide choices of income options that allow recipients to take the effects of inflation into account. For example, a full annual payout under a plan might be $8,400 per year, but if the individual chooses to receive only $5,000 per year, then the difference ($3,400) could be reinvested to produce a higher rate of income in future years. Some public pension plans for government employees also include an annual increment that may partially offset inflation. Social Security, of course, is adjusted annually for inflation.

While financial advisers outline various ways besides saving and pension contributions to make financial ends meet in retirement (i.e., smart shopping at the supermarket, part-time or temporary employment, an eye for thrift in clothing purchases, etc.), one idea frequently proposed is to "trade down" one's home. Under this plan an individual would sell a still-mortgaged larger home that was bought to house an entire family, and purchase a smaller home with no mortgage and a lower maintenance cost. If the former home was not mortgaged, or part of the funds realized from this transaction remained after purchasing the new home, then the surplus could be invested—in securities, mutual funds, an annuity, government bonds, or other sources—to produce additional cash for retirement income.

Whatever the individual's personal financial circumstances—and these vary almost infinitely—it is obvious that a well-thought-out plan for retirement income is essential. In spite of the variety of individual circumstances, attention to the few areas and principles outlined above will do much to assure a comfortable and secure retirement for most people.

Babson-United Investment Advisors. *United Mutual Fund Selector*. Vol. 21:12, Issue 516 (June 30, 1989).

Quinn, J. B., "Saying the Big Goodbye." *Newsweek* (October 9, 1989).

Luciano, L., and Fenner, E. "Having to Play Catch-Up." *Money* (June, 1991).

Tucker, E. "Annuity Fundamental." *United Retirement Bulletin* (September, 1989).

personality development Contrary to past theories, which described the adult personality as a finished product completed during childhood and early youth, many psychiatrists who work with the elderly now think that personality development continues throughout life.

Psychiatrists now believe that every phrase of development throughout the life cycle is potentially important, each making a unique contribution. The psychic structure undergoes significant change from the childhood tendency toward normality and pathology, determined by the adult experiences.

Scheier, R. L. "Development Continues in Older Adults." *American Medical News* (November 21, 1986).

pets   A variety of studies indicate that pets have a positive influence on human health and contentment. Pets can also help the elderly cope with loneliness and isolation, especially when they live alone.

Comprehensive studies conducted on coronary care patients reveal that the mortality rate of patients with pets was one third that of patients who did not have pets. Loneliness seems to contribute significantly to heart disease. Having and caring for a pet seems to ease the loneliness.

Pets seem to have a calming effect on the cardiovascular system. Blood pressure and heart rates are measurably lower when a pet is in the room. Some patients' blood pressure fell below resting levels when they gently stroked their pets. Even gazing at an aquarium of fish made a significant difference.

Hospitals, nursing homes, and psychiatric facilities are using birds and fish for their proven effectiveness in a patient's recovery from a variety of mental and physical disorders. The University of San Francisco's School of Nursing offers a course to all third-year nursing students in the care and handling of animals as a therapeutic method of treating patients.

A pet providing nonjudgmental and nondemanding friendship is perhaps the primary concern of a lonely aged person. The effects of lowered heart rates, lower blood pressure, and a calming influence are of greater interest to health-care professionals. They recognize that animal companionship makes a very real difference in a patient's chances for long-term survival.

Lynch, J. J. "Man's Best Friendly Medicine." *Creative Living* 16: 16–20 (1987).

pharmacokinetics   (see Table 10, 11) Pharmacokinetics is the action of drugs in the body over a period of time. Drugs administered orally are absorbed into the blood, distributed by circulation throughout the body and eliminated by detoxification in the liver and by excretion in the urine and bile. Drugs administered topically exert a local effect, although absorption into the blood stream may lead to an intended distant action, such as with nitroglycerin, or with an unintended action, as with systemic absorption of atropine. Parental administration (injection) bypasses gastrointestinal absorption, to be absorbed into the circulation.

Most drugs are absorbed from the gastrointestinal tract. They are usually given in tablet or capsule form, their solubility and rate of dissolution will affect absorption. Other factors that influence gastrointestinal absorption include the structure of the absorptive surface and the metabolic activity of the absorptive cells.

Age changes in gastrointestinal function influences the rate and completeness of drug absorption. Diminished gastric secretion may retard dissolving of tablets, the higher pH may reduce the solubility and absorption of some drugs such as tetracycline and reduce the effectiveness of others such as penicillin. Age-related changes that may impair drug absorption include delayed gastric emptying and reduced gastrointestinal blood flow.

The reported effects of aging on gastric emptying time are conflicting. Absorption is affected by drugs that alter the rate of gastric emptying. Many drugs prescribed for the elderly either accelerate or retard gastric emptying. Anticholinergic agents (agents that block the passage of nerve impulses) such as paracetamal, sulfamethiazole, and riboflavin retard gastric emptying and the delivery of drugs to the upper small intestine where most absorption occurs. Conversely, metoclopramide stimulates upper gastrointestinal motility, accelerating the absorptions of paracetamal, tetracycline, lithium carbonate, and levodopa. Digoxin absorption from the upper gastrointestinal tract depends upon the form in which digoxin is administered.

Some drugs are better absorbed when given together with drugs that reduce gastrointestinal motility, allowing longer contact with the absorptive surface. When multiple drugs are used, reduced absorption due to binding or inactivation may occur: antacids decrease absorption of digoxin, salicylates, and tetracycline; cholestyramine binds oral anticoagulants, cardiac glycosides, and thyroid preparations.

When drugs are given with food the possibility of food-drug interaction exists: tea and orange juice respectively decrease and increase the absorption of iron, and acidic fruit juices and carbonated beverages inactivate many drugs, such as penicillin, and mineral oil containing laxatives causes malabsorption of fat soluble vitamins.

Brocklehurst, J. C. *Textbook of Geriatric Medicine and Gerontology*. New York: Churchhill Livingstone, 1985.

ping pong See TENNIS, BADMINTON, AND PING PONG.

pituitary removal One theory of aging proposes that the pituitary gland, the main gland in the endocrine system, releases what are called "death hormones." The theory proposes that these hormones play a significant role in aging. To test the theory, scientists removed the pituitary glands of rats and gave them hormone supplements to keep them alive. If the pituitary gland is removed early in the life of the rat, the rat lives substantially longer. The treated rats show retarded aging of collagen (a main supportive protein in skin, tendon, bone, cartilage, and connective tissue) and better kidney and immune systems. However, many of the rat strains that were studied were atypical because they tend to develop pituitary tumors late in life. Also, the rats whose pituitary glands were removed weighed less than the untreated rats, which may explain their longevity. This has not been used in humans.

See also AGING, BIOLOGICAL THEORY OF.

Kurz, M. A. "Theories of Aging and Popular Claims for Extending Life," in *Aging*, Goldstein, E. C., ed. Vol. 2, Art. 1. Boca Raton, Fl.: Social Issues Resource Series, Inc., 1981.

plastic surgery See COSMETIC SURGERY.

pneumonia Pneumonia is an acute illness caused by inflammation or infection of the lungs. It can occur in any season but is most common during winter and early spring. People of any age are susceptible, but it is more common among infants and the elderly. Pneumonia is often caused by aspiration of infected materials into the distal bronchioles and alveoli. People who are highly susceptible include those whose respiratory defense mechanisms are damaged, those with chronic obstructive lung disease, influenza, and tracheostomy (opening through the neck into the windpipe) patients who have recently had anesthesia, and alcoholics. Nasocomial pneumonia (acquired in the hospital) increasingly is a cause of mortality due to an increase in the number of patients with impaired defenses resulting from certain types of therapy and an increase in the number of patients on respirators.

Pneumonia is a communicable disease. The mode of transmission is dependent on the infecting organism. Pneumonia is classified according to the offending organism rather than anatomic location.

Typical or classic pneumonia is found in those with diminished defense mechanisms, recent respiratory tract infection or viral influenza.

Symptoms include sudden onset with a shaking chill, fever, pleuritic chest pain, and productive cough. Sputum is greenish and purulent (puslike) and may be blood tinged. Respirations are rapid and shallow with fine inspiratory crackling rales (abnormal breathing sounds).

Diagnosis is made by physical examination, sputum culture and sensitivity studies, chest x-ray, and complete blood count.

Treatment is primarily supportive. It includes bed rest and fluids in large quantities. If the patient is unable to tolerate oral fluids, intravenous fluids are given.

Humidification, by a cool-mist vaporizer, of inspired air is usually helpful in liquifying secretions. Oxygen may be administered by nasal prong or mask to relieve dyspnea (shortness of breath). Coughing and deep breathing are encouraged to expand the lungs and raise sputum. Analgesics are given to reduce temperature. Codeine may be given for chest pain.

Atypical pneumonia is most commonly caused by mycoplasma pneumoniae. *Legionella pneumophila,* the organism causing Legionnaire's disease, occurs most commonly in older adults and in people who smoke. Predisposing conditions include chronic renal disease, chronic bronchitis, emphysema, diabetes, cancer, immunosuppressive medications, and smoking. About 25,000 cases of Legionnaires' disease occur annually.

Onset of symptoms is gradual. The patient experiences malaise, headache, sore throat, dry cough, and soreness of the chest wall. Patients with Legionella infections may also have abdominal pain, diarrhea, and respiratory distress. Increased temperature and shaking chills are also common.

Treatment for infection by mycoplasma pneumoniae and *Legionella pneumophila* is erythromycin or rifampin.

Aspiration pneumonia is caused by the aspiration of material into the airways. Non-infectious aspiration pneumonia is caused by aspiration of gastric acid; even a small amount can cause severe respiratory distress. If a bacterial infection occurs it usually manifests itself in 48 to 72 hours. Aspiration of large quantities of inert substances such as water, barium, and tube-feeding liquids obstruct the airway and cause respiratory distress. A secondary infection may occur in obstructed airways.

Bacterial aspiration pneumonia occurs in patients who have consciousness disorders such as anesthesia, coma, seizures, or excessive alcoholism. It occurs in other patients who also have a poor cough mechanism.

The clinical course is mild and gradual in early stages. Symptoms include a cough and low-grade fever over several days or weeks, progressing to expectoration of large amounts of foul-smelling sputum.

Aspiration pneumonia acquired in the hospital may be insidious in onset. Early symptoms may be fever and mild tachypnea.

Treatment is symptomatic and includes measures used in the treatment of classic pneumonia.

Two vaccines are available to prevent respiratory infections. They should be given to people with a high risk of developing complications of pneumonia, those with chronic heart or lung disease and people 65 or older. Strict adherence to handwashing is a major preventive measure.

Scherer, J. C. *Introductory Medical-Surgical Nursing,* 3rd ed. Philadelphia: J. B. Lippincott Co., 1982.
Steinberg, F. U. *Care of the Geriatric Patient,* 6th ed. St. Louis: C. V. Mosby Co., 1983.

pneumonia immunization See IMMUNIZATION IN THE ELDERLY.

pollutants Pollution is often believed to be a factor in premature aging. Air pollution, as a cause of chronic pulmonary disease, might speed up the decline of ventilatory performances usually associated with aging. The risk of air pollution is not limited to industrialized areas. For example, to keep warm during cold nights, the natives from the highlands of New Guinea burn fires in small closed huts. They inhale extremely high levels of smoke. As a result, in this study pulmonary disease appears at an early age and is present in 78 percent of the subjects over 40.

Brocklehurst, J. C. *Textbook of Geriatric Medicine and Gerontology.* New York: Churchill Livingstone, 1985.

polymyalgia rheumatica   Polymyalgia rheumatica is a condition found primarily in elderly women and is characterized by pain and stiffness in the proximal muscles, particularly in the upper limbs. There is usually an underlying systemic disorder with malaise, weight loss, anemia, and an elevated erythrocyte sedimentation rate (erythrocyte sedimentation rate is how fast red blood cells settle in a test tube during a certain length of time.) In about 15 percent of cases there is an association with giant-cell arteritis.

Treatment consists of daily doses of steroids. Improvement occurs within 72 hours but complete recovery of symptoms takes approximately a year.

See also ARTERITIS, GIANT CELL.

Brocklehurst, J. C. *Textbook of Geriatric Medicine and Gerontology.* New York: Churchhill Livingstone, 1985.

Polynesians   The Polynesians have a traditional diet of breadfruit, taro, pulaka, fish, and coconut, with chicken and pork on special occasions. Their major sources of activity are farming, canoe building and fishing. Fifty-six percent of their caloric intake is made up of saturated fat, yet their cholesterol intake is small. Their weight rises steadily with age until 45 to 54 and then declines. There is an increase of skinfold-thickness in both sexes. In young adults the serum cholesterol levels range from 184.5–198.2 mg.

The serum cholesterol levels rise with age until they peak between 220.4–254.4 mg— high according to recommended U.S. standards. Triglycerides also increase with age. Blood pressure rises slowly with age. Angina pectoris and myocardial infarction are also present in the population. High cholesterol, triglycerides, and blood pressure promote heart disease, and the Polynesian diet may contribute to premature death.

See also MASAI; NEW GUINEAN HIGH-LANDERS; SOLOMON ISLAND TRIBES; SOMALI CAMEL HERDSMEN; TARAHUMARA INDIANS; YANOMANO INDIANS.

Brocklehurst, J. C. *Textbook of Geriatric Medicine and Gerontology.* New York: Churchhill Livingstone, 1985.

polypharmocotherapy   Polypharmocotherapy is the use of multiple drug therapies for treatment of diseases. The elderly consume a disproportionately high amount of medication when compared to the general population. The over-65 age group represents 11 percent of the United States' population but consumes over 25 percent of all drugs prescribed. Chronic diseases that respond to drug therapy are prevalent in the elderly and multiple diseases are the rule, not the exception. Therefore, it can be expected that the elderly would take more medicines and for longer periods of time.

Health-care professionals should carefully question a patient on the medications that are being used, both prescription and non-prescription. Though multiple drug therapy is unavoidable, each drug added to a treatment program increases the potential for adverse effects, including problems from drug interaction and drug abuse by the patient. With patients being treated by several physicians and other health-care personnel, one must be extremely vigilant of a patient's current drug therapy so as to avoid any unnecessary drug exposure.

See also MEDICATION, NONCOMPLIANCE; MEDICATION, SELF.

Covington, T., and Walker, J. *Current Geriatric Therapy*. Philadelphia: W. B. Saunders, 1984.

positive attitude Contrary to popular belief, aging is not a disease. It is believed that the prescription for long life is good nutrition, plenty of exercise, adequate sleep, and a positive attitude.

Much research is currently being done about the effect of mental attitude on the course of disease. Norman Cousins is probably one of the better-known authors who advocate positive attitude and "the will to live" as essential for recovery from major illnesses. It is well known that some people can be given a placebo and get better. These people think that they are going to recover and they do. This is true for productive longevity also. A positive attitude can be a self-fulfilling prophecy; if individuals want and believe they can have a long life they will have it.

Generally, the older person who remains involved and active is healthier, lives longer, and certainly gets more out of the later years of life. The old saying "you are as old as you feel" can apply to almost every older individual.

All individuals should live each day to its fullest and dwell on what they can do instead of what they are unable to do.

The ultimate tragedy in an individual's life is not dying, but what is allowed to die while he or she is living.

See also AUTOGENIC TRAINING; BIOFEED-BACK TRAINING; GESTALT DREAM ANALYSIS; HATHA YOGA; MEDITATION; SELF-IMAGE EXERCISE; TAI CHI CHUAN.

Cousins, N. *Anatomy of an Illness as Perceived by the Patient*. New York: W. W. Norton & Co., 1979.

power-of-attorney See LEGAL REPRESENTATIVE.

premature death reduction The risks of premature death from chronic diseases can be reduced by abstaining from cigarette smoking, avoiding alcohol abuse, exercising regularly, avoiding or correcting serious obesity, and scrupulously following physicians' instructions for treatment of existing chronic conditions such as diabetes or hypertension. Accidental death can be reduced by never driving under the influence of drugs or alcohol, always using safety belts, and paying attention to safety precautions in all activities. These safety precautions include everything from installing smoke alarms in the home to following water safety rules to reading the directions before using any potentially dangerous product.

Meister, K. "The 80's Search For the Fountain of Youth Comes Up Very Dry," in *Aging*, Goldstein, E. C., ed. Vol. 2, Art. 76. Boca Raton, Fl.: Social Issues Resource Series, Inc., 1981.

premature ventricular contractions (PVCs) Premature ventricular contractions are ventricular ectopic (abnormal) beats that occur before depolarization (heart contraction) of the ventricles (two largest cavities of the heart) when an atrial impulse is due. Although premature ventricular contractions are seen in healthy people, the incidence and frequency of occurrence are higher for the elderly and those with heart disease. Premature ventricular contractions are associated with stress, acidosis (increase of hydrogen, causing an abnormal state of reduced alkalinity in the body), ventricular enlargement, myocardial infarction, digitalis toxicity, and hypoxemia (lack of oxygen in blood).

Symptoms of premature ventricular contractions include palpitations, anxiety, fatigue, and confusion.

Treatment for premature ventricular contractions are usually necessary if there are more than 5 PVCs per minute or if the PVCs are chained together.

Pharmacologic suppression of premature ventricular contractions is most often accom-

plished with lidocaine, quinidine, disopyr-
amide, or procainamide.

See also ARRHYTHMIAS, CARDIAC.

Phipps, W. J., et al. *Medical Surgical Nursing.*
St. Louis: C. V. Mosby Co., 1983.
Scherer, J. C. *Introductory Medical-Surgical
Nursing.* Philadelphia: J. B. Lippincott Co.,
1982.

prenuptial property agreement Prenuptial property agreements can have advantages for people who marry in later life. A
spouse of only a few months may become
unexpectedly burdened with enormous medical costs if the partner suddenly has a stroke
or becomes mentally disoriented and there
is no help forthcoming from the family.
Keeping "before marriage" assets in one's
own name during the marriage can make a
difference if application is made for Medicaid assistance for a spouse in a nursing
home. Should the late-life romance prove
unsatisfactory *and* end in divorce, a prenuptial agreement can assure that no one is
left without any financial resources.

Nauton, E. "Elderly Marriages . . . Till Money
Do Us Part," in *Aging,* Goldstein, E. C., ed.
Vol. 1, Art. 58. Boca Raton, Fl.: Social Issues
Resource Series, Inc., 1981.

presbycusis (hearing loss) Presbycusis
is the loss of hearing that accompanies advancing age. This nerve type hearing loss in
older people has been attributed to atrophy
of the end-organ, neural degeneration, vascular changes in the stria vascularis (fibrous
tissue that covers the cochlea duct), or other
changes in the inner ear.

Etiology of this condition has not been
clearly established but the role of circulation,
nutrition, heredity, tissue changes, climate,
accumulative exposure to daily noise, and
the stress of modern civilization all have
been suggested as contributing factors.

In some people, presbycusis may be com-
pounded by the presence of a treatable disorder such as diabetes, multiple sclerosis and

metabolic disorders, or the toxicity of the
use of certain drugs. Drugs that are known
to cause hearing loss after prolonged use are
aspirin, quinine, caffeine, aminoglycosides,
and other antibiotics and some diuretics.
Often a change in the drug will alleviate the
problem.

Symptoms are minimal for most of these
patients because of the slow progression of
the hearing loss. Loss of higher-frequency
sounds associated with high-pitched tinnitus
is an early symptom.

Family members and friends are usually
more aware of the problem than the patient
is. They have learned to speak more clearly,
loudly, and slowly to the patient. Older
people may also unknowingly have learned
to engage in face-to-face conversation, and
to eliminate as many external noises as possible.

The patient may begin to withdraw from
outside contacts and social encounters because of his or her inability to hear or understand conversation. Frequently, patients
resist rehabilitative efforts, possibly because
of the supposed stigma of a handicap created
by wearing a hearing aid. It is important for
these patients to maintain hope and realize
that hearing loss is not always progressive
and that many advances are continually being
achieved through research.

Ballenger, J. J. *Diseases of the Nose, Throat,
Ear, Head and Neck,* 13th ed. Philadelphia:
Lea & Febiger, 1985.

presbyopia Presbyopia is the gradual loss
of the ability of the lens of the eye to focus
from distance to near. This accommodation
loss occurs in everyone and is related entirely to age. As a result most people read
without difficulty until the age of 40. The
focusing ability continues to decrease until
approximately age 65 to 70, at which time
it is stabilized and subsequently changes
very little.

The chief symptom of presbyopia is an
inability to see near work. The person must

hold objects farther and farther away to see them clearly, thus, the frequent complaint is "my arms are too short." Other symptoms include headaches and ocular discomfort.

Treatment for presbyopia involves reading glasses for those people without any other refractive error or a bifocal added to the distant correction for people with distant refractive errors. One relatively new innovation is bifocals without lines. Many older people prefer this alternative as they feel bifocals with a line are reflective of their age.

See also ASTIGMATISM; HYPEROPIA; MYOPIA.

Newell, F. W. *Ophthalmology Principles and Concepts,* 6th ed. St. Louis: C. V. Mosby Co., 1986.

Slatt, B. J., and Stein, H. A. *The Ophthalmic Assistant Fundamentals and Clinical Practice,* 4th ed. St. Louis: C. V. Mosby Co., 1983.

pressure sores See DECUBITI.

preventive medicine Preventive medicine, practiced while the patient is well, can help protect health in the future. The following recommendations for check-ups and preventive activities make good sense.

For Everyone:
1. Establish relations with a primary-care physician (for physical exams and routine care).
2. Don't smoke.
3. Drink alcohol in moderation (no more than five drinks a week; two drinks at a sitting).
4. Maintain a healthy diet (low fat, low salt, high fiber).
5. Exercise regularly, within safe limits.
6. Wear seat belts.
7. Minimize stress.
8. Avoid excess weight.
9. Watch for changing skin moles.
10. Obtain tetanus-diptheria booster every 10 years.
11. Check hearing every five years.
12. Test for glaucoma every two years (unless there is a family history of glaucoma, then check yearly).
13. Check blood pressure at least every year.
14. Schedule basic physical exam every one to two years.
15. Secure a stool occult blood test every year.
16. Submit to a proctosigmoidoscopy (instrument used to view rectum and the lumen of sigmoid colon) every three to five years.
17. Undergo stress test before starting strenuous exercise program.

For Women Over Age 50:
1. Have breasts annually examined by a physician; perform breast self-exams monthly.
2. Have a mammogram every one to two years.
3. Have a digital rectal and pelvic exam every year.
4. Get a pap smear every year.
5. Discuss estrogen replacement therapy with physician.
6. Insure adequate calcium intake (1,200 to 1,500 mg per day).
7. Schedule an EKG every five years.

For Men Over Age 50:
1. Have digital rectal and prostate exam every year.
2. Schedule an EKG every five years.

Modern Maturity, AARP (Feb/March, 1987).

progeria Progeria is a genetic disorder that causes children to age at a greatly accelerated rate. Until age six months, they appear normal. Then they begin to lose their hair, including eyebrows and eyelashes, their joints bulge, bones begin to disintegrate, muscles shrivel, the skin wrinkles, and they grow thin. By early teens, the victims look as if they are in their nineties and soon die, usually of athersclerosis, a disease of the elderly.

Researchers are studying progeria cases in hope of learning what causes the aging process. Some scientists believe that aging is inevitable and is written in our genetic code. Others believe that aging is a disease of the immunological system and can be altered.

Research into aging is at a very early stage but workers in the field believe that understanding progeria will help aging research.

Dolnick, E. "Pioneering Research On the Aging Process Yields Contradictory Theories, Prospects," in *Aging*, Goldstein, E. C., ed. Vol. 2, Art. 39. Boca Raton, Fl.: Social Issues Resource Series, Inc., 1981.

prostate cancer   See CANCER, PROSTATE.

prostate hypertrophy, benign The prostate gland is an accessory organ that produces most of the seminal fluid. The prostate is located just below the outlet of the urinary bladder. The urinary stream travels through the center of the gland in the prostatic urethra. With advancing age and the influence of male sex hormones the periurethral (surrounding urethra) glandular tissues undergoes hyperplasia, with gradual enlargement of the gland. The inward encroachment of this tissue decreases the diameter of the prostate urethra.

Urinary flow is increasingly diminished as the prostate enlarges, thus these symptoms appear gradually. The patient may notice that it takes more effort to void and there is decreasing force and narrowing of the urinary stream. The residual urine remaining in the bladder accumulates, the bladder fills more quickly, and the urge to void occurs more and more frequently. Urgency, to the point of incontinence, may occur. Difficulty in starting the stream and hematuria (blood in urine) may occur. Residual urine is a good culture medium for bacteria, and if infection results, symptoms of cystitis (bladder inflammation) will be present. The combination of symptoms, i.e., hesitancy, narrowed stream, straining to void, frequency, urgency, and nocturia is known as prostat-

ism. Any obstruction in the lower urinary tract can cause these symptoms, but the most common is prostatic enlargement.

Digital examination will reveal that the gland is enlarged. Cystoscopy (examination with a scope) will show the extent of the enlargement on the urethra and the effects on the bladder. Intravenous and retrograde pyelograms (X-rays of renal pelvis and ureter) will reveal possible damage to the upper urinary tract due to the backup of urine. These X-ray dye tests help demonstrate the amount of damage present. Blood chemistry tests such as serum creatinine are ordered to determine kidney function. Prolonged obstruction at the bladder neck can result in renal damage.

Symptomatic benign prostatic hypertrophy is treated surgically by removing part of the prostate gland. A transurethral resection (TUR) is the easiest type of prostate surgery because there is no external incision. Following a prostatectomy, hematuria (blood in urine) is generally present; frank (massive) bleeding is a serious emergency and a potential complication following surgery.

See also CANCER, PROSTATE; INCONTINENCE; URINARY TRACT INFECTIONS.

Scherer, J. C. *Introductory Medical-Surgical Nursing*, 3rd ed. Philadelphia: J. B. Lippincott Co., 1982.
Steinberg, F. U. *Care of the Geriatric Patient*, 6th ed. St. Louis: C. V. Mosby Co., 1983.

pruritus (itching of the skin) Pruritus is a skin disorder with a variety of causes, including allergy, parasitic infestations, diabetes mellitus, liver disorders, and emotional distress. One type of pruritus that occurs in older individuals is caused by a degeneration of the skin. Pruritus without lesions is generally due to an internal problem such as diabetes mellitus, liver disorder, psychiatric disturbance, or the use of certain drugs such as tetracycline or alcohol.

The most common type in an older individual is pruritus with lesions, and this is caused by the skin's inability to retain water.

If pruritus occurs in the genital areas it may be caused by infection or infestation, but if these are ruled out, the abrasiveness of the dye in toilet tissue should be considered. Other causes may include allergy to detergents or soaps and the use of synthetic underwear. Cotton underwear absorbs perspiration and allows air to circulate better.

Symptoms of pruritus include dry scaly skin, itching, skin lesions, and a slight decrease of the sensation of the skin.

Treatment of pruritus should first involve determining the cause. With successful treatment of underlying systemic problems, pruritus often will disappear. Pruritus caused by drugs will usually disappear when the drugs are discontinued.

Pruritus caused by degeneration of the skin may be treated with many things. Increasing the humidity in the home environment is useful. Using a humidifier or vaporizer in homes with central heat or air is helpful. Bathing less frequently in water that is not extremely hot is usually recommended. Oil-based soaps such as Dove or Caress and bath oils or mineral oil in the bath water should be used. It is important to remember when using bath oils there is a risk of injury from slipping in the tub.

Topical applications of lotions or oils have a great therapeutic value. Sometimes antihistamines and systemic steroids will control symptoms more rapidly.

Pruritus caused by skin degeneration in the older person is not curable but is treatable. When any of the above treatments are used all symptoms may disappear, but if treatment is discontinued they may reappear.

Brocklehurst, J. C. *Textbook of Geriatric Medicine and Gerontology*. New York: Churchhill Livingstone, 1985.

pterygium   A pterygium is a fibrovascular wing-shaped connective tissue growth encroaching on the cornea from the nasal conjunctiva in the interpalpebral fissure (opening between eyelids). There is no evidence to pinpoint a specific cause of a pterygium but people who seem to be the most susceptible are those who spend most of their lives outdoors in sunny, dusty, sandy, and windy areas. Pterygium is probably an irritative phenomenon due to ultraviolet light. A pterygium progresses as a person ages, developing slowly through years of exposure to sunlight, wind, and dust.

Initially there may be signs of chronic conjunctivitis, thickening of the conjunctiva, and symptoms of a mild conjunctivitis. The cosmetic appearance is usually the only complaint.

In the temperate zone of the United States pterygia seldom progress rapidly and usually require no treatment. If surgery is needed, it responds well to any surgical procedure. In tropical areas pterygia progress rapidly, are commonly thick and vascular, and have a tendency to recur irrespective of the type of surgery.

Treatment consists of surgical excision of the pterygium if it encroaches on the cornea. After surgical intervention, antibiotic ointment is instilled, and a firm patch is applied to eliminate any bleeding. A Beta radiation application can be given if it appears that it will regrow.

Boyd-Monk, H., and Steinmetz, C. G. *Nursing Care of the Eye*. Los Altos, CA: Appleton & Lange, 1987.
Newell, F. W. *Ophthalmology Principles and Concepts*, 6th ed. St. Louis: C. V. Mosby Co., 1986.

ptosis (blepharoptosis, droopy lid)
Ptosis is the relaxation of the upper lid and narrowing of the palpebral fissure (opening between eyelids). Senile ptosis is most frequently caused by a decreased muscle tone and relaxation of the skin.

Symptoms of senile ptosis include a decrease in the visual field, a foreign body sensation if the lashes are pushed onto the cornea (trichiasis), and the cosmetic aspect of a droopy eyelid.

Treatment involves surgical shortening of the levator palpebrae muscle of the upper eyelid. If the pupils are not covered by the eyelids, surgery may be delayed for a period of time.

Newell, F. W. *Ophthalmology Principles and Concepts,* 6th ed. St. Louis: C. V. Mosby Co., 1986.
Slatt, B. J., and Stein, H. A. *The Ophthalmic Assistant Fundamentals and Clinical Practice,* 4th ed. St. Louis: C. V. Mosby Co., 1983.

pulmonary disease, drug-induced   The elderly are at greater risk for pulmonary complications from drugs because they are more likely to be suffering from diseases that require treatment with drugs that can produce pulmonary toxicity. They are also more likely to have decreased pulmonary function due to aging or progressive respiratory disease.

The most common drug-induced respiratory complication is asthma (bronchospasm); aspirin and Beta blockers are most commonly the responsible drugs. Many of the anticancer drugs are likely to produce pulmonary responses, as are central nervous system depressants. The degree of respiratory depression is primarily dose-related.

To prevent or lessen drug-induced pulmonary depressions, health-care personnel need to be aware of the possible complications of a given drug and carefully monitor the patient who may be at risk. The lowest possible dose that will provide the desired response should be employed.

Covington, T., and Walker, J. *Current Geriatric Therapy.* Philadelphia: W. B. Saunders, 1984.

pulmonary edema, acute   Acute pulmonary edema is the accumulation of excessive fluid in cells, tissues, or serous cavities.

Acute pulmonary edema is an acute emergency condition most often associated with heart disease. It can also be caused by inhalation of an irritant and too rapid an administration of plasma or intravenous fluids.

In pulmonary edema, cardiac output is decreased, causing an increase in left atrial pressure. This results in an increase in pulmonary vein and capillary pressure. As the pulmonary capillary pressure exceeds the intravascular osmotic pressure, serous fluid is rapidly forced into the lung. The person literally begins to drown in his or her own secretions.

Symptoms of acute pulmonary edema include profound dyspnea (shortness of breath), pallor, cyanosis (bluish color due to deficient oxygen of blood), tachycardia (rapid heart beat), wheezing, anxiety, restlessness, productive cough (pinkish, frothy sputum), and moist respirations (gurgling).

The goals of treatment for pulmonary edema include physical and mental relaxation, improvement of cardiovascular function, relief of hypoxemia (lack of oxygen in arterial blood), and decreased venous return. Morphine or Demerol is given intravenously to provide relaxation. Supplemental oxygen is administered and aminophylline may be used to dilate the bronchi and make breathing easier. Measures to retard venous return to the heart include a wet phlebotomy (the removal of blood from a vein), or a dry phlebotomy (rotating tourniquets). The purpose of rotating tourniquets is to pool blood in the extremities, causing a reduction in cardiac load. The tourniquets are placed on three extremities and rotated every 15 minutes.

Since acute pulmonary edema is frequently a complication of congestive heart failure, the treatment for congestive heart failure is also necessary. This treatment includes the administration of diuretics and digoxin, bed rest, and a salt-restricted diet.

See also CONGESTIVE HEART FAILURE.

Phipps, W. J., *et al. Medical Surgical Nursing.* St. Louis: C. V. Mosby Co., 1983.
Steinberg, F. U. *Care of the Geriatric Patient,* 6th ed. St. Louis: C. V. Mosby Co., 1983.

pulmonary embolus   Pulmonary embolism is the lodgement of a foreign substance such as a clot or particle of fat in a pulmonary arterial vessel. The source of the embolism may be a thrombi (clot) originating in the iliac, femoral, or pelvic veins. They are common in older people who are confined to bed. Predisposing conditions to pulmonary embolism are recent surgery, fracture, or trauma of the lower extremities, and a debilitating disease.

Pulmonary emboli almost always occur suddenly. The size of the pulmonary artery and number of emboli determine the severity of the symptoms. If the embolus blocks the pulmonary artery or one of its main branches, immediate death may occur.

Symptoms of a pulmonary embolism include severe chest pain, dyspnea, cyanosis, tachycardia, and shock. When a smaller area of the lung is involved, symptoms are less severe and may include pain, tachycardia, and dyspnea. Fever, cough, and blood-streaked sputum may also be present.

The diagnosis is made by the clinical history, chest film, lung scans, and pulmonary angiography. In addition, EKGs and serum enzymes may assist in the diagnosis.

Treatment of a pulmonary embolus will depend on the size of the area involved. Intravenous heparin is started to prevent extension of the thrombus and to prevent the formation of additional thrombi. Placing the patient in high Fowler's position usually helps his or her breathing. This position is elevation of the head of the bed and placement of the patient in a semisitting position.

A pulmonary embolectomy (cut made in an artery to remove a blood clot) using a cardiopulmonary bypass may be necessary if the clot is lodged in a main pulmonary artery.

Prevention includes exercises to strengthen leg muscles and prevent venous thrombus formation and early ambulation after surgery.

Scherer, J. C. *Introductory Medical-Surgical Nursing*. Philadelphia: J. B. Lippincott Co., 1982.

purpura, senile   See BRUISES.

PVCs   See PREMATURE VENTRICULAR CONTRACTIONS.

pyorrhea   See PERIODONTAL DISEASE.

R

radiation, ionizing   Although it has been claimed that radiation causes accelerated aging, there is no evidence to support it. In laboratory animals, chronic radiation causes an increased mortality rate. Although there is an increase in mortality rates, there does not seem to be an acceleration of the aging process. The laboratory animals did not show any of the physiological changes of aging before they died. People who are born and live permanently in areas with radioactivity do not appear to age more quickly than others.

Brocklehurst, J. C. *Textbook of Geriatric Medicine and Gerontology*. New York: Churchhill Livingstone, 1985.

radio   Seventy-five percent of the older population listens to the radio one to four hours per day, suggesting that this is a favorite medium for many older people. Radio stations tend to target their programming to smaller audiences and this allows a person to choose a favorite, whether it be classical music, religious, ethnic, 24-hour news or talk show stations. Many older listeners enjoy the interviews and may phone in questions and responses to the talk shows regularly. Some radio stations provide programs during which books are read, congressional hearings are covered, and dramatic works are aired. National Public Radio broadcasts ''From the Bookshelf'' five days a week, an excellent way to ''read'' current best sellers.

Shortwave reception is better than ever, although it does require special equipment. Older individuals can enjoy conversing with people in Moscow, London, Paris, or other cities around the world.

Fromme, A. *Life After Work*. Glenview, Ill.: AARP, 1984.

Gillies, J. *A Guide to Caring for and Coping with Aging Parents*. Nashville: Thomas Nelson Publishers, 1981.

reading Books have always been excellent ways to deal with isolation, depression and curiosity. Reading may be a good activity to help fill the days of older individuals.

For older people with decreased vision, libraries have hundreds of books in all categories printed in large type. The *Reader's Digest* and *The New York Times Magazine* both have large-print editions and are available both at libraries or through subscription.

Libraries also lend tapes and records while National Public Radio provides excellent access to best sellers with the program "From the Bookshelf" five days a week. The Library of Congress supplies cassette players and tapes and pays postage costs to mail these to people who are visually limited. Lists of such "talking books" can be obtained from state agencies for the visually handicapped.

Fromme, A. *Life After Work*. Glenview, Ill.: AARP, 1984.

Gillies, J. *A Guide to Caring for and Coping with Aging Parents*. Nashville: Thomas Nelson Publishers, 1981.

reality orientation Reality orientation is a widely used treatment primarily for confused and disoriented hospitalized people and residents of nursing homes. When employed by staff in such facilities, the treatment involves reminding the patient of the day of the week, the name of the institution, their own names, the date, the weather, current news, and so on. While research has not convincingly demonstrated improvement in individuals subject to such treatment, visitors to institutionalized relatives and friends may find use of the technique worthwhile. Mentioning one's own name and the name of the person, referring to the season, the place, city, day of the week, date and relying on visual aids like a large wall calendar for marking off days can all be useful. Talk about current events and family occurrences supported by pictures of family members to help establish time and relationships.

Kohut, S., *et al. Reality Orientation for the Elderly*. Oradell, N.J.: Medical Economics Books, 1987.

rectal cancer See CANCER, COLON AND RECTAL.

refractive errors The normal condition of the eye in which, with no accommodation, parallel light is focused on the retina is emmetropia. Any optical departure from this condition is called a refractive error.

Refractive errors cause a decrease in visual acuity and include presbyopia, myopia, astigmatism, and hyperopia. Of these the first three may occur at any time in life although their incidence tends to increase with age. The refractive error that is seen almost universally with aging is presbyopia.

See also ASTIGMATISM; HYPEROPIA; MYOPIA; PRESBYOPIA.

Newell, F. W. *Ophthalmology Principles and Concepts*, 6th ed. St. Louis: C. V. Mosby Co., 1986.

Slatt, B. J., and Stein, H. A. *The Ophthalmic Assistant Fundamentals and Clinical Practice*, 4th ed. St. Louis: C. V. Mosby Co., 1983.

Reisburg's global deterioration scale (see Table 15) Reisburg's Global Deterioration Scale consists of the seven stages of Alzheimer's disease.

Reisburg's cognitive rating scale measures five areas of deterioration; concentration, recent memory, past memory, orientation, and self-care. The first two stages on the scale are virtually indistinguishable from normal aging. In the third stage, also called the borderline stage, the victim begins to experience diminished performance on the job.

The fourth stage, early Alzheimer's, is when many patients are diagnosed. In this stage, the victims exhibit a decreased ability to do things such as planning dinner, handling finances, and shopping. The fifth stage of the illness is called the moderate stage. During this stage the patient can no longer survive without assistance for dressing, eating, and mobility.

The sixth and seventh stages of the disease are called the late stages. During the sixth stage the victims can only speak five or six words and can walk. In the seventh stage the victim can only sit up and smile.

See also ALZHEIMER'S DISEASE.

Roach, M. "Reflection in a Fatal Mirror," in *Aging,* Goldstein, E. C., ed. Vol. 2, Art. 83. Boca Raton, Fl.: Social Issues Resource Series, Inc., 1981.

relationships without marriage   Be-
cause Social Security benefits in the past could be reduced if an individual remarried in later life many individuals interested in a spousal relationship were confronted with the choice of breaking up, living with their partner without marriage, or living apart but maintaining dating and intimacy.

Amendments to the Social Security Act in 1977 provided that widows and widowers over 60 years of age could remarry and not suffer a reduction in their Social Security survivors benefits. Remarried persons are entitled to receive benefits on their deceased spouses' account equal to the benefit their spouse would have received if still alive. If the new spouse receives Social Security benefits, the other partner may elect to take a dependent's benefit on the new spouse's work record if that benefit would be larger than the one received from the former spouse.

This rule does not apply to people under 60 or to those receiving benefits as a surviving divorced spouse.

Relationships without marriage may still represent a practical choice for some people. Some couples share apartments and living expenses in an effort to stretch limited incomes or simply for companionship. For others sexuality, companionship, intimacy,

and warmth—which can remain important needs in old age—are the motive.

Deedy, J. *Your Aging Parents.* Chicago: The Thomas More Press, 1984.

remarriage   Practical tips on remarriage
in late life concern especially the case of widowhood. Grief over the loss of a former spouse, whether by death or divorce, needs to work itself out. Quick remarriage because of loneliness, economic instability, or sexual needs (rebound syndrome) may lead to negative consequences, especially when the new spouse does not live up to the former spouse's image. Any new spouse cannot be a simple replacement for the deceased, but is an individual in his or her own right with a unique personality.

In choosing a person for remarriage late in life the considerations differ somewhat from those in youth: backgrounds and tastes, habits, and values, will probably have become ingrained and approval of children may become part of the picture.

Remarrying can be strongly opposed by adult children. Frequently, children view their parents as asexual creatures and therefore disapprove of any remarriage. They may also object from selfishness, overprotectiveness, jealousy, concern for inheritance, or because of their own experience of grief from loss of their parent. Because adult children often must take a responsible role following the death of a parent their own grief process may be delayed. Many problems of remarriage can be worked out by having the future partners and all their children look at the issues honestly.

Most later marriages turn out to be meaningful to both parties. Perhaps success is built on the experience that older people bring to the new marriage, but the common practice of selecting a spouse from a group like one's own may also be a factor.

See also DATING; RELATIONSHIPS WITHOUT MARRIAGE.

Deedy, J. *Your Aging Parents.* Chicago: The Thomas More Press, 1984.

Loewinsohn, R. J. *Survival Handbook For Widows*. Glenview, Ill.: AARP, 1984.

reminiscence (structured life review)

Reminiscence, which was once considered merely a "natural" process of nostalgic storytelling by old people, was first recognized as a valuable psychological life review process by Dr. Robert N. Butler, a psychiatrist, former head of the National Institute on Aging, and now chief of geriatric services at Mt. Sinai Hospital in New York. Apparently related to the late-life task of developing "ego-integrity," described by developmental psychiatrist Erik Erikson, the process of reminiscence may be related to the effort of individuals to see their lives as a whole—as having had value—and therefore to maintain self-esteem. In therapeutic situations the Structured Life Review is guided by a formal set of questions, which ask about life events and family of the individual; what experiences were unpleasant and what pleasant; work done; things he or she might change or leave unchanged; and so on. Family members can lend support to a life review process if they ask similar kinds of questions and then take time to listen to the responses. This may have reciprocal value for family members—it can help to give them their own sense of rootedness in the past.

Haight, Barbara K. "The Therapeutic Role of a Structured Life Review Process in Homebound Elderly Subjects." *J. of Gerontology* Vol. 43, No. 2. p. 40–44 (1988).

Lester, A. D. and Lester J. L. *Understanding Aging Parents*. Philadelphia: The Westminster Press, 1980.

Western, Leone Noble. *The Gold Key to Writing Your Life History*. Port Angeles, Wash.: Peninsula Publishing Inc., 1981.

renal failure

Aging has a variety of effects on the kidneys and renal function. The diagnosis of renal failure is complicated by the presence of other systemic diseases that produce similar symptoms or by symptoms that are nonspecific.

Management of fluid and electrolyte balance is of the utmost importance to guard against dehydration and cardiovascular overload. Dialysis may be necessary for proper management. Mortality in acute renal failure is as high as 55 percent to 60 percent and is due primarily to infection.

Chronic renal failure can result from any cause of acute renal failure. The nephrotic syndrome is characterized by edema, albuminuria (excess of serum proteins in urine), decreased plasma albumin, and usually increased blood cholesterol. The diagnosis is often obscured in elderly patients for various reasons, including cardiovascular disease. The nephrotic syndrome may be associated with primary renal disease or with other systemic disease involving the kidney. Malignant tumors, renal vein thrombosis, amyloidosis (protein in tissue and organ), and diabetes mellitus are frequent secondary causes of nephrotic syndrome.

Improvement may often be seen with treatment of the underlying cause. Bed rest and restriction of salt and water intake may decrease edema formation. Patients who do not respond to conservative measures may respond to diuretic therapy. Elderly patients, however, may be more sensitive to shifts in vascular fluids; thus, therapy should be initiated gradually and assessed frequently.

Since the nephrotic syndrome eventually results in end-stage renal failure, the patient should be managed conservatively to avoid further renal damage prior to dialysis.

Covington, T., and Walker, J. *Current Geriatric Therapy*. Philadelphia: W. B. Saunders, 1984.

representative payee   See LEGAL REPRESENTATIVE.

residential choice and design for the elderly

The vast majority of older Americans prefer to live independently with their spouse, or alone, rather than to live with other people. Less than 10 percent of males and 20 percent of females over 65 who are not living with a spouse live with someone else. The General Social Survey, conducted annually by the National Opinion Research Center at the University of Chicago, shows that the majority of the older population is unenthusiastic about living with others, and that less than 25 percent even favors living with their own children.

Over 70 percent of the elderly own their own homes, and, whether they own or rent, 80 percent prefer to remain in their own familiar surroundings rather than to move. Forty percent of the adult U.S. population changes residence annually, but only 20 percent of the elderly do so. This latter group does not always seek out warm weather locations in the south, but instead often looks for other amenities, such as family and friends, church locations, low tax rates, and the like, in choosing a residence area.

The great majority of older Americans prefers to stay in place out of choice rather than out of inertia. Still, because residential options are numerous and an appropriate residence may be more critical in old age than at any other time in life, a number of studies have given considerable attention to the residential choices of the elderly. Typically older Americans address several major questions when they consider residential plans. Does one's present residence—which may have been purchased to house a large family—suit one's present life circumstances, or is the home too large and difficult to maintain? Is a move to a warmer climate desirable, or does staying near children, family members, friends, neighbors, and in familiar surroundings seem preferable? If one does decide to move, what part of one's income can one afford to spend for housing (the usual standard is not more than 30 percent)? Does the new location, or even one's present location, enable access to shopping areas, health facilities, transportation, recreation, entertainment, opportunities for socializing, and leisure activities (hobbies, sport, volunteer work, or a part-time job)? Suppose that sometime in the future it becomes necessary to restrict one's physical activities due to health problems, several factors in home design, remodeling, and location should be considered: whether all rooms are on the ground floor to avoid use of stairs; railings are on stairways; pull bars are in bathrooms; there's good lighting; friendly neighbors or family live nearby; safety and security services are within call; and access is available to restaurants and home meal delivery services.

No one answer to these questions can suit everyone because the tastes and needs of America's elderly vary widely. For instance, the 100,000 or more who live in single room occupancies (SROs) located in residential hotels and elsewhere in inner cities, obviously have very different attitudes and perceptions of life and their retirement needs than someone who lives in a retirement community in the south.

The residential options available to older Americans can satisfy a wide variety of tastes and requirements. Today over a million people live in retirement communities which range from the vast Sun City, Arizona, with over 45,000 residents, to the modestly sized Avery Heights life-care center in West Hartford, Connecticut, that houses a few hundred people. These elderly residential communities usually designate a minimum age for permanent tenancy, and they offer numerous appealing options for older people—buildings and grounds maintenance, room cleaning services, food services, nearby shopping malls, recreational facilities, and so forth.

Another alternative chosen by an estimated 300,000 older persons is the mobile home, or trailer home, often located in a trailer park. While this type of residential setting has sometimes been criticized for shabbiness and run-down conditions, a number of parks maintain high standards and offer quality environments. Other people live in "Granny flats," a name probably borrowed from England to describe an attached but separate apartment located in or on the same lot as the residence of an adult child, or situated in a trailer on a family member's property.

Recently home sharing has been advocated for older people. In this arrangement a pair, or group, of older individuals, jointly occupy a residence, dividing expenses for mortgage and taxes or rent, insurance, utilities, heat, and air conditioning. The advantage of such an arrangement for lowering living costs is obvious, but it also offers shared living, which many elderly find beneficial.

One instance of home sharing in a 27-room mansion in Florida captured national attention because the dozen tenants who were sharing this home successfully sought relief in court from a local zoning rule against multiple tenancy. They won their case by gaining recognition as a "family," which entitled them to continue to occupy the mansion together and to employ people as their home managers.

As life advances housing needs may change because illness or disability may interfere with an individual's capacity to carry out the routine chores of daily living in a present residence. In such cases it may be possible to adapt an existing home to accommodate a disability, or to secure support services to help remain in an existing residence or even a resort type community.

For individuals who remain physically independent, however, moving into "congregate housing" is becoming increasingly popular. Private as well as public housing for the elderly often provides "congregate" living arrangements, so called because they include common facilities, such as a dining room for meal service, lounges, and recreation areas, shared by all residents. The residents live in one- or two-room apartments equipped with light cooking facilities, and they use the common facilities as occasion warrants, or according to some predetermined plan, such as taking a daily meal in the common dining room.

Yet another variant is the "life-care community," which combines condominium units or apartments for independent living; nearby hotellike units for those who need some assistance with daily tasks, such as help with bathing, or moderate nursing supervision; and, if needed, a nursing home facility. Many life-care communities are nonprofit and run by fraternal organizations (Masonic homes, for example) or church groups. They commonly charge a major one-time entry fee, similar to a payment for purchasing a condominium, with a monthly rental charge based on the level of service required—the rates increase depending on whether one is residing in the independent living apartments, the hotel-like facility, or the nursing home.

In the past special residential facilities for older people were considered undesirable because it was thought that residential separation of the older generation would deprive them of the stimulation of living with younger people. People spoke of separate housing for the elderly with contempt, calling it "age-segregated."

For many years the federal government accepted this negative view, and federal policy for public housing supported only age-integrated facilities. In the early 1960s an age-segregated facility was constructed for the first time in San Antonio, Texas, and subjected to intensive study by psychologists, who were retained to determine the impact of such a specialized living environment on older people. The research showed beyond question that a specialized residence for older people not only provides better services, but that the residents thrive in the environment—socializing more than they would normally, engaging in stimulating activities, and eventually surviving beyond normal life expectancy.

Some experts have proposed that the "life-care" residence, which has proven very successful in meeting the needs of older adults, might well serve as the normal pattern for future elderly living. Whether or not the older generation ever abandons its present preference for autonomous living in its own separate home or apartment, it is clear that the alternative of living in a retirement community or other special facility already has wide appeal and is satisfying the needs of a growing segment of the older population.

Gillies, J. *A Guide to Caring for and Coping with Aging Parents.* Nashville: Thomas Nelson Publishers, 1981.

Russell, C. M. *Good News About Aging.* New York: John Wiley and Sons, 1989.

U.S. Bureau of the Census, *Statistical Abstract of the United States: 1989,* 109th ed. Washington, D.C.: U.S. Government Printing Office.

Ward, R. *The Aging Experience,* 2nd ed. New York: Harper and Row, Publishers, 1984.

retinal detachment   Retinal detachment is the separation of the sensory retina from the underlying pigment layer. Retinal detachment can be caused by a hole in the retina that allows fluid to seep behind the retina and strip it off (rhegmatogenous detachment) or by traction on the retina caused by fibrous tissue shrinkage (traction detachment). Retinal detachments are seen more frequently in people who have had eye surgery, especially cataract surgery, or who have diabetes, myopes, or following ocular trauma. The occurrence of retinal detachments increases approximately 200 times after removal of the natural lens of the eye. Thus, a large portion of retinal detachments are seen in people over age 65 who have had cataract extractions.

Symptoms of retinal detachment include light flashes, floaters, and a decrease in side vision. This is described as a curtain pulled in from the side, or a cobweb appearance, which later may lead to a decrease in central vision when the macula is involved.

Treatment of retinal detachment involves prompt surgery. A flat detachment, in which a hole is present with little fluid behind the retina, may be treated with transpupillary laser therapy around the hole. With elevation of the retina the usual form of treatment consists of cryotherapy applications to promote adhesions between the retina and choroid drainage of the subretinal fluid, and placement of an encircling band.

It is important to recognize early symptoms of retinal detachment. If a retinal detachment is detected before the central vision is impaired, surgery generally can restore good vision. If the central area is affected, surgery may not be as beneficial and may not be suggested.

Newell, F. W. *Ophthalmology Principles and Concepts,* 6th ed. St. Louis: C. V. Mosby Co., 1986.

Slatt, B. J., and Stein, H. A. *The Ophthalmic Assistant Fundamentals and Clinical Practice,* 4th ed. St. Louis: C. V. Mosby Co., 1983.

Retired Senior Volunteer Program
See RSVP.

retirement, preparing for   Retirement is a time of change and adjustment for older people. No longer are there pressures of work, and the demands and deadlines that had become almost routine parts of daily life have passed. Even with these changes retirement comes as a long-awaited goal for most. For a rare few, however, leaving work is a traumatic experience involving loss of status, aimlessness, lowered self-esteem, and a feeling of no longer being needed.

While the retirement transition is usually made quite easily, a fully satisfying life after leaving the workplace does require anticipation and planning. Failure to plan and prepare for retirement results in having an inadequate income unprotected from inflation, poorly conceived late-life goals, and boredom caused by inactivity.

A number of major business corporations now conduct preretirement planning programs for their employees, and a host of books and "how-to" manuals are available to assist individuals in independently educating themselves for maintaining an active, interesting, and successful life. These sources suggest a step-by-step process for designing a retirement plan. The major elements of the process involve:

1. Assembling needed background information on financial matters, housing, fitness and health, and use of leisure time
2. Talking things over with others, such as present retirees and professional counselors, who can contribute ideas and perspectives
3. Defining a realistic, specific, and personal set of goals for retirement income, health and fitness maintenance, housing, and use of leisure time
4. Putting goals and plans into writing, and reviewing these from time to time.

Many people feel that having leisure, freedom, and independence are the best features of retirement. Not only does life after work allow time for amusement, recreation, and travel, but it offers new opportunity to exercise talents and engage in hobbies. Volunteer work may also become possible for the first time, opening new areas for motivation and personal satisfaction.

People who profit from retirement view this period as a bridge from one stage of life to another, building upon past experience to face a new and challenging phase of life. They succeed in making the retirement years have as much purpose, meaning, and joy, as any stage of life.

Atchley, R. C. *Social Forces and Aging,* 4th ed. Belmont, Calif.: Wadsworth Publishing Company, 1985.
Deedy, J. *Your Aging Parents.* Chicago: The Thomas More Press, 1984.
Fromme, A. *Life After Work.* Glenview, Ill.: AARP, 1985.

Harris, I., and Associates, *The Myth and Reality of Aging.* Washington, D.C.: The National Council on Aging. 1975.

retirement age, history of   The age of 65 was originally selected as the time for retirement by the "Iron Chancellor," Otto von Bismark of Germany, when he introduced a social security system to appeal to the German working class and combat the power of the Socialist Party in Germany during the late 1800s. Somewhat cynically, Bismark knew that the program would cost little because the average German worker never reached 65, and many of those who did lived only a few years beyond that age.

When the United States finally passed a social security law in 1935 (more than 55 years after the conservative German chancellor introduced it in Germany), the average life expectancy in America was only 61.7 years. Of course, people who did reach 65 had a considerable number of years to live and to enjoy SOCIAL SECURITY benefits (see also LATER LIFE EXPECTANCY.)

Initially Social Security was limited in its coverage to workers in commerce and industry, but over the years the program was expanded and liberalized to cover widows, virtually the entire working population, and certain disabled people under age 65. The most dramatic change came in the early 1970s when the program was indexed to inflation—a plan whereby benefits are adjusted upward annually in accord with rising prices.

During the early 1980s, however, planners realized that the rampant inflation then underway and the growing older population, demanded reform of the system. Under pressure from the near-bankruptcy of the Social Security trust fund (reserves for benefit payments were down to three months), Congress found it necessary to raise the Social Security withholding taxes and to schedule increases in the age of elegibility for full retirement benefits—beginning in the year 2000 the retirement age for full benefits will be raised at intervals until it will reach 67 in the year 2027.

At the same time as Social Security benefits were becoming more generous, many large companies and government employers were using a variety of plans to encourage early retirement by their employees. Some of the inducements offered under these plans included payments of: lump sums equivalent to a year or more or post-retirement salary; part or full salary along with retirement benefits for a period of months or years; full retirement benefits for a specified retirement age before the individual actually reached that age.

No precise figures are available to show how many people have taken advantage of these early retirement plans, but almost half of all male and over half of female employees retire before age 65—and, it is possible that many of these people did so by taking advantage of company and government employee incentives to retirement. Social Security itself, of course, adds to company inducements by allowing people to retire at age 62 with 80 percent of the benefit that they would receive at age 65.

While it is well established that the overwhelming majority of the population retires willingly (some studies show that 98 percent or 99 percent of the population retires willingly, and others show that at most only 7 percent do so unwillingly), mandatory, or forced, retirement at specific ages has been considered highly objectionable. As a result, Congress in 1977 passed the Age Discrimination in Employment Act, barring forced retirement for nonfederal employees prior to age 69, and eliminated compulsory retirement for federal employees at any age. In 1986 the Age Discrimination in Employment Act was strengthened to terminate forced retirement at any age in all but small businesses (fewer than 12 employees), and for a few categories of workers—police officers, fire fighters, prison guards, airline pilots. College professors were excluded from its coverage for seven years.

There are now reasons to believe that the early retirement trend, quite contrary to all past expectations, may possibly reverse in the next few years. The reason is that the U.S. may experience a labor shortage beginning about the year 2000, when the large bulge of working age population brought on by the baby boom will begin to decline as Baby Boomers age and retire. Just how this will affect the long-term trend to early retirement is not yet certain, but it is quite possible that business and government will have such great needs for workers that they will be obliged to offer potential retirees special inducements—such as high pay, part-time work, and special benefits—to remain at work. Should this come about, the days of incentives for early retirement may become a thing of the past, and work combined with leisure turn into the pattern of life in the senior years.

Schulz, J. H. *The Economics of Aging*, 4th ed. Dover, Mass.: Auburn House Publishing, 1988.

retirement living patterns, women's

Because women live longer than men and normally marry men older than themselves, the majority of women spend part of their lives as widows, and many spend part of their last years living by themselves. Three-quarters of men over age 65 are married, but over half of women in that age group are widowed. At age 75 close to 70 percent of women are widows, while close to 70 percent of men are still married. In terms of living alone, from age 65–74 about 35 percent of women dwell solo compared to 15 percent of men, and at 75+ more than half of women do so compared to less than one-quarter of men.

Women's life patterns have changed dramatically since the 1950s when motherhood and homemaking were still the norm. Because women in past times spent comparatively little time in the paid work force, many of them in the current older generation have experienced financial disadvantages in late life—without pensions of their own and reduced benefits from their spouse's pension after his death.

Greater participation by women in the paid work force has brought some improvement in recent years, but the statistics still show that women over age 65 have a median income of less than $7,000 compared to $12,000 for men. This is true in spite of a relatively greater increase in the average income for older women, up 87 percent since 1962 compared to 72 percent for men.

Factors that have contributed to the improvement of the financial circumstances of older women have included Congressional reform of the Social Security Act and, in 1984, the adoption of the Retirement Equity Act. The original Social Security Act was designed for families and provided benefits for wives alone at age 64. Benefits were later extended to divorced former wives, and a special minimum benefit was introduced for long-term, low-wage workers—a category that fitted many women.

The Retirement Equity Act also included a section designed to counter the too-frequent practice where husbands took a full pension benefit during their lifetimes rather than taking a reduced benefit that would have continued payments to their wives after their death. Under the Retirement Equity Act men in government or private industry pension programs must secure the consent, written and witnessed, of their wives to any decision to bypass pension income options that provide income to a surviving wife on the death of the husband.

Today, 70 percent of women between age 25 and 54—the period of life when employment is most typical—participate in the paid workforce, and this figure is expected to rise to 80 percent by the year 2000. Because of this, women's late-life financial circumstances should improve—most women are now building up their own independent Social Security and private pension plans.

In general, women today need to think seriously about re-entering the paid work-

force if they discontinue their employment to raise families during part of their lives. Their probable status as widows also suggests that they need to plan for a period of active and independent living during their senior years.

Gardner, M. "Now Retirement Is a Women's Issue, Too," in *Aging,* Goldstein, E. C., ed. Vol. 2, Art. 14. Boca Raton, Fl.: Social Issues Resource Series, Inc., 1981.

Schulz, J. H. *The Economics of Aging,* 4th ed. Dover, Mass.: Auburn House Publishing Company, 1988.

retirement residence   (see Table 24)   In recent years retirement centers, which may be a cluster of individual units or high-rise apartment-type dwellings, have become increasingly available and popular.

Some advantages of retirement centers include around-the-clock security, stimulating activities, companionship, and privacy. Many retirement centers provide a dining room where meals are served, transportation to nearby stores, churches, and doctors, and planned activities that interest most active older citizens. Retirement centers free older people from yard upkeep and maintenance of their homes.

There are three main types of retirement centers: federally funded, private, and private nonprofit run by church groups, fraternal organizations, etc. The federally funded retirement centers usually have no down payment and the rent is determined by income. Privately owned centers usually require a down payment, monthly rent, and maintenance fees as do private non-profit centers.

Entry in a center is normally by contract, and such a move requires full understanding of financial obligations, terms, and conditions. Decisions to enter a retirement center need to go beyond a printed brochure, a telephone conversation, or someone's recommendation. A visit to the facility with observation of activities, dining rooms, recreation and hobby areas, including, if possible, an overnight stay is desirable.

Retirement centers are not as spacious as a private home so a move to one may require disposal of furniture and other personal property. Pets and gardens may not be permitted, and fees may be substantial. While some centers may include a medical clinic, personal assistance and nursing services are not provided and residents must be ambulatory or at least self-sufficient.

Though the popularity of retirement communities is increasing, some people prefer other living arrangements because they feel that being with older people constantly reminds them of their age, or that the lack of intergenerational contact will diminish intellectual and psychological stimulation. While studies show that such concerns are generally unfounded, commitment to living in a retirement center needs to take such concerns into account.

Deedy, J. *Your Aging Parents*. Chicago: The Thomas More Press, 1984.

Gillies, J. *A Guide to Caring for and Coping with Aging Parents*. Nashville: Thomas Nelson Publishers, 1981.

retirement states   (see Tables 25, 26) States with the largest percentage of people over age 65 include Florida (17.6 percent), Arkansas (14.3 percent), Rhode Island (14.3 percent), Iowa (14.1 percent), and Pennsylvania (14.1 percent). Eight states account for half of the nation's more than 30 million persons aged 65 and over. California, New York, and Florida each have upwards of 2 million retirees, while Pennsylvania, Ohio, Illinois, Michigan, and Texas each have upwards of 1 million retirees.

AARP/AOA *A Profile of Older Americans; 1990.* AARP: Washington, D.C.: 1990.

Dickson, P. *Sunbelt Retirement and Retirement Edens*. Washington, D.C.: AARP, 1986.

rhinitis   Rhinitis is an inflammatory disease of the nose, frequently caused by viral infections or the common cold. In older individuals, rhinitis is often due to atrophic changes in the nose.

Congestion, discharge (rhinorrhea), and postnasal drainage are common symptoms with anosmia (loss of smell) an occasional complaint. In some individuals the nasal mucosa is particularly reactive to commonplace substances, such as dust and cigarette smoke, causing chronic rhinitis. Septal deformity and nasal polyposis (development of multiple polyps) are also contributing factors in chronic rhinitis.

Cyrosurgery may be used to reduce excess mucosa and control rhinorrhea. Cauterization, especially electrocauterization, is also effective. In atrophic rhinitis where crusts commonly form and offensive nasal breath is present, nasal hygiene is most important. Frequent irrigation and gentle removal of the crusts is essential. Use of a bland ointment helps prevent the reformation of the crusts.

See also ACUTE RESPIRATORY DISEASE; EPISTAXIS; SINUSITIS.

Ballenger, J. J. *Diseases of the Nose, Throat, Ear, Head and Neck*, 13th ed. Philadelphia: Lea & Febiger, 1985.

rhinoplasty   See COSMETIC SURGERY.

rhytidectomy   See COSMETIC SURGERY.

ribonucleic acid   See RNA.

right-to-die laws   See LIVING WILLS.

RNA (ribonucleic acid)   Ribonucleic acid, RNA, is found in all body cells, where it plays a critical role in translating the genetic code. There have been claims that RNA can rejuvenate old cells, improve memory and alertness, prevent wrinkling of the skin, and slow down the aging process. However, the RNA in a cell is made in that cell and can not be imported into the cell. RNA that is consumed orally is broken down by digestion. High levels of RNA in the diet can be harmful to people who have kidney disease or a hereditary predisposition to gout.

The House Select Committee on Aging consultants agree that there is no scientific basis for claims that RNA can reverse aging.

Meister, K. A. "The 80's Search for the Fountain of Youth Comes Up Very Dry," in *Aging*, Goldstein, E. C., ed. Vol. 2, Art. 76. Boca Raton, Fl.: Social Issues Resource Series, Inc., 1981.

role reversal   The terms *role reversal* and *sandwich generation* are somewhat misleading because they refer to a situation that is relatively rare. They have come into use to describe instances in which children with older parents take a similar kind of responsibility toward their parents as their parents took toward them in infancy. The idea of role reversal goes beyond simple help with routine daily tasks to mean that adult children become parents to their own parents.

The term *sandwich generation* is applied to people who are still taking responsibility for their own children, for instance by putting them through college or helping them to get started with a young family, and who are also making decisions and caring for their elderly parents. The implication is that many adults in the sandwich generation are shouldering unwanted burdens.

While there are cases of role reversal, it is by no means true that it is common for adult children to assist their parents to a point of complete role reversal. Federal government statistics on income distribution indicate that parents of young adults are likely to have greater financial resources than their children, and research has shown that older parents assist their adult children personally and financially more frequently than their children assist them.

Studies of intergenerational exchanges also show that help with daily activities flows quite copiously from parents to their adult children. Indeed, a national poll carried out by Harris Associates showed that people under 65 considered one of the values of

Social Security to be that it would be too difficult to support older parents without it—suggesting that adult children are generally not helping their parents financially now, and that they feel they might have to do so in the absence of Social Security.

While there are instances in which older parents experience a period of helpless dependence on their children, these are usually relatively brief times that constitute a prelude to death. The vast majority of older people maintain their independence until the time when death brings their lives to a rapid close and they pass their property and wealth on to the next generation. The terms *role reversal* and *sandwich generation* are not indexed in standard gerontological sources. Rather, they are part of the folklore generated by the media and popular, overdramatized accounts of the burdens imposed by the old on the young.

See also SANDWICH GENERATION.

Harris, D. K., and Cole, W. E., *Sociology of Aging*. Boston: Houghton Mifflin Company, 1980.
U.S. Bureau of the Census, *Statistical Abstract of the United States: 1989*, 109th ed. Washington, D.C.: U.S. Government Printing Office.

RSVP (Retired Senior Volunteer Program)   The Retired Senior Volunteer Program (RSVP) is a federally financed community volunteer program utilizing the services and talents of senior citizens in a variety of programs determined by local need. It is based on a pilot program begun in 1967 in Staten Island, New York.

In 1971, the federal government launched the RSVP program nationally under the auspices of ACTION, the federal voluntary agency that includes Senior Companion, the Foster Grandparent program, the National Center for Service Learning, VISTA (Volunteers in Service to America), and the Peace Corps. It began with 11 projects and a budget of $500,000. By 1981, the budget was in excess of 26 million dollars with more than 26,000 volunteers in 707 projects in all

50 states, the District of Columbia, Puerto Rico, the Virgin Islands, and Guam.

Thousands of agencies and community organizations engage the services of RSVP in meeting their goals of delivering assistance to those in need. Many roles are available for the older citizen depending on physical capacity, experience, and need. Volunteers are engaged in providing companionship to the lonely, child care, tutoring, crime prevention, home energy repairs, transportation, and many other services. With significant increases in life expectancy and greater emphasis on preventive health care, the older population will continue to be a dynamic, productive force in the future.

For more information write or call:
RSVP
c/o ACTION
806 Connecticut Ave., N.W.
Washington, DC 20525
(202) 289-1510

S

safety   See SECURITY, ADVICE ON.

salt intake   Sodium intake is a major variable influencing the aging of the cardiovascular system. High salt intake seems to cause higher blood pressure, therefore increasing the chances of coronary diseases. People who consume very little sodium have lower blood pressure and thus reduced cases of coronary disease.

See also SOLOMON ISLAND TRIBES; YANOMAMO INDIANS.

Brocklehurst, J. C. *Textbook of Geriatric Medicine and Gerontology.* New York: Churchhill Livingstone, 1985.

sandwich generation   The *sandwich generation* is an inaccurate and overworked term that presumably describes people 50 to 60 years of age caught between the need to assist their aging parents as well as their children in college or starting family life. Presumably members of the sandwich generation are ready to relax and travel because their children are grown, but they find that they must now take on a new guardianship, becoming, in a sense, parents to their parents. Thus this middle generation is thought to be burdened with coping with the health, housing, financial, and emotional problems of their parents, and with feelings of guilt and resentment. Research on intergenerational family relations, however, shows that older people assist their children as much as their children help them, and that care of parents, though it may become a burden in some cases, is usually managed without undue difficulty when it does become necessary.

See also CAREGIVERS; ROLE REVERSAL.

Brozan, N. "The Sandwich Generation," in *Aging,* Goldstein, E. C., ed. Vol. 1, Art. 52. Boca Raton, Fl.: Social Issues Resource Series, Inc., 1981.

scalp care   See HAIR CARE.

scheduled time   When faced with living alone or with retirement, some older people may be tempted to not dress, eat, or sleep on a regular schedule.

A fairly strict daily routine has a positive effect on the health of the older person. Some continue schedules they have followed when young, but others need to make new schedules to include new needs. Exercising on a regular schedule and eating at a specific time help to assure an orderly and healthier life.

It is advisable for older people to make an effort to get out as often as possible. Walking, shopping, beauty appointments, or even appointments with physicians all offer useful ways to get out of the house. While scheduled activity has value, it can result in sheer "busy-ness," so scheduling time for relaxation also makes sense.

Gillies, J. *A Guide to Caring for and Coping with Aging Parents.* Nashville: Thomas Nelson Publishers, 1981.

SCORE (Service Corps of Retired Executives) The Service Corps of Retired Executives association, or SCORE, is an organization of volunteers made up of retired business executives and professionals who offer free counseling services to small businesses. Within the association there are some members still actively engaged in business or a profession, and they are known as the Active Corps of Executives or ACE.

The volunteers provide counseling to small businesspeople on a one-to-one basis, or through seminars designed for those seeking advice about going into business. Typically, their clients need help in finding solutions to business problems, or they wish to expand their businesses but lack the knowledge to take the necessary steps.

SCORE was started almost 25 years ago by the U.S. Small Business Administration and now has offices in approximately 400 communities across the United States. SCORE members are all volunteers and serve without compensation but do receive reimbursement from federal funds for approved out-of-pocket travel expenses and for a modest level of clerical support.

For additional information write or call:
SCORE
c/o Small Business Administration
6th Floor, 1111 18th St. N.W.
Washington, DC 20036
(202) 634-4950

SCP See SENIOR COMPANION PROGRAM.

security, advice on (safety) Security and safety are important in providing a pleasant environment. Because recovery from injuries is more difficult in later life and weakened muscles and poor vision increase the danger, older people need to take greater precautions than they did in youth. Rugs in homes should have rubber undercoats to keep them from sliding. Chairs should be easy to get into and out of. Steps and staircases should have sturdy railings. A rail clamped to the bathtub or bed may also be useful.

Avoiding the possibility of criminal victimization is also wise. If the person's hearing is decreased, it may be useful to install a burglar alarm that will frighten an intruder and wake the person instantly. A dog may also provide protection. Doors should be locked, even during the day, with a good deadbolt lock. Older people should not open their door to strangers even if they have a chain on the door. They should keep their phone in an easily accessible area and have important numbers, such as fire, police, ambulance, and the nearest neighbor, handy. Older individuals should know and care about their neighbors because keeping an eye out for neighbors and their property can be a good deterrent to crime—a proposition that has contributed to the growth of neighborhood watch programs nationally.

Older people should avoid giving information to strangers over the phone, on the street, or at home. Fraud, through a large variety of con games and other schemes, is used against the elderly frequently. The consequences may be only the loss of a small amount of pocket change, but it can result in the loss of life savings. A basic piece of advice includes avoiding sidewalk, door-to-door, and telephone solicitations.

Older people should not keep large sums of money or valuables in their homes—the bank is a safer place. Having Social Security checks sent directly to a bank and paying bills by check or direct withdrawal can be useful. It is common knowledge, especially in the criminal community, that Social Security and other pension checks arrive during the first days of each month, and crime against the elderly escalates during this time. If a person does not use a direct deposit method, he or she may want to consider a locked mailbox, since nearly 20,000 Social

Security checks are stolen each year, usually from mailboxes. The older person should keep any valuables such as stocks, bonds, or jewelry in a safe deposit box or a locked area in the house.

When older individuals leave their homes, it is a good idea to leave the television, radio, or a light on. If they are going to be gone for a day or more they should put their lights and radio on an automatic timer that will allow the lights to go on and off, inform their friends and neighbors about their absence, and stop paper and mail deliveries until they return.

When older people are on the streets, they should pay attention to their surroundings, walking with confidence and purpose. They should keep to lighted streets, preferably go out with companions, and avoid doorways and alleys where an attacker could be lurking. To avoid purse snatching, women should carry shoulder bags, which can also be secured under their arm, with the opening next to their body. Carrying large amounts of money should be avoided, and men should place their wallets in the front pocket of their trousers instead of the hip pocket. Keys should be carried separately from purse or briefcase. It is safer not to struggle if one is physically attacked. The attacker will generally take the purse or wallet and run if there is no resistance, thus leaving the victim uninjured. It is a good idea for older people to carry a whistle to use as an alarm if they are in trouble. When using public transportation, it is best to ride as closely as possible to the driver.

In recent years religious cults have begun to target the elderly. While some cults are authentic and well-meaning, many are not. These indulge in deception, demand unquestioning loyalty to their leader, and require that material possessions be turned over to the cult. Cults hold out the promise of a caring community, which may seem attractive to older people and cause them to join. As long as the older individual works and can contribute to the cult, they remain acceptable; but when they become too old or incapacitated they may be expelled without any financial resources.

Deedy, J. *Your Aging Parents*. Chicago: The Thomas More Press, 1984.

seizures   Seizures occurring for the first time in later life are almost always due to clearly defined pathology with cerebral arterial disease being the major cause. Brain tumors, whether primary or metastatic, must be excluded through appropriate testing. Meningocerebral scarring (scarring of the lining of the brain from convulsion) secondary to head trauma is also a possible cause.

If no apparent lesion can be found, management with anticonvulsant drugs must be initiated. Phenytoin (Dilantin) is widely used and effective in a broad range of seizure disorders. Since it is metabolized in the liver, the elderly should be monitored closely for symptoms of toxicity. Phenytoin may inhibit insulin release and may therefore complicate the management of diabetes. Its interaction with other drugs should also be closely watched.

Phenobarbital is an anticonvulsant drug used alone or in conjunction with other drugs, especially phenytoin. It should be used with caution in patients who are depressed or suicidal. It should be used with extreme caution in the elderly with renal failure since it is excreted partially unchanged in the urine. Reduced dosages are usually indicated in those patients with reduced renal or hepatic function.

Primidone (Mysoline) is especially useful in psychomotor (impaired consciousness followed by a series of bizarre, useless acts) seizures. Carbamazepine (Tegretol) is used in both grand mal (preceded by aura with loss of consciousness, and convulsion) and focal (attack consisting of aura without convulsion) seizures while Valproic acid (Depakene) and Ethosuximide (Zarontin) are used primarily for petit mal (sudden momentary loss of consciousness with only minor jerking) seizures. The use of all anticonvulsant drugs should be carefully monitored for interaction with other drugs, since the elderly are frequently taking multiple medications.

Covington, T., and Walker, J. *Current Geriatric Therapy*. Philadelphia: W. B. Saunders, 1984.

selenium   Selenium is an essential nutrient that some people believe may have an anti-aging effect on the body. Selenium is a potentially dangerous remedy for aging because excess amounts of selenium are toxic. The difference between the level of selenium needed in the human diet and the level that is considered toxic is not large. There is no evidence either clinical or in experimental animals that demonstrates that selenium can retard, much less reverse, the aging process.

See also AGING, BIOLOGICAL THEORY OF.

Meister, K. A. "The 80's Search for the Fountain of Youth Comes Up Very Dry," in *Aging*, Goldstein, E. C., ed. Vol. 2, Art. 76. Boca Raton, Fl.: Social Issues Resource Series, Inc., 1981.

self-esteem   See DIGNITY IN LATE LIFE.

self-image exercise   In self-image exercises, participants are asked to imagine themselves in front of a full-length mirror. Each participant imagines his or her body from all sides and is asked to imagine undressing in front of the mirror. After everyone has had time to imagine this, the participants are asked to open their eyes and discuss feelings about what they saw or felt. Usually, the older people express negative feelings, and the group leader tries to show that these feelings come from social values and are not inherent in the aging process. In this exercise, elderly people can remove themselves from the cultural image of aging and this helps them increase respect for themselves.

See also AUTOGENIC TRAINING; BIOFEEDBACK TRAINING; GESTALT DREAM ANALYSIS; HATHA YOGA; MEDITATION; POSITIVE ATTITUDE; TAI CHI CHUAN.

Fields, S. "Sage Can Be a Spice in Life," in *Aging*, Goldstein, E. C., ed. Vol. 1, Art. 26. Boca Raton, Fl.: Social Issues Resource Series, Inc., 1981.

Senior Companion Program (SCP)
The Senior Companion Program (SCP) is a volunteer program under the auspices of ACTION. It was established in 1974 to link the low-income elderly with adults who have special needs.

Volunteers are all low-income individuals over age 60. They serve approximately 20 hours a week and receive a tax-free stipend funded through a grant from ACTION. Funding is also obtained through the private sector. Senior Companions also receive transportation assistance, meals on service days, annual physical examinations, accident and personal liability insurance, and special recognition at annual events.

Senior Companions serve through a variety of local and state organizations, agencies, and institutions. Approximately 80 percent are assigned to the chronically homebound, a program that was established in 1986 as a three-year demonstration program and is still active, emphasizing services to the terminally ill, homebound people dwelling alone, respite care, and assistance to the mentally ill. The 1986 change was noteworthy because it marked the first time Congress specifically authorized SCP funds for the homebound.

See also ACTION.

For additional information write or call:
Senior Companion Program
c/o ACTION
806 Connecticut Ave., N.W.
Washington, DC 20525
(202) 606–4851

Senior Corporation of Retired Executives   See SCORE.

sexuality Sexuality is important to the quality of life of the older adult, and, quite contrary to what many believe, most elderly people have sexual desires—they are not asexual. In fact, one study of a sample of 800 persons age 60–90 found that age may have advantages for sexual expression. In this study, 36 percent of the respondents said that their sex life had improved since they were young, whereas only 25 percent said that it was less satisfactory.

Eighty percent stated that they remained sexually active, most had intercourse once a week or more, and people who were active sexually felt that sex was more spontaneous because they were free of the pressures and interruptions of family obligations. Having leisure time available for lovemaking was also considered an advantage. The majority concurred that sex was an important part of life for older couples.

An enjoyable, active sex life in earlier years increases the likelihood of continued positive sexual expression in later years. Sex in age is recreational rather than reproductive, and sexual arousal and behavior need not necessarily be aimed at achieving orgasm because it may simply fulfill the human need for warmth, physical closeness, and intimacy.

While researchers observe that lack of a partner is the greatest restraint on sexual activity in late life, health problems (rather than any inherent lack of interest) can cause sexual difficulties in both older men and women. Diabetes may cause impotence; cardiac disease can make intercourse exhausting; hypothyroidism may diminish libido; arthritis may make sexual contact painful; senile vaginitis may cause pain during intercourse and itching in the vaginal area; pelvic relaxation may interfere with sexual function. Other factors, such as a prostatectomy, mastectomy, hysterectomy, or simple fear that intercourse will harm or kill the sex partner can also hinder activity. Frequently, too, sexual difficulties have no physical or-igin, but result from the abuse of alcohol, drugs, or tobacco.

Most of these problems can be treated. Hypothyroidism and vaginitis can generally be medically treated. Pelvic relaxation can be corrected surgically, and a heart-attack (myocardial infarction or congestive heart failure) victim can generally resume sexual activities within four to six weeks. Psychological problems can be more difficult to treat, but a variety of therapies are available for treating them.

Experts disclaim the still-prevalent myths about asexuality in aging. Sexual expression through intercourse, touching, stroking, embracing, or even masturbating can have broad therapeutic benefits in age as well as in earlier life. Experts insist that older people are not physically unattractive and undesirable, that sex in age is not shameful or perverse, and that masturbation, which has been naively thought by some to cause brain damage, may be the only release available to the elderly.

People who consider sexual activity to have value in age urge a change in public attitudes. They call for greater acceptance of sexual behavior and expression in the older generation—terms like D.O.M. (dirty old man) or D.O.W. (dirty old woman) are out of place in modern times—and feel that public displays of affection (holding hands while walking down the street, for example) by older people have charm as well as value for demonstrating the revival of intimate love in late life.

See also DYSPAREUNIA.

Atchley, R. C. *Social Forces and Aging,* 4th ed. Belmont, Calif.: Wadsworth Publishing Company, 1985.

Rossman, I. *Clinical Geriatrics,* 3rd ed. Philadelphia: J. B. Lippincott Co., 1986.

Starr, B. D., and Weiner, M. B. *The Starr-Weiner Report on Sex and Sexuality in the Mature Years.* New York: McGraw-Hill, 1981.

Steinberg, F. U. *Care of the Geriatric Patient,* 6th ed. St. Louis: C. V. Mosby Co., 1983.

sexual relations, painful   See DYSPA-
REUNIA.

shingles   See HERPES ZOSTER.

shock   Shock is a condition of acute circulatory failure resulting in low blood pressure extensive enough that the body cannot
maintain normal functions.

Symptoms of shock include cold hands
and feet; fast, weak pulse; disorientation or
confusion; skin that is pale, moist, and sweaty;
shortness of breath and rapid breathing; lack
of urination; and low blood pressure.

Causes of shock include sudden loss of
blood from injury, bleeding peptic ulcer, or
ruptured aneurysm; fluid loss as in severe
burns, fluid and electrolyte imbalance, or
peritonitis; impaired heart pumping function;
blood poisoning; endocrine diseases such as
Addison's disease or diabetes mellitus.

Treatment depends on the underlying disorder. If shock is from blood or fluid loss,
blood transfusions or intravenous fluids are
administered. If blood pressure is at a life-
threatening low level, drugs to raise the
blood pressure are given. If infection is present, antibiotics are used.

Risk of complications increase with serious injury, surgery, if infection is present,
in cases of anemia and cancer, or with an-
aphylactic (allergic) shock to drugs such as
penicillin and local anesthesia.

In the elderly, mortality from shock is
high, approximately 30 percent. Mortality
from shock caused by intestinal obstruction
and fecal peritonitis have the greatest risks
with a mortality rate between 45 percent and
70 percent.

Brocklehurst, J. C.: *Textbook of Geriatric Med-
icine and Gerontology.* New York: Churchill
Livingstone, 1985.
Griffith, H. W. *Complete Guide to Symptoms,
Illness and Surgery.* Tucson: The Body Press,
1985.

sinusitis   Sinusitis is inflammation of one
or more of the sinuses. Since the paranasal
sinuses are directly continuous portions of
the upper respiratory tract, they are usually
involved in infections originating there. Sinusitis is common among the elderly and
other adults. Any anatomic or physiologic
feature that obstructs free drainage from the
sinuses can lead to infection. Other causes
are tooth infections, nasal polyps, allergy,
smoke, and air pollutants.

Symptoms of sinusitis include a headache
over the affected sinus, nasal discharge, fever, sore throat, dizziness, and sometimes
difficulty in breathing.

Treatment includes decongestion of the
nasal mucosa by analgesics and by local
applications of heat. Vasoconstrictor medication (a drug that causes narrowing of blood
vessels) is better given systemically by mouth
early in the course of acute sinusitis rather
than locally as nose drops. A constant, hu-
midified environment and bed rest are also
important to speedy recovery. After initial
inflammation and edema have partially sub-
sided, displacement irrigation may be used
to clear the sinuses of debris.

The use of an air conditioner or humidifier
can reduce the number and severity of sinus
attacks. Avoiding irritants such as dust and
smoke may also be helpful. Occasionally a
change in climate may be necessary to avoid
conditions known to precipitate sinus attacks.

See also ACUTE RESPIRATORY DISEASE;
ANOSMIA.

Ballenger, J. J. *Diseases of the Nose, Throat,
Ear, Head and Neck,* 13th ed. Philadelphia:
Lea & Febiger, 1985.
Steinberg, F. U. *Care of the Geriatric Patient,*
6th ed. St. Louis: C. V. Mosby Co., 1983.

skin cancer   See CANCER, SKIN.

skin care   See BATHING.

smell   Although the senses of smell and
taste are related chemical senses, complaints
of malfunction are more frequently centered

around a loss of olfaction. The sense of smell decreases with aging due to the diminution in the number of olfactory nerve endings in the nose.

A decreased sense of smell can be caused by viral infections, high doses of aspirin, hepatitis, hyperthyroidism, head trauma, nasal polyps, and smoking.

Defects in the sense of smell may be more important with respect to the eating habits of the older person than is the loss of the sense of taste. An inability to discriminate food odors can change the older person's food preferences and eating patterns.

See also ANOSMIA.

Steinberg, F. U. *Care of the Geriatric Patient,* 6th ed. St. Louis: C. V. Mosby Co., 1983.

smell, loss of   See ANOSMIA.

Social Security, application for   Payment of Social Security benefits is not automatic; every individual must apply when he or she reaches the required age. Benefits reduced by 20 percent are available as early as age 62. Full benefits begin when the individual reaches age 65. To assure prompt payment of benefits individuals should apply for Social Security three months before the date when they become eligible. Individuals can also apply for Medicare when they apply for Social Security. In most Social Security offices it is necessary to apply in person unless it is impossible. Social Security offers an option of having monthly checks sent as a direct deposit to the individual's bank or saving institution, a convenience that has the added value of eliminating the risk that monthly checks will be stolen from the mailbox. Individuals who take advantage of this option need not go out to make a deposit, and this can be especially useful for people who have difficulty getting about.

See also MEDICARE, RETIREMENT AGE.

Deedy, J. *Your Aging Parents.* Chicago: The Thomas More Press, 1984.

Gillies, J. *A Guide to Caring for and Coping with Aging Parents.* Nashville: Thomas Nelson Publishers, 1981.

Social   Security,   history   of   The Congressional act that created Social Security was signed into law by President Franklin D. Roosevelt on August 14, 1935, a major milestone in American history. The act at first provided income only to retired workers, and was titled Old Age Insurance (OAI). In 1939, before the first benefits were paid, the act was extended to survivors and dependents, with the title now becoming "Old Age and Survivors Insurance" (OASI). In 1956 persons under age 65 with serious disabilities became eligible for benefits (OASDI). In 1965 Medicare was added, and the Act now provided Old Age, Survivors and Dependents, and Health Insurance (OASDHI). As a result of these additions and other modifications, spending for Social Security has grown from $1 billion in 1950, 10 years after the first payments under the act were made, to more than $300 billion per year at the present time.

Initially the act excluded the self-employed, farm, and domestic workers, employees of charitable, educational, and religious organizations, clergy, employees of state and local government, military personnel, federal employees, Americans working for foreign governments or international organizations, and railroad employees who were covered by the Railroad Retirement Act. Congress extended eligibility successively to each of these groups, so that today virtually all American workers and self-employed persons have coverage.

Wages withheld from pay checks and Social Security payments made by the self-employed are put into the Social Security Trust fund. The money in this fund can be used only for two purposes: to pay benefits to eligible persons; or, for loans to the U.S. Treasury, which the Treasury can in turn loan to government departments (such as Education or Defense), with the interest and principal to be paid back into the fund. In this respect the Social Security Trust Fund is rather like a public savings account on which the federal government can draw like a credit card.

From the early days of the program and until the mid-1980s, a substantial part of the withholding taxes were paid directly over to beneficiaries, representing a sort of "pay-as-you-go" plan. Today, however, the trust fund is large and growing, and many experts think that the interest earned from loans to the federal Treasury and to government departments may eventually become large enough to cover the costs of retiree benefit payments.

Numbers of potential Social Security beneficiaries change each year because of the addition of new persons who meet the minimum qualifications for benefits (10 years of employment and payment into the program), but by 1990 approximately 180 million persons had been covered. The first person to receive benefits was Mrs. Ida Fuller, who retired from a secretarial post in a law firm in 1940 and received a monthly payment of $22. Because she lived to reach age 100 in 1975, Ida Fuller did remarkably well with her investment in Social Security—she paid in $100 but she eventually received $21,000, a rate of return that would cause great joy to most investors in annuities or the stock market. Today about 38 million persons receive benefits that average about $525 per month per retiree. As noted above, total benefits for all workers and Medicare recipients exceed $300 billion annually.

In 1972 Social Security benefits were indexed to inflation, with annual cost-of-living adjustments paid to beneficiaries annually since then. In the early 1980s, inflation combined with the growing number of beneficiaries to raise fears over the possible bankruptcy of the system, a state that came to be known as "Social Security insecurity." Congress and the President acted promptly to correct the deficiencies in the system by increasing the payroll tax and by other re-

forms, and today reserves in the Social Security trust fund are building up at a rate of more than $40 billion per year.

Economists like James Schulz of the Heller Center at Brandeis University in Massachusetts warn against complacency about the system. They note especially that recessions will erode payments into the trust fund because the fewer people at work the less that will be withheld from wages for payment into the trust fund. Further, they warn that the future of the system depends on the will of the American people to support it, and that tampering with withholding rates or overreliance by public officials on Social Security to loan to the Treasury for relending to government departments—which is as a way of avoiding tax increases to pay government expenses—could bring about disaster.

Still, the size of the trust fund is expected to reach $2.5 trillion early in the next century. When the crest of the Baby Boom generation reaches old age in 2030, the trust fund should be over $12 trillion, making a reserve which experts think will be sufficient to meet the needs of the 60 million persons then over 65—the largest number of older persons in American history.

Nordlinger, S. E. "The Social Security System at Work," in *Aging*, Goldstein, E. C., ed. Vol. 2, Art. 95. Boca Raton, Fl.: Social Issues Resource Series, Inc., 1981.

Russell, C. H. *Good News About Aging.* New York: John Wiley and Sons, 1989.

Schulz, J. H. *The Economics of Aging,* 4th ed. Dover, Mass.: Auburn House Publishing Company, 1988.

U.S. Bureau of the Census, *Statistical Abstract of the United States: 1989,* 109th ed. Washington, D.C.: U.S. Government Printing Office.

sodium chloride   See VITAMINS.

SOD   See SUPEROXIDE DISMUTASE.

Solomon Island tribes   The Solomon Islands were known to cook their vegetables by long boiling in sea water, and studies have been made to determine the dietary effects of this practice. The results showed a daily salt intake of 130 to 230 milliosmoles a day. Both sexes and nearly all age groups in the Solomon Islands have high systolic and diastolic blood pressures. Blood pressures greater than 140/90 have been found in 7.8 percent of the men and 9.9 percent of the women. While this seems to support the theory that a diet high in sodium can cause high blood pressure in the elderly, there were no ECG abnormalities—not even those associated with coronary diseases.

See also BUSHMEN OF THE KALAHARI DESERT; MASAI; NEW GUINEAN HIGHLANDERS; POLYNESIANS; SOMALI CAMEL HERDSMEN; TARAHUMARA INDIANS; YANOMANO INDIANS.

Brocklehurst, J. C. *Textbook of Geriatric Medicine and Gerontology.* New York: Churchill Livingstone, 1985.

Somali camel herdsmen

The Somali camel herdsmen have made a remarkable adaptation to a high-fat diet. The herdsmen drink up to five liters of camel milk per day. Five liters of camel milk contains about 335 g of fat and a calorie intake of 6,247 calories, yet serum cholesterol levels among the Somali do not exceed 153 mg. Nor do their body weight, serum cholesterol, and beta-lipoproteins increase significantly with age. Although the Somali showed a moderate rise in blood pressure from age 21–70, none of the subjects had any symptoms of artherosclerosis. Contrary to what one might expect with this high-calorie, high-fat diet, the Somali herdsmen do not seem to be affected by heart disease.

See also BUSHMEN OF KALAHARI DESERT; MASAI; NEW GUINEAN HIGHLANDERS; POLYNESIANS; SOLOMON ISLAND TRIBES; TARAHUMARA INDIANS; YANOMANO INDIANS.

Brocklehurst, J. C. *Textbook of Geriatric Medicine and Gerontology.* New York: Churchill Livingstone, 1985.

spouse, relationships with

Over 70 percent of men and 36 percent of older women in the 65+ age group are married, and in the youngest segment of this group—the 65–69 year olds—half the women and about 85 percent of the men are married. Because the normal phases of family life usually involve launching the children when couples are in their forties and fifties, older married people are likely to find themselves together and alone just as they were in youth, when they were courting and first married. This state, along with entry into retirement during this period, provides the leisure and opportunity to renew an intimate relationship. According to marriage and family specialists, this state often brings about a pleasant revival of romance.

Marital happiness later in life, however, is no more automatic than it is at any other time. If, for example, the wife has been a homemaker and living fairly independently during the day while the husband was away at work, the husband's constant presence at home after retirement will affect her independence—she may have less opportunity to get together with her friends, to chat on the phone, to watch favorite TV soap operas, and to carry out housekeeping routines at her own pace.

Studies show that marital adjustments need not create serious problems, however, and that successful, happy marriages in late life tend to have a set of characteristics that reflect a degree of wisdom and conscious planning by the spouses. For one thing, the husband looks on his wife as an indispensable pillar of strength. For another, the couple become partners in many activities, and there is an egalitarianism between them that blurs the usual sex roles—for instance, the husband may take on more cooking and cleaning, participate with his wife in grocery shopping, and the pair may do gardening together. As gerontologist Robert Atchley has noted in his comprehensive book, *Social Forces and Aging,* "Happy couples tend to remain sexually active in later life," adding that marital satisfaction is a central influence in overall life satisfaction in age just as it is throughout all the years.

Contrary to ballyhoo about a rampant growth in late life divorce, the incidence of divorce among older married couples remains far below what it is at earlier ages. Between age 25 and 34 there are over 35 divorces per 1,000 married persons, and at age 45–49 the rate is still around 15 per 1,000 married couples. By age 60 to 64, however, the rate has dropped to about three per 1,000, and after age 65 it falls to two per 1,000—making the occurrence of divorce in the most advanced years from seven to 15 times less likely than at earlier ages. Though the foregoing figures do not include enough information to prove it, it is possible that marital satisfaction actually increases with the years.

Health alone appears to have a greater influence on life satisfaction than marriage. As noted in the article on sexuality, ill health is the most common reason for a decline in sexual activity over the years, and ill health can also make one of the partners in a marriage into the caregiver to the other.

In spite of a limited number of studies of the impact of ill health on marriage, it appears that most spouses nurse and help their partners willingly and devotedly even when the problems involved are severe—the caregiving partner may be frail while the other is confined to a wheelchair, suffering from organic brain syndrome, and the like. Some spouses struggle on even when in ill health themselves, but illness of both partners is the most frequent precipitating cause of moving of one or both of the partners to a nursing home. In general, however, late-life marriages are tranquil and satisfying, and the partners remain together mutually supporting one another until death does them part.

Atchley, R. C. *Social Forces and Aging,* 4th ed. Belmont, Calif.: Wadsworth Publishing Company, 1985.

U.S. Bureau of the Census, *Statistical Abstract of the United States: 1989,* 109th ed. Washington, D.C.: U.S. Government Printing Office.

SSI   See SUPPLEMENTAL SECURITY INCOME.

stamp collecting   Stamp collecting is considered the world's most popular hobby. Stamp collecting probably started when the first adhesive postage stamp, the Penny Black, was issued in 1840. In 1886 collectors banded together and formed the American Philatelic Society. The Postal Guide to U.S. stamps can offer guidelines for people interested in starting a stamp collection.

Stamp collecting, like many other hobbies, is a good outlet for the elderly. It does not require strenuous activity and the elderly may enjoy reminiscing with the commemorative stamps.

Gillies, J.: *A Guide to Caring for and Coping with Aging Parents.* Nashville: Thomas Nelson Publishers, 1981.

stomach cancer   See CANCER, STOMACH.

stress   See ANXIETY.

stress of life   The stress of life has long been known to accelerate the rate of aging. So far, the most solid evidence supporting this view comes from comparative epidemiology. Studies have been conducted in which people of different cultures with the same factors for coronary risk, such as smoking habits and blood pressure levels, have been studied. The people who lived in a more traditional and stable society had three times fewer cases of coronary disease. The people who lived in the more modern society had three times more cases of coronary disease. This study helps establish that stress plays a very important role in a person's health.

See also JAPANESE AMERICANS.

Brocklehurst, J. C. *Textbook of Geriatric Medicine and Gerontology*. New York: Churchill Livingstone, 1985.

stroke   See CEREBRAL VASCULAR ACCIDENT.

suicide   Suicide is the act of purposely killing oneself. The incidence of suicide increases greatly with age. In countries where 10 percent to 15 percent of the population is over 65, 25 percent to 30 percent of all suicides occur among the elderly. Elderly people, unlike many younger people, do not make suicidal gestures and attempts to seek attention or to get help. Suicidal attempts and completed suicide by the elderly almost always happen during persistent depressions, and repeat attempts at suicide more often have fatal results among the elderly than among younger people. Preoccupation with suicide should always prompt attempts at treatment.

While the male suicide rate is from three to five times the rate for women up to age 44, the difference between the sexes widens dramatically in the later years of life. At age 55–64 there are 26–27 suicides for every 100,000 males in the United States and 8.4 for every 100,000 females. At 65–74 there are 35.5 male suicides per 100,000 and 7.2 female. At 75–84 the rate is 54.8 suicides for males compared to 7.5 for females, and at 85 + the difference between the sexes reaches a peak when there are over 12 times as many male suicides—a rate of 61.6 for men but 4.7 for women. No one has fully analyzed and supported with statistics the reason for the lifelong and growing difference in male-female suicide rates, but the greater frequency of obviously terminal illness and disabling heart and stroke conditions among men are suspected reasons.

See also DEPRESSION.

Brocklehurst, J. C. *Textbook of Geriatric Medicine and Gerontology*. New York: Churchill Livingstone, 1985.

sunstroke   See HYPERTHERMIA.

supergenes   Dr. Roy Walford of the University of California at Los Angeles School of Medicine believes that he has identified a single supergene that controls much of the aging process. Since 1970, he has been studying a small segment of the sixth chromosome in humans called the major histocompatibility complex. This is the master genetic control center for the body's immune system and is a logical suspect in the aging process.

Tests with mice show that those who lived longest had a high rate of DNA repair and "good" genes. It is believed if DNA repair rates could be boosted, the human life span would be extended.

See also AGING, BIOLOGICAL THEORY OF.

Coniff, R. "Living Longer," in *Aging*, Goldstein, E. C., ed. Vol. 1, Art. 8. Boca Raton, Fl.: Social Issues Resource Series, Inc., 1981.

superoxide dismutase (SOD)   Superoxide dismutase is an enzyme naturally present in all body cells that protects against the destructive effects of superoxide, a byproduct of the cell's use of oxygen. It has been suggested that the level of this enzyme present in a cell is an important factor in influencing that cell's rate of aging. This idea is controversial within the scientific community. Research has been conducted on mice with SOD dietary supplements. Dietary supplements did not influence the SOD level in cells.

See also AGING, BIOLOGICAL THEORY OF.

Meister, K. A. "The 80's Search for the Foundation of Youth Comes Up Very Dry," in *Aging*, Goldstein, E. C., ed. Vol. 2, Art. 76. Boca Raton, Fl.: Social Issues Resource Series, Inc., 1981.

Supplemental Security Income (SSI)

Supplemental Security Income (SSI) is a federal program administered through the local Social Security office that guarantees a minimum monthly income to those in need. It is designed to supplement the limited income and assets of older, blind, or disabled individuals. Those who are age 65, blind, or disabled can qualify even if they have never worked. A home, personal goods, a car, and insurance policies may not necessarily be included to determine eligibility. Information on eligibility can be obtained through a local Social Security office.

Averyt, A. *Successful Aging.* New York: Ballantine Books, 1987.

survivors' guide for financial arrangements   The death of a spouse or a parent can be very difficult for a survivor. During this period of grief some very important financial arrangements must be made.

Collecting the papers needed to file for various benefits and to finalize the estate should be the first step in arranging finances. One will need copies of the death certificate to send to many companies. Certified copies can be obtained from the funeral director or the county health department for a few dollars. One will also need copies of all insurance policies. There are many types of policies to be on the lookout for, such as life insurance, mortgage or loan insurance, accident insurance, auto insurance, credit card insurance, and employer-supplied insurance. One will also need the Social Security number of the deceased, of the spouse, and of any dependent children. If the deceased was a war veteran, one will also need a copy of honorable discharge, an item which can be obtained from the Department of Defense's National Personnel Record in Washington, D.C. A copy of the marriage certificate will be needed if the spouse is claiming any benefits. These copies can be obtained at the office of the county clerk where the marriage license was issued. Copies of the birth certificates of dependent children, if they are claiming benefits, should also be acquired. A copy of the will and a complete list of all property, including real estate, stocks, bonds, savings accounts, and personal property may be useful. After these papers have been collected it is necessary to determine what one is eligible for.

The deceased is covered by Social Security if he or she has paid in for at least 40 quarters. There are two types of benefits available if the deceased is eligible.

1. A death benefit to be used for burial expense. This payment is made to an eligible spouse or a child entitled to survivor benefits.
2. Survivor benefits for a spouse or children
   a. Spouse age 60 years or older.
   b. Disabled widows age 50 or older.
   c. Spouse of deceased who is younger than 60 but who cares for dependent children under 16 or cares for disabled children.
   d. The children of the deceased who are under 18 or those who are disabled.

These are only some of the guidelines for survival. For a comprehensive booklet write:
AARP Fulfillment
P. O. Box 2400
Long Beach, CA 90801

For additional information write or call:
AARP
Consumer Affairs, Program Department
1909 K Street, N.W.
Washington, DC 20049
(202) 872–4700

suspicion   See ANXIETY.

Swedish elderly   The Swedish elderly benefit from what many consider to be the most generous social system in the world. The national pension plan provides a basic pension that is payable regardless of previous working income; a supplementary pension based on income from gainful employment; and a partial pension that allows people between 60 and 65 to combine part-time work with their pension. The health plan for the Swedish elderly is far more sweeping than Medicare. All citizens are entitled to medical care benefits, dental care, hospital care, and related travel. Prescribed drugs can be purchased for greatly reduced prices and in some cases are entirely free. The aged are also entitled to social home help, a service that offers home visits by nurses and aides who come by two or three times a week and do whatever they can to assist the older person. For the elderly who cannot be treated at home, there are long-term care wards, central and local nursing homes, and a semi-outpatient care system known as "day medical care." For the elderly who live in rural areas, the government pays the postal workers to run errands for them, pay bills, or to just stop by and chat.

Green, P. S. "Marquis Childs on Sweden," in *Aging*, Goldstein, E. C., ed. Vol. 1 Art. 98. Boca Raton, Fl.: Social Issues Resource Series, Inc., 1981.

swimming   Swimming is good exercise— a simple, healthy way to relax that strengthens muscles—including the heart—and relieves the discomfort of back ailments and swollen joints. Even severely handicapped individuals can learn to swim and benefit from the activity. As a strenuous sport, however, swimming should be initiated or continued only with medical approval.

Opportunities for swimming activity are readily available in most American cities and towns. Health spas and the YMCA frequently offer indoor pools that allow year-around participation in swimming. There are frequent local, statewide, and regional meets for those who enjoy competitive swimming. The national meet for Masters (above the age of 25) helps make swimming one of the most popular sports for seniors, but vigorous daily training is essential to join the ranks of the master swimmers.

Gillies, J. *A Guide to Caring for and Coping with Aging Parents*. Nashville: Thomas Nelson Publishers, 1981.

T

tachycardia, sinus   Sinus tachycardia is a cardiac arrhythmia that is characterized by an atrial and ventricular rate of 100 beats per minute or more. On an EKG the P waves, which are sinus in origin, are more peaked and followed by a QRS wave. Sinus tachycardia is common among many age groups but it more prevalent in the elderly. Eighty-eight percent of people over the age of 70 have experienced sinus tachycardia.

Sinus tachycardia is a normal response with strenuous exercise, fever, pain, hyperthyroidism, hemorrhage, shock, strong emotion, and anemia. Sinus tachycardia can also be associated with the ingestion of alcohol, tea, coffee, tobacco, atropine, epinephrine, or isoproterenol.

Sinus tachycardia is usually a benign rhythm, although it may be the first sign of heart failure. Symptoms of sinus tachycardia include palpitations, dizziness, and possible chest pain.

Treatment of sinus tachycardia should be aimed at controlling the underlying cause. Occasionally sedatives may be prescribed to reduce anxiety.

See also ARRHYTHMIAS, CARDIAC.

Phipps, W. J. *et al. Medical Surgical Nursing*. St. Louis: C. V. Mosby Co., 1983.
Scherer, J. C. *Introductory Medical-Surgical Nursing*. Philadelphia: J. B. Lippincott Co., 1982.

Tai Chi Chuan   Tai Chi Chuan is a set of exercises that combine mental concentration, coordination of breathing, and movement. The movements are done very slowly, as if the person were floating, so they require great concentration and balance. By performing just a few of these exercises on a regular basis the older person can improve balance, grace and strengthen his or her self-confidence.

See also AUTOGENIC TRAINING; BIOFEEDBACK TRAINING; GESTALT DREAM ANALYSIS;

GROUP BREATHING; HATHA YOGA; MEDITA-
TION; POSITIVE ATTITUDE; SELF-IMAGE EX-
ERCISE.

Fields, S. "Sage Can Be a Spice in Life," in
Aging, Goldstein, E. C., ed. Vol. 1, Art. 26.
Boca Raton, Fl.: Social Issues Resource Series,
Inc., 1981.

Tarahumara Indians   The Tarahumara
Indians live in the mountains of northern
Mexico. These Indians have long been known
by anthropologists for their remarkable
physical accomplishments. They are, for instance, famous for their method of hunting
deer by running after an animal until it drops
from exhaustion, sometimes a day or two.
Scientists studied a group of these Indians
between the ages of 18 and 48 during a 45.7
km race. The winner ran this distance in
four hours and 55 minutes. All the runners
were checked at the three-quarter mark and
at the end of the race. They showed declines
in systolic and diastolic blood pressures. No
abnormalities were found on electrocardi-
ograms. It appears that this type of balanced,
sustained physical activity may enable physically fit adults to make best use of their
physical abilities.

See also MASAI; NEW GUINEAN HIGHLAN-
DERS; POLYNESIANS; SOLOMON ISLAND TRIBES;
SOMALI CAMEL HERDSMEN; YANOMANO IN-
DIANS.

Brocklehurst, J. C. *Textbook of Geriatric Medicine and Gerontology*. New York: Churchill
Livingstone, 1985.

taste   Decreased taste sensation is a common complaint of older individuals. This is
usually due to the loss of taste buds in the
tongue, a natural aging process. It may be
related to smoking. Taste sensitivity to sweet,
sour, and bitter is lost before the sensitivity
to salt. A reduced saliva flow may cause
difficulty swallowing. It may be beneficial
for the person to season food more and sip
a drink as he or she eats.

Steinberg, F. U. *Care of the Geriatric Patient*,
6th ed. St. Louis: C. V. Mosby Co., 1983.

taxes   For the most part federal taxes for
the older generation are similar to those for
the rest of the population. There are, however, a few points that taxpayers over age
65 should keep in mind, and one of these
concerns tax credits that may be available
under specified circumstances. These include: the credit for dependent care expenses, the earned-income credit, and the
senior tax credit. A tax credit directly reduces the amount of tax owed, whereas a
tax deduction reduces the amount of income
on which the tax is based. Generally, there
is more benefit from a tax credit than a tax
deduction.

Under 1986 tax laws, the following requirements qualify for dependent credit:

One's expenses for a dependent, such as an
incapacitated parent or spouse, must be to
allow one to work or look for work

One must have income from work during
the year. Unpaid volunteer work or volunteer
work for a nominal wage does not qualify

One (and one's spouse, if one is married)
must keep up a home that one lives in with
at least one qualifying dependent parent or
spouse

One must file a joint return if one is married,
and

One's payments for dependent care must be
made to someone other than a person whom
one claims as one's dependent, although one
may include payments made to relatives for
care even if they live in one's home, provided the relatives are over 19 years of age.

The tax code places specific restrictions
on the amount of the work-related expenses
that qualify for the dependent care tax credit
and also limits the amount of expenses that
can be used to calculate the credit. Therefore, it is essential to carefully examine the
IRS rules.

The earned-income tax credit (EITC) has
been traditionally used only by low-income
workers who have dependent children and

maintain a household. But adults who are caring for both a dependent child under age 19 and a frail parent may also qualify if their income is under $10,000. Information about this credit is on the standard federal income tax form 1040. The IRS office can help to determine eligibility.

The senior tax credit is available to:

Anyone 65 or older who received less than $5,000 a year in Social Security income ($7,500 for a married couple).

Anyone under age 65 who is permanently or totally disabled and receives taxable disability payments.

It is important to make the most of deductions and to obtain all the credits to which one is entitled. Everyone over age 65 should have a copy of "Tax Benefits for Older Americans" (#554). Call or write the local IRS office to obtain a free copy.

The American Association of Retired Persons provides a free tax preparation service through its Tax-Aide program. Local IRS offices and offices of Area Agency on Aging can help locate the nearest Tax-Aide office.

When moving to another state, tax rates should be investigated since property taxes, income taxes, inheritance taxes, and sales taxes vary from state to state. State tax structure can have a significant impact on an individual's financial situation and estate.

In addition to these credits, older taxpayers who are married should note that they get an additional standard deduction for each person if they do not itemize deductions, and that couples do not need to file for income tax payments if their income is below $10,400. The Internal Revenue Service also provides free tax assistance for the elderly, and questions that reflect status as a single person and variations in dollar amounts of the standard deduction can be answered through this service.

Under the present law, no taxes are assessed on the Social Security income of single people whose gross adjusted income

is less than $25,000, while for married couples, Social Security income becomes taxable only when the adjusted gross income is $32,000 or more. In a home sale, people over age 55 may exclude from taxation any gain of $125,000 or less if they have owned and occupied the home for three out of the last five years; residents of nursing homes need to have owned and occupied the home for one out of the last five years. As with other taxpayers, elderly people have a tax exemption of $2,000 for the taxpayer and each dependent (in 1989 people filing a joint return with an income that exceeds $155,320 and single people with an income of $93,130 have the amount of the deduction reduced as income rises).

Averyt, A. *Successful Aging.* New York: Ballantine Books, 1987.

TB See TUBERCULOSIS.

teeth See CARIES, SENILE; ORAL HYGIENE; PERIODONTAL DISEASE.

television Television is often criticized for being an "electronic sitter" for older people. Although the older person must be selective, there are many good programs and features on television. Cable television may offer some variety not available on the three major broadcasting networks—ABC, CBS, and NBC. Cable News Network, Christian Broadcasting Network, and ESPN sports network are some of the favorite cable stations of older individuals. Educational networks present many programs, such as National Geographic specials, historical series, and old movies, that older people seem to enjoy.

Televisions with smaller screens have sharper pictures. If the older person's vision is failing, he or she may want to consider purchasing a television with a smaller screen and good color to help sharpen the picture. People who are handicapped or just have trouble getting up and down may also consider a remote control device that allows them to change channels and adjust volume from their seats.

Fromme, A. *Life After Work*. Glenview, Ill.: AARP, 1984.
Gillies, J. *A Guide to Caring for and Coping with Aging Parents*. Nashville: Thomas Nelson Publishers, 1981.

tendonitis   See BURSITIS.

tennis, badminton, and ping pong
Tennis is a strenuous sport that can be continued as an individual becomes older if the person has developed stamina over a period of years of consistent involvement. Generally, tennis should not be taken up anew after the age of 65 without thorough physical conditioning. Playing doubles rather than singles tennis is one way to play the enjoyable sport with lower physical stress. Those who have developed the stamina for tennis find it is an excellent way to keep their bodies in good physical condition. Badminton and ping pong offer alternative physical activity of a less strenuous nature.

Gillies, J. *A Guide to Caring for and Coping with Aging Parents*. Nashville: Thomas Nelson Publishers, 1981.

tennis elbow   See BURSITIS.

tetanus immunization   See IMMUNIZATION IN THE ELDERLY.

throat cancer   See CANCER, MOUTH, THROAT, AND LARYNX.

thromboembolism   See THROMBOPHLEBITIS.

thrombophlebitis (thrombosis, thromboembolism, blood clot)   Thrombophlebitis is an inflammation of veins that may result in clot formation. Thrombophlebitis has increased in the elderly population due to longer survival of critically ill people

and more extensive surgical procedures. It is a well-established fact that a person's age has a profound influence on the susceptibility to thromboembolism.

Thromboembolism is an obstruction of a blood vessel by a blood clot that has broken loose from its site of formation.

Thrombosis is the formation of blood clots inside a blood vessel or in one of the chambers of the heart. Many factors predispose a person to the development of a blood clot. These include inactivity, congestive heart failure, chronic illness, and prolonged bed rest.

There may be no subjective symptoms at first, but a vague ache may be noticed in the affected leg.

The classic symptoms of thrombophlebitis, however, include pain, tenderness, swelling, fever, increased heart rate, slight cyanosis (skin blueness), and slight prominence of veins in the affected area.

Treatment of thrombophlebitis includes rest, elevation of feet, local heat application, and administration of anticoagulants. Hospital admission is usually necessary for intravenous administration of anticoagulants and bed rest. Elastic support stockings may be helpful. Surgical intervention may be necessary if the thrombosis is extensive and recurrent or if embolization is recurrent. With danger of a pulmonary elbolism, vena cava surgery may be useful.

Prevention of thrombosis is important. Early ambulation, elevation of the foot of the bed, and active and passive exercises of the legs in bed are effective. Elastic support of the legs also is of value.

The most feared complication of deep thrombophlebitis is pulmonary embolism, which can cause sudden death.

Scherer, J. C. *Introductory Medical-Surgical Nursing*, 3rd ed. Philadelphia: J. B. Lippincott Co., 1982.
Steinberg, F. U. *Care of the Geriatric Patient*, 6th ed. St. Louis: C. V. Mosby Co., 1983.

thrombosis   See THROMBOPHLEBITIS.

thyrotoxicosis See HYPERTHYROIDISM.

TIA See TRANSIENT ISCHEMIC ATTACK.

tinnitus (ringing in ears) Tinnitus is an auditory sensation subjectively noted by the older person as a ringing or roaring in the ears. It may vary in intensity and may be continuous or intermittent.

Tinnitus is associated with hearing loss arising from disorders of the sound conduction system, the cochlea (temporal bone forming one division of inner ear), or neural pathways of the cochlear nerve. Tinnitus is caused by a variety of factors, including impacted ear wax, ear infection, usage of certain drugs, or systemic diseases such as hypertension and central nervous system disease. The sounds range from low frequencies (like a ventilating fan or seashell sound) to a rushing sound common in Meniere's disease to high-pitched noise (like whistles or insect sounds).

Conductive hearing loss produces a low-pitched steady sound that becomes pulsating if inflammation is present. High-tone hearing loss produces high-pitched continuous or intermittent tinnitus and is an important early sign of drug toxicity (aspirin, digitalis, quinine, etc.). Tumors of the inner ear can be indicated by low pitched tinnitus without hearing loss.

Other than relieving a conductive hearing loss, there is no specific medical or surgical therapy for tinnitus. If it is secondary to a hearing loss, it often will become less of a problem with the passage of time. However, it may reoccur at times of fatigue, stress, or respiratory infection. Reassurance is important in these instances.

People with tinnitus are most bothered at night, when external noises are low. The use of a bedside radio may sufficiently overshadow the tinnitus so the patient can fall asleep. Occasionally, mild sedatives are prescribed for insomnia, but barbituates and tranquilizers are rarely indicated since in most instances patients are able to adapt to the presence of tinnitus and ignore it. Recently, relaxation training has had some excellent results.

Ballenger, J. J. *Diseases of the Nose, Throat, Ear, Head and Neck,* 13th ed. Philadelphia: Lea & Febiger, 1985.

touch Some older individuals experience a decrease in tactile sensitivity, primarily in areas of hairless skin such as the palms of the hands and soles of the feet. The ability to sense vibrations also declines, primarily in the lower extremities.

While it appears that the elderly are less sensitive to pain, it may be that they are less willing to report actual pain and that pain thresholds remain essentially unchanged throughout life.

Older individuals may misjudge the firmness of their grasp. Thus, heavier plates, glasses, and utensils will be easiest to handle. Older people also may have difficulty turning pages easily. Glancing at page numbers while reading helps to prevent missing pages.

Steinberg, F. U. *Care of the Geriatric Patient,* 6th ed. St. Louis: C. V. Mosby Co., 1983.

transient ischemic attack (TIA, carotid obstruction) Transient ischemic attacks are short-term losses of blood to the cerebral area with temporary episodes of neurologic dysfunction. They last less than 24 hours and usually only for a few minutes.

TIAs may be caused by thrombus, emboli, hemorrhage, generalized hypoxia, or localized hypoxia. They commonly precede cerebral thrombosis. Drugs are often responsible, particularly thiazide, diuretics, reserpine compounds, and promazine derivatives because of their hypotensive effects. Anemia is often overlooked in the elderly as a cause of TIAs. Physical exertion or even standing for any length of time produces signs of TIAs if hemoglobin is below normal.

Symptoms of TIAs include dizziness, diplopia (double vision), headache, weakness, vomiting, nausea, mental changes, loss of consciousness, and amaurosis fugax (transient loss of vision in one eye).

Treatment of TIAs should include the determination of its cause. Vasodilators, anticoagulant therapy, or drugs that inhibit platelet aggregation are alternatives for the treatment of TIA. Anticoagulant therapy, including aspirin, decreases the number of attacks. Surgical correction is possible if an isolated extracranial arterial lesion is found. If the TIAs persist and the risk of stroke outweighs the risk of surgery, a carotid endarterectomy may be performed. Education is an important part of the treatment. Since TIAs often precede a stroke it is essential that the person understands the symptoms and their importance.

Phipps, W. J. *Medical Surgical Nursing.* St. Louis: C. V. Mosby Co., 1983.

tretinoin (Retin-A)   Tretinoin is a dermatologic cream marketed as Retin-A, which has been traditionally used as a treatment for acne. Recent studies have shown tretinoin effective in the reduction of wrinkles, roughness, and mottled pigmentation (age spots). Caucasians can be helped within a four-month period by daily topical application of the cream. Whether this benefit can be maintained after discontinuation of the tretinoin therapy or during continued therapy is not yet determined. The most impressive improvement occurs in fine wrinkling, while little or no improvement is observed in more advanced changes.

Tretinoin has some negative side effects. Initially almost all people treated with tretinoin will experience a dermatitis, which will last two weeks to three months. As the dermatitis begins to subside, improvement in the fine wrinkling and hyperpigmentation becomes evident. This dermatitis includes xerosis, peeling, and subjective irritation. Pinkness of the skin tends to have an onset of one week to two months of therapy. Generally, people view the pinkness as a desired effect of the therapy.

Gilchrest, B. A. "At Last! A Medical Treatment for Skin Aging." *JAMA* 259: 569–570 (1988).

Weiss, J. S., *et al.* "Topical Tretinoin Improves Photoaged Skin." *JAMA* 259: 527–532 (1988).

trichiasis   Trichiasis is a condition in which the eyelashes are directed toward the globe of the eye, causing irritation of the cornea and conjunctiva. It may result in a secondary infection. This condition usually follows blepharitis (eyelid infection) but may also be associated with trachoma, cicatricial pemphigoid, alkali burns, and injuries. Trichiasis frequently occurs in the elderly because orbital fat diminishes and the eyelids become loose.

Treatment is usually directed toward the destruction of the irritating lashes, although the cornea and conjunctiva may be temporarily protected by a soft contact lens. Eyelashes removed by epilation (pulling out) regrow to full size in 10 weeks. Electrolysis is an electrical method used to remove lashes permanently but it is seldom practical for more than a few lashes. Liquid nitrogen applied to the anesthetized palpebral conjunctiva may be used to treat extensive trichiasis. Small areas are treated with direct application to the cilia. The cornea and skin must be protected when using liquid nitrogen.

Newell, F. W. *Ophthalmology Principles and Concepts,* 6th ed. St. Louis: C. V. Mosby Co., 1986.

trusts   See LEGAL REPRESENTATIVE.

tuberculosis (TB)   Tuberculosis is a highly infectious disease transmitted most commonly by direct contact with a person who has the active disease, through the inhalation of droplets from coughing, sneezing, and spitting. The disease is primarily airborne.

Resistance to the disease varies considerably with age, but generally the older the individual the less resistance they have. Tuberculosis has been a decreasing problem in the United States over the last 20 to 30 years, because of effective chemotherapy and public health programs. Presently, the greatest risk group is the population over 45 years of age. Overcrowding and poor hygienic conditions make the spread of disease more likely. The spread of the disease is on the rise in homeless people and other groups who suffer from a lack of nutrition and live in poor hygienic conditions as well. The highest morbidity and mortality rates occur in the most densely populated areas.

Factors that can lead to the development of tuberculosis are fatigue and poor nutrition, which lower resistance. Onset of symptoms is insidious. They may not appear until the disease is well advanced. This emphasizes the need for routine examinations. Early symptoms are vague and include fatigue, anorexia (loss of appetite), weight loss, and a slight nonproductive cough. Increased temperature in the late afternoon and evening and night sweats are frequent as the disease progresses. A productive cough, a mucopurulent (combination of mucus and pus) blood-streaked sputum (material coughed up from the lungs) and hemoptysis (coughing up of blood from the respiratory tract) may occur. Marked wasting and weakness, dyspnea (difficulty breathing), and chest pain are symptoms of the later stages of the illness.

Diagnostic tests consist of a tuberculin skin test, chest X-ray, and sputum examination. Serial sputum specimens may be necessary because the tubercle bacilli may not be recovered in a single specimen. Gastric lavage (washing out of stomach) or gastric aspiration may be useful to determine the presence of the organism.

Chemotherapy is the treatment of choice. Isoniazid (INH), streptomycin, ethambutal, and rifomipin are primary medications in the treatment of tuberculosis. Drug therapy usually lasts for 18–24 months. It must be stressed to the patient the necessity of taking the prescribed medications without interruption on a regular basis. Side-effects of drug therapy are toxicity and the tendency of the

tubercle bacillus to develop resistance to the drugs. Combined therapy with two or more drugs decreases drug resistance and increases the tuberculostatic action of the drugs. Rest and a nutritious diet are also important.

Surgical treatment may be required for patients with advanced disease or those who do not respond to medical treatment. When the disease is located in one section of the lung, a segmental resection or wedge resection may be performed. If the diseased area is larger, a lobectomy (surgical removal of lobe of lung) may be done. If the entire lung is diseased a pneumonectomy (removal of all or part of a lung) is performed.

Phipps, W. J., et al. Medical Surgical Nursing. St. Louis: C. V. Mosby Co., 1983.
Scherer, J. C. Introductory Medical-Surgical Nursing. Philadelphia: J. B. Lippincott Co., 1983.

U

---

ulcer, gastric   See ULCER, PEPTIC.

ulcer, peptic (gastric ulcer)   A peptic ulcer is an ulceration of the mucosa and deeper structures of the upper gastrointestinal tract. Ulcers may be acute or chronic. An acute peptic ulcer is usually superficial, involving only the mucosal layer. It usually heals within a short time but may bleed, perforate, or become chronic. A chronic peptic ulcer involves both the mucosa and submucosa.

Duodenal ulcers (ulceration located in the uppermost portion of the small intestine) are more frequent in people 25 to 50 years of age, where peptic ulcers occur more frequently in people over 50 years of age. Peptic ulcers are caused by the digestive action of the acidic gastric juices and pepsin on the mucosa.

Symptoms include pain such as a "burning" or "gnawing" in the epigastric region, usually occurring within several hours after meals. Bleeding may be the fist sign of the ulcer, presented as hematemesis (vomiting of blood) or melena (dark tarry stools due to blood altered by intestinal juices). Diagnosis is made by the history and the gastrointestinal X-ray series.

Duodenal ulcers are always benign, whereas gastric ulcers may be either benign or malignant. The combined use of X-ray, gastric analysis, gastric washings, and gastroscopy are helpful in differentiating between benign and malignant lesions. Failure to heal, which may indicate a malignancy, is the usual reason to operate.

Neutralizing the acid so that it does not irritate the ulcer and decreasing the hypermotility (spastic movement) and secretions of the stomach are treatment objectives. A bland diet may be recommended, omitting spicy foods, alcoholic beverages, coffee, or other foods that cause gastric distress. Drugs such as aspirin can also be irritating to the gastric mucosa.

Antacids are given to neutralize hydrochloric acid. Cholinergic blocking agents such as tincture of belladonna and atropine may be given to decrease the gastric motility. Adverse effects of these drugs include dilation of the pupils, blurring of the vision, and difficulty voiding. Cholinergic blocking agents are avoided in persons with narrow angle glaucoma or prostatic enlargement. Cimetedine, which decreases the production of hydrochloric acid, is used in the treatment of duodenal ulcers. Ulcers usually heal within eight weeks with the use of Cimetedine therapy. Carafate has been introduced as an alternative to Cimetedine. Rest and relaxation are important, thus sedatives may be prescribed to promote rest.

Hemorrhage is a frequent complication. Bleeding occurs when a blood vessel is eroded by the ulcer. Examining the stool for occult blood may detect bleeding. Faintness, weakness, and dizziness may result from large losses of blood. When bleeding cannot be controlled, immediate surgical intervention is necessary.

The ulcer may penetrate the tissues and perforate, resulting in the gastrointestinal tract contents seeping out, causing peritonitis. The abdomen becomes rigid, extremely painful, and tender. This is an emergency condition requiring immediate surgical closure.

Peptic ulcers that do not respond to medical treatment may require gastric surgery. This consists of subtotal gastrectomy with gastroenterostomy. Vagotomy (division of the vagus nerve) is done to decrease the secretions of hydrochloric acid and gastric motility. Nutritional problems that follow gastric resection are related to the amount of the stomach removed.

The dumping syndrome can be a complication of gastric surgery. Sensations of weakness and faintness are accompanied by profuse perspiration and palpitations. This is due to rapid emptying of large amounts of food and fluid through the gastroenterostomy into the jejunum.

See also DUMPING SYNDROME; GASTRITIS; VITAMIN B$_{12}$ DEFICIENCY.

Phipps, W. J. *Essentials of Medical-Surgical Nursing.* St. Louis: C. V. Mosby Co., 1985.
Reichel, W. M. *Clinical Aspects of Aging.* Baltimore: The Williams & Wilkins Co., 1979.

ulcerative colitis   Ulcerative colitis is an inflammation and ulceration of the colon. The mucosa of the colon becomes hyperemic (engorged with blood), thickened, and edematous. The ulceration can be so extensive that large areas of the colon are denuded of mucosa.

The etiology of the disease is obscure. Some physicians believe that ulcerative colitis is a disease of multiple causative factors, which may include infection, allergy, autoimmunity, and emotional stress. The term *idiopathic,* meaning of unknown cause, is often used to describe this disease.

Ulcerative colitis is most common during young adulthood and middle life, but it can occur at any age. It affects both men and women. Ulcerative colitis is especially dangerous in the elderly.

Its onset may be gradual or abrupt. The patient has severe diarrhea (12–20 or more bowel movements per day) and expels blood and mucus along with fecal matter. Weight loss, fever, severe electrolyte imbalance, dehydration, anemia, and cachexia (constitutional disorder, general ill health, and malnutrition) may follow. The patient may experience anorexia (loss of appetite), nausea, and vomiting, as well as extreme weakness. The urge to defecate is so abrupt that the patient may experience incontinence.

This disease may be present in a mild form for years, or it may be rapid and cause death from hemorrhage, peritonitis (inflammation of the membrane lining the abdomen), or debility. The patient may experience a sudden dramatic recovery and remain free of the disease for years or have a recurrence.

Diagnosis is made by history and physical examination, proctoscopy, sigmoidoscopy, X-ray examination, and examination of the stool. Diseases such as cancer, amebic dysentery or diverticulitis, which could cause the same symptoms, should be eliminated with the studies.

Treatment is supportive and includes providing rest for the bowel, giving it an opportunity to heal, and correcting anemia and malnutrition. Some patients can be managed medically and helped into remission and others require a total colectomy and permanent ileostomy.

A bland diet is prescribed and foods such as raw fruits and vegetables or highly seasoned foods are usually eliminated. A nourishing diet of protein foods, such as meat and eggs served in small frequent meals are important. A record is kept of the quantity and type of food intake and output and the number and character of bowel movements.

Blood transfusions and iron are given to correct anemia. Parenteral fluids and electrolytes may be prescribed. Supplementary vitamins to correct diet deficiencies may be given.

Drugs that slow peristalsis (rhythmic contraction of smooth muscle) such as atropine or tincture of belladonna, or drugs used to coat and soothe the mucosa, such as kaolin and pectin, may be ordered. Sedatives and tranquilizers help the patient to relax and rest. A sudden onset of abdominal distention should be reported at once.

Corticosteroid drugs may be given if the patient does not respond to other measures. Dramatic relief of symptoms often occurs following their use. The patient must be maintained on as low a dosage as possible to maintain the remission.

Rossman, I. *Clinical Geriatrics,* 3rd ed. Philadelphia: J. B. Lippincott Co., 1986.
Scherer, J. C. *Introductory Medical-Surgical Nursing,* 3rd ed. Philadelphia: J. B. Lippincott Co., 1982.

upper respiratory infection See ACUTE RESPIRATORY DISEASE.

urban/rural elderly Studies have found differences between the attitudes and habits of elderly living in urban environments as compared to those living in rural areas. Access to services and goods that the elderly need and to activities and people they enjoy are easier in cities. It has also been found that the elderly who live in cities are more ready to become involved in life and have a more positive attitude than those living in rural areas. Eighty-five percent of the aged living in urban areas read the newspaper whereas only 48 percent of those in rural areas read a daily newspaper. Interest in politics was expressed by 53 percent of those living in an urban area and by 17 percent of those living in a rural area. In general, the aged living in urban areas have more life satisfaction because of the opportunities for involvement that are offered to them in a city. However, those people who have spent their entire life in a rural area may be most happy remaining there into old age.

Brocklehurst, J. C. *Textbook of Geriatric Medicine and Gerontology*. New York: Churchill Livingstone, 1985.

URI   See ACUTE RESPIRATORY DISEASE.

urinary retention   The most common causes of urinary retention in elderly patients are bladder-neck obstruction, posterior-urethral stricture, and neurological abnormalities. The majority of cases of acute retention occur in men as a result of bladder-neck obstruction due to prostatic hypertrophy.

People with a stricture of the posterior urethra can undergo a reconstruction procedure with excellent results. In temporary acute paraplegia, a catheter can be left in for up to six weeks. Antibiotics should be given continuously during this time. In people with permanent neurological damage, division of the external urethral sphincter may remove the necessity for permanent catheterization.

See also PROSTATE HYPERTROPHY, BENIGN.

Brocklehurst, J. D. *Geriatric Medicine and Gerontology*, 3rd ed. New York: Churchill Livingstone, 1985.

urinary tract infection (UTI)   Urinary tract infection is a major problem in old age. These infections can be caused by residual urine in the bladder, which may be due to a flaccid bladder, increasing immobilization, and poor nutrition.

Symptoms include urinary frequency, painful urination, incontinence, fever, lower back pain, urgency, hematuria (blood in urine), and confusion. Many urinary tract infections, however, may be totally asymptomatic.

Treatment for urinary tract infection is generally medical and antibiotics may be prescribed. Medications commonly used in the treatment of urinary tract infection include urinary antiseptics such as Gantrisin, Furadantin, and Bactrim. Sulfonamides are the usual systemic antibiotic of choice. The people that have urinary tract infections or are prone to UTI should be encouraged to increase their fluid intake and improve their general nutrition. Increasing fluids helps to dilute the urine, which lessens irritation and burning and provides a continual flow of urine to discourage stasis and multiplication of bacteria in the urinary tract. Some individuals with chronic urinary tract infections take urinary antiseptics prophylactically. Females should be instructed on good hygiene habits, including proper toilet tissue handling (wiping front to back).

It is important that urinary tract infections are identified and treated promptly. These infections contribute to illness during the acute infection and are also significant in the development of chronic renal failure.

Steinberg, F. U. *Care of the Geriatric Patient*, 6th ed. St. Louis: C. V. Mosby Co., 1983.

U.S. National Institute on Aging (NIA)   The National Institute on Aging in Bethesda, Maryland, part of the National Institutes of Health, was created more than a decade ago through the efforts of the scientific and medical communities. In recent years the NIA budget has been about $140 million annually. In addition to studying the care and social problems of the elderly the NIA is in the forefront of medical research. In its pilot program, the NIA has focused on three prime areas of interest: genetics, neuroscience, and psychosocial factors. The foundation's purpose in genetic research is to discover which genes might cause the aging process. The second prime area of interest, neuroscience, focuses on the ability of the aging brain to repair damage from injury or disease—and in recent years Alzheimer's disease has been a major focus. The third area of research, psychosocial factors, deals with factors such as the impact of stress and retirement on the elderly. Although the NIA primarily works on these three areas, they also conduct research in many other fields of medicine.

Roessing, W. "Aging Well," in *Aging,* Goldstein, E. C., ed. Vol. 3, Art. 6. Boca Raton, Fl.: Social Issues Resource Series, Inc., 1981.

uterovaginal prolapse The supports of the uterus and vagina are closely related and should be considered together. Uterine prolapse may predominate but is usually associated with some degree of vaginal wall laxity. Uterovaginal prolapse may be caused by congenital weakness of the pelvic organ supports, following childbirth, stemming from hormone deficiency, or be brought on by the natural aging process. With aging, the hormonal changes, combined with the stress of childbirth many years before, cause the muscles in the pelvis that support the uterus and vagina to start to relax.

Because of the proximity of the bladder, bladder symptoms may occur such as incomplete emptying and urinary infection.

Management of uterovaginal prolapse depends on the severity of symptoms. Insertion of a pessary (instrument placed in the vagina to support uterus or rectum) for support may be used. However, in some cases surgery may be indicated.

See also URINARY RETENTION, URINARY TRACT INFECTION.

Brocklehurst, J. C. *Textbook of Geriatric Medicine and Gerontology.* New York: Churchill Livingstone, 1985.

uterine cancer See CANCER, UTERINE.

UTI See URINARY TRACT INFECTION.

V

vaginal bleeding Vaginal bleeding can be serious after a woman has gone through menopause. Any vaginal bleeding one year or more postmenopause is considered abnormal. There are several factors that may cause vaginal bleeding, including vaginitis, cervicitis (inflammation of uterine cervix), ovarian cancer, endometrial (lining of the uterus) cancer, and the use of drugs, such as digoxin, Coumadin, and estrogen.

Treatment depends on the cause of the bleeding. A dilation and curettage (d&c) or a biopsy may be necessary to determine the cause. If it is a benign condition, it will usually respond to the appropriate treatment. If it is a malignant condition, a hysterectomy or radiation therapy or both may be recommended.

If the bleeding is caused from drug usage, it will be necessary to alter, or stop the medications.

See also CANCER, OVARIAN; CANCER, UTERINE; VAGINITIS.

Steinberg, F. U. *Care of the Geriatric Patient,* 6th ed. St. Louis: C. V. Mosby Co., 1983.

vaginitis (vaginitis, senile) Vaginitis is inflammation of the vagina and is the most common gynecological problem of older females. The most common cause is a progressive atrophy of tissue, which decreases normal moisture, shrinks the structures, and allows invasion of pyogenic bacteria.

Symptoms include itching, burning, dryness, possibly a pinkish discharge, and painful intercourse.

Treatment for vaginitis includes a culture to determine the causative bacterial agent. If no bacteria is identified, the vaginitis is usually treated with warm douches of a weak acid solution such as vinegar and water. An estrogenic preparation, given orally or applied intravaginally as an ointment, may help to restore the epithelium to a normal state.

If painful intercourse is the major problem, water-soluble lubricants during intercourse may be suggested. If a bacterial infection is isolated, sulfa, or other antibiotic treatment may be necessary, in either cream or oral form.

Scherer, J. C. *Introductory Medical-Surgical Nursing,* 3rd ed. Philadelphia: J. B. Lippincott Co., 1982.
Steinberg, F. U. *Care of the Geriatric Patient,* 6th ed. St. Louis: C. V. Mosby Co., 1983.

vaginitis, senile   See VAGINITIS.

varicose veins   Varicose veins are dilated tortuous veins, usually in the lower extremities. The valves of these veins are incompetent, allowing the blood to seep backward. The seepage causes congestion and further distention of the veins. Although the saphenous veins (veins running down leg) are most commonly affected, the rectum and esophagus may also be affected. Hemorrhoids are varicose veins around the rectum and anus.

Factors that contribute to varicose veins include obesity, thrombophlebitis, familial tendency, pelvic tumors, pregnancy, and prolonged standing. Men, as well as women, suffer from varicose veins.

Symptoms of varicose veins include fatigue in the legs, leg cramps, leg pain, and swelling of the ankles. If varicose veins are left untreated the vein becomes thick, hard, and painful.

Treatment of mild varicose veins may include rest periods with the legs elevated, bathing in warm water, exercise, and changes in routine so that there are no extended periods of time when the person is sitting or standing without movement. Sometimes support or elastic stockings are recommended.

Varicose veins are usually treated surgically if leg fatigue, cramps, and edema are pronounced. One method that is used frequently is ligation and stripping. The affected veins are severed from their connections and removed. The patient may be instructed to continue wearing elastic bandages or stockings following the surgery.

General instructions include elevating the leg while sitting, avoiding long periods of time standing, and weight reduction for the obese.

The major complication caused by varicose veins is reduced circulation to the leg, which can lead to sores that will not heal, infection, and possibly gangrene.

See also HEMORRHOIDS.

Narrow, B. W., and Buschle, K. B. *Fundamentals of Nursing Practice,* 2nd ed. New York: John Wiley and Sons, Inc., 1987.
Scherer, J. C. *Introductory Medical-Surgical Nursing,* 3rd ed. Philadelphia: J. B. Lippincott Co., 1982.

vasopressin   A drug in the experimental stage that shows promise of improving memory is vasopressin, a naturally occurring neurotransmitter found in the hypothalamus. Its use as a drug was developed at the National Institute of Mental Health.

Used as a nasal spray, vasopressin permeates the nasal membranes and reaches directly into the brain. Some studies show that the drug increased learning and memory in normal college students by 20 percent.

If tests prove it safe and effective, vasopressin may offer new hope to the elderly who experience faltering memories.

See also FORGETFULNESS; MEMORY PILL.

Martin, P. "Good News About Growing Older," in *Aging,* Goldstein, E. C., ed. Vol. 2, Art. 41. Boca Raton, Fl.: Social Issues Resource Series, Inc., 1981.

ventricular fibrillation   Ventricular fibrillation is a cardiac arrhythmia in which the ventricles twitch and there are no recognizable waves on the ECG tracing. Ventricular fibrillation is seen with electrocution, drowning, drug toxicity, and most often myocardial infarction. The prevalence of ventricular arrhythmias increase with age. Arrhythmias are also more serious in elderly because they may further compromise vital organs whose intrinsic function has been reduced by aging and disease.

Symptoms of ventricular fibrillation include no blood pressure, pulse, or audible heart beat and respirations that quickly cease.

Ventricular fibrillation is a fatal arrhythmia that must be treated immediately. Treatment involves instituting CPR (cardiopulmonary resuscitation), defibrillation (using electric shock to the heart to stop the rapid contractions), and administering epinephrine, sodium bicarbonate, and isoproterenol (Isuprel). The most effective treatment for ventricular fibrillation is defibrillation. CPR should be given immediately before and after defibrillation and should never be stopped for longer than five seconds, until the medication begins to take effect.

See also ARRHYTHMIAS, CARDIAC.

Phipps, W. J., *et al. Medical Surgical Nursing.* St. Louis: C. V. Mosby Co., 1983.
Scherer, J. C. *Introductory Medical-Surgical Nursing.* Philadelphia: J. B. Lippincott Co., 1982.

vertigo (dizziness, dysequilibrium, fainting)   Vertigo is one of the most common symptoms in old age. Vertigo may be caused by changes in blood pressure, diagnostic tests, vascular lesions, poorly fitted hearing aid or eyeglasses, inner ear defects, heart disorders, drug reactions, or Meniere's disease (disease characterized by vertigo, nausea, vomiting, tinnitus, and progressive deafness).

Symptoms of vertigo include light-headedness, diminished vision and hearing, nausea, headache, vomiting, and difficulty sitting up from the prone position, walking, and making quick turns. Faintness or loss of consciousness may indicate cardiac disorders.

Treatment for vertigo should include determining the cause of the dizziness and then appropriately treating it. The person who is experiencing dizziness should be instructed to sit on the edge of the bed before getting up to walk and to make use of handrails whenever possible. If drugs are determined to be causing the dizziness, the drug or dosage should be altered. Antihypertensive drugs (drugs to lower blood pressure) and sedatives are the drugs most likely to cause dizziness. If cardiac disorders are found, the person may require hospitalization to determine the proper treatment.

Phipps, W. J. *Medical Surgical Nursing,* 2nd ed. St. Louis: C. V. Mosby Co., 1983.
Steinberg, F. U. *Care of the Geriatric Patient,* 6th ed. St. Louis: C. V. Mosby Co., 1983.

vision   As an individual ages, light does not reach the retina as readily due to decreased pupil size, loss of lens transparency, and the thickening of the lens and lens capsule. Thus, a 65-year-old needs twice as much illumination to see as does a 20-year-old, and the 75-year-old needs three times as much. If the eyes adapt slowly to changes in illumination, wearing dark glasses until the person just steps into the doorway will enable him or her to overcome this problem. A small pocket flashlight will enable him or her to read restaurant menus or theater programs. If the person has decreased side vision, he or she should turn his or her head further to the right or left, especially when driving or crossing streets.

Visual acuity, the ability to see details at a distance, has a more rapid decline in the sixties and seventies. Most elderly people need glasses to correct this loss of vision.

When decreased vision occurs, it is helpful to simplify the environment. Suggest that the person discard items that are not needed in cupboards, bookshelves, and closets. Small bright red, pressure-sensitive markers can be put on items that are hard to see and often needed.

Increased far-sightedness, or presbyopia, occurs due to the loss of elasticity of the lens of the eye. If not corrected with eyeglasses, near objects will not be in focus.

The lens of the eye also tends to yellow with increasing age, affecting color discrimination. Blue and violets are filtered out and are more difficult to identify than colors at the red end of the color spectrum.

In almost 95 percent of the people over 65 years of age, opacification of the lens, a cataract, occurs. If the cataract causes sufficient visual difficulty to interfere with the patient's lifestyle, it can be removed in a surgical procedure done as an outpatient. The vast majority of patients have an artificial lens implanted at the time of surgery, thus avoiding the difficulties and inadequacies of cataract glasses or contact lenses.

Impairments such as macular degeneration, diabetes mellitus, multiple sclerosis, or a stroke greatly affect the eyes. Often, rehabilitative services are needed to enable the patient to cope with the effects of these changes. Low-vision clinics and numerous private and public agencies work with the ophthalmologist and other professionals to assist the visually handicapped. Some aids that are available include lighted magnifiers, large-type print, talking books, as well as assistance in filing for special Social Security benefits and tax benefits.

See also CATARACT; MACULAR DEGENERATION; PRESBYOPIA.

Reichel, W. M. *Clinical Aspects of Aging*. Baltimore: The Williams & Wilkins Co., 1979.
Steinberg, F. U. *Care of the Geriatric Patient*, 6th ed. St. Louis: C. V. Mosby Co., 1983.

vision, transient loss of   See AMAUROSIS FUGAX.

visiting homebound and institutionalized elderly   Often individuals who visit the elderly, whether out of a sense of duty or because they enjoy it, find that they do not know what to do during such events. Fortunately experience has shown that there are particular ways to create pleasant and meaningful times for the visitor as well as for homebound or institutionalized persons.

Taking snapshots of family, friends, and events of past times can be pleasant and helpful in keeping the individual in touch with reality (reality orientation), and, when left behind, these can continue to be a source of entertainment for the older person. Bringing a gift of a small craft to work on together can be fun, especially so if the older person is withdrawn or unable to talk. Flowers, or perhaps small plants, are always appropriate and can serve as a topic of conversation.

Taking along small, unobtrusive pets (like a cat or small dog) can be desirable if appropriate in the surroundings, as can sharing exercise either by going out of doors or walking up and down hallways. Getting acquainted with a roommate, if there is one, and other visiting friends creates an atmosphere of sociability.

If an older person has difficulty with chatting, then taking along a book, or letters new and old, to read aloud can help. Reading the same book from visit to visit can provide structure and substance to times passed together. Games and card playing are also suitable.

Gifts do not have to be limited to birthdays or to holidays. Even bringing needed items of clothing or other practical articles brightly wrapped in packages can provide excitement for the visitee. Planning ahead with regard to conversational topics, having in mind a list of interesting family news items, or asking about favorite TV programs, sports shows, and current news events can also contribute. Tactile communication, as in giving a massage, brushing hair, embracing, and kissing, is gratifying.

Generally, short, frequent visits are much better than long occasional ones. Regularity is important too. The elderly tend to be more content if they know that visits will occur with consistency—an observation that holds true for telephone calls, letters, or mailed cassette tapes.

A positive attitude during a visit is highly important—everyone experiences days when everything goes wrong, and it is best not to visit when one has had one of those days. It is unwise to overload the older person with unnecessary concerns, and discussion of one's personal problems should usually be avoided because there is little that the older person can do about them but grieve. Avoiding criticism of the institution (as well as the person being visited) is wise, as problems should be addressed in contexts where solutions are possible, not where anxieties will simply increase.

When dealing with a confused individual, it is often not what is said or done that is important. The visit itself is the message—the reality of one's physical presence is enough. If nothing is said or done, but one is simply there, perhaps holding hands or lightly touching the individual, one conveys a message of care and consideration. One's silent presence, after all, may be all that is needed by homebound or institutionalized people.

Gillies, J. *A Guide to Caring for and Coping with Aging Parents*. Nashville: Thomas Nelson Publishers, 1981.

Kohut, S., *et al. Reality Orientation for the Elderly*, 3rd ed. Oradell, N.J. Medical Economics, 1987.

VISTA (Volunteers In Service To America)

Volunteers in Service to America (VISTA) is a service project under the auspices of ACTION. It was established in 1964 and is the oldest program in ACTION.

VISTA volunteers work and live among the poor, establishing programs that focus on hunger, unemployment, homelessness, illiteracy, drug and alcohol abuse, domestic violence, and the needs of the elderly, handicapped, and low-income youth. Though the average age of volunteers is 37, 18 percent are 55 years of age or older.

Nearly all VISTA volunteers are recruited by local sponsors. They serve full time for one to two years and receive allowances for food, lodging, travel, and medical insurance as well as a small stipend. Much of the funding for VISTA is generated through the private sector.

See also ACTION.

For additional information write or call:
VISTA
% ACTION

806 Connecticut Avenue, NW
Washington, DC 20525
(202) 606-4845.

visual limitations   Frequently, valuable information, instructions, and warnings can not be read and understood by those with impaired eyesight because of poor selection of print size or visual contrasts.

The most visible printing combination is black ink letters on white paper. Any print lighter than black or paper darker than white decreases the contrast. As people age, the need for contrast increases because of the discoloration of the lens of the eye. Contrast is not the only problem. The size of the print is very important. Help wanted ads generally appear in 6-point type, hampering job hunting efforts by the elderly. Newspapers are often printed in 8- or 9-point type. Most pamphlets and brochures on community services use typewriter type of 10-point size. The minimum recommended size type for the general population is 11 points. Twelve-point size type is suggested for the elderly, while 14 point is the minimum approved for the severely visually handicapped.

The use of these recommended type sizes are often ignored by government agencies, businesses, and manufacturers. The size print for medication warnings is smaller than the print in telephone directories. Room air fresheners packed in aerosol cans display warning that puncturing or exposure to high heat can cause explosions—but the print is below 11-point size and is often a chrome reflective paint on white background, offering no visual contrast. The use of colored ink on colored paper makes it almost impossible for most elderly to read.

Better Communications, Inc., a nonprofit organization, has been formed to research and promote better visual communications for the visually impaired, blind, deaf, and those with poor reading skills.

Ralph, J. "Visual Booby Traps for Aging Population," in *Aging*, Goldstein, E. C., ed. Vol.

2, Art. 58. Boca Raton, Fl.: Social Issues Resource Series, Inc., 1981.

vital capacity   Vital capacity measures the volume of air a person can blow out of the lungs after a deep breath. William B. Kannel and Helen Hubert of Boston University School of Medicine report that vital capacity can predict both long-term and short-term mortality. They say, "This pulmonary function measurement appears to be an indicator of general health and vigor and literally, a measure of living capacity."

Vital capacity falls with age, though the reason for the decline is not clear. It had been thought that vital capacity reflected how well the lungs function. But Kannel says his studies indicate it has more to do with chest size, how well the muscles work, and how healthy a person is. The ease with which the chest wall can expand and contract is an important factor.

A person whose vital capacity is always low is not going to do as well as someone whose level is always high. Many people believe that vital capacity can pick out people who are going to die 10, 20, or 30 years from now. So far, exercise or physical training does not seem to increase vital capacity. Efforts are increasing to learn what controls this characteristic and how to manipulate it.

Miller, J. A. "Making Old Age Measure Up," in *Aging,* Goldstein, E. C., ed. Vol. 2, Art. 12. Boca Raton, Fl.: Social Issues Resource Series, Inc., 1981.

vitamin A   See VITAMINS.

vitamin B-complex   See VITAMINS.

vitamin B$_{12}$ deficiency (pernicious anemia)   Pernicious anemia is the most common type of megaloblastic (abnormal blood cells) anemia. It is caused by a vitamin B$_{12}$ deficiency secondary to the lack of intrinsic factor secretion due to gastric atrophy. It occurs most frequently in later life.

The onset is insidious so that the anemia may be severe by the time the patient is first seen. The symptoms often can be mistaken for other illnesses, especially in the elderly. Inflammation of the tongue is an important sign. Liver enlargement is common, especially if there is cardiac failure, and mental changes seem to predominate. Other symptoms include anorexia (loss of appetite), nausea, vomiting, flatulence, dyspepsia (discomfort under the breastbone after eating), and diarrhea.

Pernicious anemia may occur over a period of eight to 12 years in patients who have had a partial gastrectomy (surgical removal of all or part of the stomach). After a total gastrectomy, B$_{12}$ stores are depleted in two to three years and pernicious anemia follows about nine months later.

Vitamin B$_{12}$ therapy is necessary for life in confirmed cases of pernicious anemia. In the elderly, this is administered by injection and rarely by oral therapy. Clinical improvement is observed almost immediately after the start of therapy. However, neurological symptoms are slower to respond unless they have been present for less than six months.

Ham, R. J. *Geriatric Medicine Annual—1987.* Oradell, N.J.: Medical Economics Books, 1987.
Reichel, W. *Clinical Aspects of Aging.* Baltimore: Williams & Wilkins Co., 1979.

vitamin C   See VITAMINS.

vitamin D   See VITAMINS.

vitamin E   See VITAMINS.

vitamin K   See VITAMINS.

vitamins (minerals; vitamins A, D, E, K, B-complex and C; calcium; iron; sodium chloride)   The need for vitamins increases with age. There are two types of vitamins: fat soluble and water soluble. The fat-soluble vitamins (A, D, E and K) can be stored in the body and may build up to toxic levels if consumed in large doses. The water-soluble vitamins (B-complex and C) are not stored well in the body, so they must be eaten daily. Mineral oil inhibits the absorption of fat-soluble vitamins and heat and air will destroy water-soluble vitamins.

Vitamin A helps prevent night blindness and is good for healthy skin and protection against infections. It is found in green vegetables, deep yellow vegetables, fortified milk, butter, and liver.

Vitamin D is necessary for the absorption and utilization of calcium in the body. It is found in green leafy vegetables, sardines, salmon, yogurt, fortified milk, and liver.

Vitamin E helps transport oxygen to the blood cells and also helps protect the red blood cells. It is found in nuts, seeds, eggs, sweet potatoes, leafy vegetables, and whole grains.

Vitamin K is necessary for normal blood clotting, and it helps maintain liver function. It also aids in the absorption of food in the intestines. It is found in green leafy vegetables, cauliflower, soybeans, fortified milk, yogurt, egg yolks, and sunflower oil.

Vitamin B-complex group is necessary for healthy nervous system, skin, appetite, and digestion. It is found in poultry, liver, dairy products, eggs, oatmeal, rice, nuts, seeds, whole-grain breads, cereals, and vegetables.

Vitamin C is necessary for healthy cells in all parts of the body. It is found in citrus fruits, broccoli, cabbage, peppers, tomatoes, and baked potatoes.

Common symptoms of vitamin deficiency are muscle cramps, nerve irritability, fragile bones, exhaustion, depression, poor appetite, constipation, skin disorders, and insomnia.

If the older person's diet is found to be adequate, the person does not need vitamin supplements. Once a deficiency is found, however, it is very difficult to correct. Calcium, iron, and sodium chloride are minerals that are vital to the older adult but may be poorly absorbed through the gastrointestinal tract.

Calcium is needed for muscles to contract and relax as well as maintain bone strength. It also helps the blood to clot. It is important to have adequate amounts of calcium because the body will take the needed calcium from bones when it is lacking.

Iron is found in all tissue cells of the body. It is stored in the liver and used to make hemoglobin. When an older person has an iron deficiency, it is usually caused by a disease. A diet that includes leafy vegetables, flour, eggs, whole grains, and meat will adequately supply the needed iron.

Sodium chloride is needed for the transmission of nerve impulses, the relaxation of muscles, and to maintain the balance between body fluids and cells. The U.S. Recommended Daily Allowance (RDA) is about a teaspoon of salt each day. Needless to say, the problem with sodium chloride is that of taking in excessive amounts. Studies have shown that hypertension and abnormal fluid retention are associated with high sodium diets. Therefore, it is very important for the person to regulate the amount of sodium intake.

Having a balanced diet is very important for an elderly person. Vitamin and mineral supplements are not necessary unless the diet is found to be inadequate.

Scherer, J. C. *Introductory Medical-Surgical Nursing,* 3rd ed. Philadelphia: J. B. Lippincott Co., 1982.

Steinberg, F. U. *Care of the Geriatric Patient,* 6th ed. St. Louis: C. V. Mosby Co., 1983.

Volunteers In Service To America   See VISTA.

volunteer work   The wisdom and expertise of many elderly people is a vast resource, many charitable and philanthropic organizations gladly receive older individuals who wish to offer volunteer services. When older individuals engage in volunteer work they often find that they become deeply engaged in the organization's activities even though they may not have been particularly interested at first.

Politics is another field of endeavor that is open to older individuals. Because approximately 20 percent of the voters in national elections are older than 65, the older age group can be a potent force in politics for the well-being of the nation. Robert Binstock, editor of *The Handbook of Aging and The Social Sciences,* holds that the elderly have in the past not wielded independent political power in their own interests, but this could change in the future. At present the number of elderly voters grows yearly, and volunteer opportunities abound.

Groups that need volunteers include foster grandparents for the mentally retarded, sitters in day-care centers or churches, Retired Senior Volunteer Program (RSVP) (which coordinates volunteer opportunities), and Service Corps of Retired Executives (SCORE), an organization that provides free management counseling to small businesses. Local AARP offices can help to identify specific volunteer opportunities.

See also RSVP; SCORE.

Gillies, J. *A Guide to Caring for and Coping with Aging Parents.* Nashville: Thomas Nelson Publishers, 1981.
Loewinsohn, R. J. *Survival Handbook for Widows.* Glenview, Ill.: AARP, 1984.

volvulus   See BOWEL OBSTRUCTION.

W

walking   Walking is one of the best ways for older people to keep fit. Establishing a routine of walking and sticking to it can assist with digestion, elimination, and circulation.

Many older people prefer walking to jogging because it is safer. Most elderly people in good health walk as well as they did in youth and middle age, although with more deliberation. Some tend to walk more slowly, eyeing the ground for unevenness and pitfalls. Many older people may need the assistance of a cane or a person when walking. For the older person who is unsteady or has a visual handicap, having someone to point out curbs or holes in the sidewalk can be quite helpful.

Many older individuals find it easier to walk in a mall or indoor shopping center than out of doors. In a mall, it never rains or snows, the surface is level, and the environment is pleasant, frequently including music, temperature control, and seasonal decor. Neighborhood parks or streets with little traffic may also be a pleasant place to walk. If none of these places are convenient for walking, an inexpensive treadmill with sturdy rails can be purchased or rented.

Many older individuals have become involved in the competitive sport of race walking for both recreation and exercise.

Rossman, I. *Clinical Geriatrics,* 3rd ed. Philadelphia: J. B. Lippincott Co., 1986.
Yanker, G., and Burton, K. *Walking Medicine.* New York: McGraw-Hill, Inc., 1990.

water, hard   A relationship between the hardness of drinking water and the aging of the cardiovascular system has been proposed often over the past 20 years. The study on three matched communities in Los Angeles appears to rule out that hypothesis. Mortality from cardiovascular diseases was not related to water hardness.

See also AGING, BIOLOGICAL THEORY OF.

Allweight, S. P., *et al. Mortality and Water-hardness in Three Matched Communities in Los Angeles.'' Lancet* 2: 860-864 (1974).
Brocklehurst, J. C. *Textbook of Geriatric Medicine and Gerontology.* New York: Churchill Livingstone, 1985.

wearing out theory   The oldest theory of aging is the ''wearing out'' theory. This theory proposes that the body wears out just as a car does. Molecules and cells within the body that are meant to last a lifetime and are not usually replaced begin to degenerate. Nerve cells do not regenerate and nor do the collagen molecules that hold the body's skin and organs together. When these are damaged, their function is lost.

The body has compensatory mechanisms. For example, when brain neurons, or nerve cells, die, adjacent nerves send out branches to fill in the space and make new connections. These compensatory responses have limits, however. Eventually, too many nerve cells are lost for adjacent ones to take over lost connections.

See also AGING, BIOLOGICAL THEORY OF.

Maranto, G. "Aging: Can We Slow the Inevitable," in *Aging,* Goldstein, E. C., ed. Vol. 2, Art. 78. Boca Raton, Fl.: Social Issues Resource Series, Inc., 1981.

Thompson, L. "After Age 30, Survival Is Infinite," in *Aging,* Goldstein, E. C., ed. Vol. 3, Art. 17. Boca Raton, Fl.: Social Issues Resource Series, Inc., 1981.

wheelchair management   As individuals grow older, the likelihood of being confined to a wheelchair increases. The nature of the disability may be temporary, such as postsurgery or following a fracture. The disability may be permanent, including such conditions as frailty or arthritis. Regardless of the reason for the disability, it may be necessary at some point to manage a wheelchair.

Transfers   Transfers from wheelchair to car, bed, and toilet are made according to the disability.

If the person is a hemiplegic (paralyzed on one side of the body—without use of that arm or leg) he or she should be assisted to a standing position, provided with underarm support and held onto at the waist, by gripping the belt or side. The person should be helped to turn or pivot and assisted with seating. The paralyzed leg should be lifted and placed in a comfortable position. Trans-

ferring back to the wheelchair is the reverse of this procedure.

If the person is a paraplegic (paralyzed from the waist down) frequently he or she develops enough upper body strength to transfer from the wheelchair with little or no assistance. If necessary, a transfer board (a plastic board placed between a wheelchair and a car seat or a chair) can be used to make the maneuver easier, as the person can slide his or her body across the board.

If the person is a quadriplegic (paralyzed from the neck down) a transfer can be made by one strong person, who places one arm under the knees and the other arm around the back and under the shoulders of the quadriplegic, but usually this maneuver is performed by two people. The transfer board can be utilized in this instance also. Some quadriplegics learn to transfer without assistance.

If the person in the wheelchair is disoriented, it may be necessary for the assistant to repeat instructions about when to stand, pivot, etc.

When making transfers into chairs, one should choose stationary chairs with arms if possible. During transfers wheelchair wheels should be locked, so the wheelchair cannot roll away.

Accessibility   Once in a wheelchair, the person or the companion will become very aware of architectural barriers. Architectural barriers are structural designs that prevent wheelchair access. Stairs, narrow doorways, curbs, revolving doors, and restrooms are some of the barriers. If there is a low curb or a step, the companion can tilt the wheelchair back to its pivot point and ease the wheelchair up. If the person in the wheelchair is able, he or she can push the wheels at the same time making this an easier maneuver.

Planning ahead by calling or writing the establishment one wishes to visit and asking about accessibility is wise. Federal and state governments have made barrier-free access a requirement in government subsidized construction. They have offered certain tax advantages to private owners, who make their businesses accessible. Because of this many newer facilities and businesses are accessible now. This gives the person in a wheelchair the choice of not patronizing establishments that are not barrier-free.

Transportation   Airlines are cooperative and helpful with handicapped passengers. An airport attendant will usually assist the disabled person to board early. In major airports the person can usually be wheeled to the door of the plane in his or her own wheelchair. Large airplanes may be able to accommodate boarding into first class in one's own chair; smaller planes may require a transfer to a specially designed airline wheelchair. A person should be sure to make it clear that his or her own chair will be needed immediately upon landing. Many airlines will place the wheelchair into the baggage compartment last for this reason.

Many metropolitan bus systems offer special transportation to the disabled. The vehicles are usually specially adapted vans, with raised roofs and hydraulic chair lifts. Fares for these buses will usually be higher than the normal bus fare because the service provided is door to door. These charges are still lower than taxi fares.

Most cars, except for the smallest compacts, are large enough to carry a wheelchair. The wheelchair can be carried on the floor in front of the back seat or in the trunk. A foldable, light-weight wheelchair makes loading and unloading more convenient. The light-weight wheelchairs, however, are not as durable. The amount of travel versus durability should be considered before purchasing a wheelchair.

If the person is in an electric or nonfolding wheelchair, a specially equipped van may be necessary for transportation. These vans may have hydraulic or electric lifts that raise the person in the wheelchair from ground level to van floor level and allow the person to remain in his or her wheelchair. They may be equipped with a folding ramp. With either the lift or the ramp, extra space is required for parking. Designated handicapped parking spaces offer this extra space. It is also important to remember that when parking it is necessary to leave enough space between cars for the car door to open fully so the person can transfer or be transferred into and out of the wheelchair.

Gillies, J. *A Guide to Caring for and Coping with Aging Parents.* Nashville: Thomas Nelson Publishers, 1981.

widowhood, preparing for   One of the most difficult adjustments in becoming a widow is learning to live independently. Formerly shared decisions must now be made alone. Chores and jobs never done before now become one's responsibility and learning to cope can be a painful process. Relying on the experience of someone who has been through the process can be helpful, and one widow, Anna Averyt of Mobile, Alabama, offers the following interesting advise.

1. Learn to manage your finances—balance your budget, learn to write checks, and balance your bank statement. Don't let outgoing funds exceed income.
2. Get an idea of what your monthly bills are and also how seasonal bills, such as utilities, vary from month to month.
3. Put some money aside for emergencies—medical bills, car repairs, or home maintenance.
4. Look at your payments for the year, including bills that come quarterly, such as home and auto insurance, health and life insurance, and property taxes. Plan for them in your budget.
5. List those months when you can expect to receive additional income, such as dividend checks or interest on certificates of deposit or stocks. This will help you know your real annual income and help you plan for the extra expenses listed above.
6. Keep a list of reputable repairmen and their phone numbers. When major re-

pairs are necessary, check with the Better Business Bureau or a local consumer protection office before hiring a worker.
7. Establish credit in your own name.
8. Appoint someone to sign checks in emergency.
9. If you do not already know how to drive, learn. Friends will take you places, but it makes you dependent.
10. When you go out with friends, don't let anyone "foot" the bill. Even if you're on a fixed income, pay your own share. This way you'll get more invitations.
11. Let your neighbors know your routine: what lights are usually on at night, whether you generally keep your shades up, and so forth. Also, let them know when you will be out of town, so that they can keep an eye out for anything suspicious.
12. Have a peephole put into the door and use it before opening to strangers.
13. Don't list your first name in the telephone book. Strangers will know you're a woman living alone. Use your first initial instead.
14. Keep in your wallet at all times: name, address, telephone number (home and business) of someone to contact in case of an emergency; health insurance card; and if desired, a card that says "In Case of Emergency, call minister" and phone number.
15. Keep a phone, a flashlight, and emergency numbers by your bed.
16. Keep items such as soup and Jell-O in the house in case you are sick and can't get out to the store.

Averyt, A. *Successful Aging.* New York: Ballantine Books, 1987.

wills   Many older people avoid making a will because they feel it is morbid or unnecessary, and in fact, only one out of eight people die with a will. Some people think that wills are only for the wealthy, not realizing that the costs and complications caused by not having a will can be especially heavy when small amounts of property are involved.

Every person needs a will to avoid unnecessary costs and difficulties when distributing property to heirs and assignees. While one can prepare a will oneself, a will drawn up by an attorney, recorded, witnessed, and kept in a safe place (most often a safe deposit box) is usually advisable. Wills should be reviewed and updated every two to three years to conform to periodic changes in family structure, business, and state or federal laws.

If there is no will, the property of the deceased is distributed among relatives in accordance with the current state laws. But, if there are no relatives and no will, property may go to the state.

Wills help to guarantee fewer family squabbles after death, provide opportunity to explain one's wishes, and most often tend to unify families.

See also ESTATE PLANNING.

Gillies, J. *A Guide to Caring for and Coping with Aging Parents.* Nashville: Thomas Nelson Publishers, 1981.
Lester, A. D. & Lester, J. L. *Understanding Aging Parents.* Philadelphia: The Westminster Press, 1980.
Soled A. J. *The Essential Guide to Wills, Estates, Trusts, and Death Taxes.* Glenview, Ill.: AARP, 1984.

wind chill   The combined effects of low temperature and wind speed make cold weather seem colder to exposed skin. This is known as the wind chill index. A very strong wind combined with temperatures only slightly below freezing can have the same chilling effect as a temperature nearly 50 degrees lower in a calm atmosphere.

The elderly and those in high-risk groups should remain indoors during winter storms or cold snaps. Only those in good physical condition should venture outdoors. If it is necessary to go outdoors, clothing should be loose-fitting, light-weight, and worn in several layers. Outer garments should be tightly woven, water repellant, and hooded. The mouth should be covered to ensure warm breathing and protect the lungs from the cold air. Mittens provide better protection than gloves.

Shoveling snow can bring on a heart attack, a major cause of death during winter storms, and should be avoided except by those in peak physical condition. Furnaces, heaters, fireplaces, and stoves should be maintained in good working condition to prevent fire hazards.

See also HYPOTHERMIA.

U.S. Department of Commerce, National Oceanic and Atmospheric Administration. *National Weather Service Pamphlet NOAA/PA* 79018 (Rev. 8/83). 1986

wisdom   Wisdom has been attributed to older people in nearly all world societies from ancient times, but modern research on the psychology of aging has paid little attention to this quality of the late years. Instead, studies of the psychology of aging have frequently focused on decline, comparing the mental performance of old people with young people on such tasks as the speed of learning new information, speed of senses in registering stimuli, ability to see patterns, measuring IQ, and the like. Older people have also been compared with themselves on performance tests as they advanced in years (longitudinal studies).

The results of comparisons between young and old, many of which have shown lower levels of performance by older groups, are ambiguous because it is by no means clear that the differences demonstrate decline— that is, the differences between young and old may simply reflect the higher levels of education of the younger generation. Further, repeated long-term studies with the same individuals show that normal changes are quite minimal. In spite of this, the tone of many reports about the psychology of aging imply major declines in competence,

and the term *decrement* is commonly used to describe the psychology of later life.

A number of researchers, however, have assessed the psychology of aging quite differently. Instead of measuring decline, their aim has been to measure the unique and special characteristics of mind possessed by older people. Among these scholars are psychologist James Birren, former dean of the Andrus Gerontology Center at the University of Southern California and now Brookdale Distinguished Scholar at UCLA; Gary Kenyon of St. Thomas University, Brunswick, Canada; Giselle Labouvie-Vief of Wayne State University in Detroit; and S. Holliday and M. Chandler, authors of *Wisdom: Explorations in Adult Competence*. Other scholars include Paul Baltes and F. Ditman-Kohli, who authored ''Wisdom as a Prototypical Case of Intellectual Growth'' in a volume entitled *Beyond Formal Operations: Alternative Endpoints to Human Development;* and K. Warner Schaie and Sherry L. Willis, who published an extensive survey of studies in the psychology of aging in their book *Adult Development and Aging,* now in its second edition.

These researchers might typically define wisdom as Kenyon did when he described it as ''the ability to exercise good judgement about important but uncertain matters of life''—where ''uncertain matters'' refers to problems that may not have come up before, or to which there are competing or conflicting solutions, and so forth. These researchers describe the old as having ''self-creating'' powers because they seem to be more independent in their decisions, and less subject to external influences like the fads and trends that sweep over the young.

They propose also that the old are better able to live with contradictions in life and that they quickly see the essentials of situations because of their greater experience. Wisdom, they observe, includes the intent to do good, which in turn depends on holding favorable attitudes toward other people.

In looking at the issue of decline in mental skills in age, these researchers are aware of the increase of organic brain disorders and of lower mental agility often occurring in the later years, but they also note that so-called crystalized intelligence and certain other mental powers can remain stable and even increase. Knowledge of vocabulary words, for example, declines very little and may actually improve at any age.

Besides this, these researchers have demonstrated that lack of mental skill may be due to lack of practice, and that training improves performance of mental tasks. Relatedly, they observe that many people who perform mental tasks less rapidly and remember less well than in the past manage to compensate for these losses.

Current efforts by these psychologists to characterize the special features of mental competence in age, where speed seems to be replaced by depth and quality, are relatively recent. In the future people can anticipate great progress in defining the now ineffable, and little understood, dimensions of the older mind. Even now sources such as the General Social Survey suggest the validity of the new thinking.

For example, one of the questions interviewers for the General Social Survey ask, "Would you say that most of the time people try to be helpful, or that they are mostly just looking out for themselves?" The elderly more than any other age group respond that people are helpful—from age 75 on, about 62 percent of the women and 52 percent of the men say people are helpful, but from age 18–24 only 43 percent of the women and 37 percent of the men think so.

When asked, "Do you think most people would try to take advantage of you if they got the chance, or would they try to be fair?" about 70 percent of the women and 60 percent of the men over 75 said that people would be fair, compared to only about 48 percent of both men and women 18–24 years old who think so.

Answers to two questions like these are important because they come from a national poll that accurately reflects the opinion of the American public, but a great deal of research is still needed to determine what such responses mean and what the special mental features of older people may be. Understanding the quality of wisdom in the old is one of the important agendas for future research in the psychology of aging.

Kenyon, Gary. "Basic Assumptions in Theories of Human Aging," in Birren, J. and Bengtson, V., *Emergent Theories of Aging.* New York: Springer Publishing Co., 1988.

Schaie, K. W., and Willis, S. L. *Adult Development and Aging,* 2nd ed. Boston: Little, Brown and Company, 1986.

withdrawal See DENIAL.

work after retirement A survey reported in *Modern Maturity,* the magazine of the American Association of Retired Persons, suggests that people who work beyond retirement age do so most often in jobs that give them freedom, challenge, and creative opportunities. Statistics show that nearly half the men working past age 65 are in occupations that the U.S. Labor Department labels as "sales," 16 percent are in executive positions, 15 percent in administrative and managerial capacities, and 14 percent in professions. Women in the present 65+ generation generally did not have the opportunity to enter professions or the managerial and administrative ranks, so most who continue to work occupy service-oriented jobs.

According to this article, the trend toward automation will replace jobs that are stressful, boring, or repetitive with more interesting work. Future job growth will occur most rapidly in human service fields, financial areas, health care, retailing, and restaurant work. Older workers who work in these capacities may be especially welcome simply because they will often be providing services to people in their own age group.

Recent trends have also seen a partial reversal of Social Security policies respecting pre- and postretirement work. Individuals in the future will gain more by delaying retirement and will be able to earn more after age 65 than they have in the past.

For example, people now add an additional 3 percent in Social Security benefits for each year worked between age 65 and age 70. While the amount of earnings permitted without reduction in Social Security benefits is now $1 for every $3 earned, the level of earnings on which this rule applies increases with growth in average wages (the $8,440 allowed in 1988 rose to $8,800 in 1989 and $9,360 in 1990), and a group in Congress has introduced The Older Americans Freedom to Work Act, which aims to remove all earnings limits for persons age 65 and older. Further, to conserve the valuable human capital resources of the older generation, government and private employers are beginning to increase training opportunities for those nearing retirement.

Under a provision of the Employee Retirement Insurance Security Act, pensions must become portable (transferable with individuals when they leave an employer), and it is expected that some older workers will leave career jobs to start their own companies; or, they may search out opportunities in job markets where the monetary benefits are less but the work is more satisfying.

"The Advent of the Gold-Collar Worker." *Modern Maturity* (October–November, 1986).

Y

Yanomamo Indians   The Yanomano Indians, who inhabit the tropical rain forests of northern Brazil and have little contact with modern cultures use no salt in their diet. Their major food is the plantain *Musa paradisiaca,* supplemented by game, fish, insects, and wild plants. Studies show that their average daily sodium excretion is about one mmol. Further, their blood pressure does not increase after the thirties but actually declines slightly. This supports the theory that sodium intake is a major variable influencing the aging of the cardiovascular system.

See also BUSHMEN OF THE KALAHARI DESERT; MASAI; NEW GUINEAN HIGHLANDERS; POLYNESIANS; SOLOMON ISLAND TRIBES; SOMALI CAMEL HERDSMEN; TARAHUMARA INDIANS.

Brocklehurst, J. C. *Textbook of Geriatric Medicine and Gerontology.* New York: Churchill Livingstone, 1985.

APPENDIXES

Appendix I
Tables and Graphs

Appendix II
Sources of Information

APPENDIX I

Tables

243

Graphs

Table 1 Adult Children: Methods Used to Control Their Elderly Parents

Methods	Percent
Screamed and yelled	40
Used physical restraint	6
Forced feeding or medication	6
Threatened to send to nursing home	6
Threatened with physical force	4
Hit or slapped	3

SOURCE: Steinmetz, S. K. "Elder Abuse," in *Aging*, Gold-stein, E. C., ed. Vol. 2, Art. 3. Boca Raton, Fl.: Social Issues Resource Series, Inc., 1981.

Table 2 Aging Body (Women) Calories per Day Needed to Maintain a Weight of 125 Pounds

Age	Calories
20 years	2,000
30 years	1,900
40 years	1,800
50–60 years	1,700
70–80 years	1,500

SOURCE: Borst, B. "How Women Age," in *Aging*, Gold-stein, E. C., ed. Vol. 2, Art. 33, Boca Raton, Fl.: Social Is-sues Resource Series, Inc., 1981.

Table 3 Annual Costs of Living for Retired Couple for Retirement Decision

City	Food	Housing	Transportation	Other	Total
Atlanta, GA	$3,969	$3,595	$1,227	$3,712	$12,503
Austin, TX	$3,534	$4,153	$1,313	$3,675	$12,675
Bakersfield, CA	$3,669	$3,963	$1,322	$3,593	$12,547
Baton Rouge, LA	$3,993	$3,162	$1,296	$3,578	$12,029
Dallas, TX	$3,636	$3,918	$1,355	$3,602	$12,511
Durham, NC	$3,919	$3,885	$1,268	$3,838	$12,908
Honolulu, HI	$4,876	$4,910	$2,462	$3,953	$16,199
Los Angeles, CA	$3,813	$4,529	$1,412	$3,809	$13,563
Orlando, FL	$3,523	$4,285	$1,331	$3,599	$12,738
San Diego, CA	$3,739	$4,350	$1,359	$3,720	$13,168
URBAN U.S.	$3,997	$4,582	$1,205	$3,730	$13,514

SOURCE: Dickinson, Peter. *Sunbelt Retirement*. Glenview, Ill.: Scott, Foresman and Company, 1986.

Table 4 Annual Costs for Retired Couple in Major Sunbelt Cities
(all figures in dollars)

City	Food	Housing	Transportation	Other	Total
Atlanta, GA	4,763	4,314	1,472	4,454	15,003
Austin, TX	4,241	4,984	1,576	4,410	15,211
Bakersfield, CA	4,403	4,756	1,586	4,312	15,057
Baton Rouge, LA	4,792	3,794	1,555	4,294	14,435
Durham, NC	4,703	4,662	1,522	4,606	15,493
Honolulu, HI	5,851	5,892	2,957	4,744	19,444
Los Angeles, CA	4,576	5,435	1,694	4,571	16,276
Orlando, FL	4,228	5,142	1,597	4,319	15,285
San Diego, CA	4,487	5,220	1,631	4,464	15,802
URBAN U.S.	4,796	5,498	1,446	4,476	16,216

SOURCE: Census Bureau, Tax Foundation

Table 5 Body Composition with Age, Changes in

Compound Change	Approximate Change Between Ages 25–65
Total body water	15%–20% decrease
Extracellular fluid	35%–40% decrease
Body fat/body weight	25%–45% increase
Body fat	
Males	18%–36% increase
Females	33%–48% increase

SOURCE: Covington, T., and Walker, J. *Current Geriatric Therapy.* Philadelphia: W. B. Saunders Co., 1984.

Table 6 Climatic Data for Leading American Cities

State and City	Average Temp., F		Sunny Days	Humidity, (%)	Precipitation (in.)		Average Wind (mph)	Elevation (ft)
	Winter	Summer			Rain	Snow		
Alabama (Montgomery)	55.1	76.0	233	71.8	47.1	0	1.5	183
Alaska (Juneau)	25.8	49.1	100	77.2	53.7	150.2	8.2	114
Arizona (Phoenix)	60.5	96.4	289	33.5	10.87	0	7.3	1,117
Arkansas (Little Rock)	41.3	82.1	212	69.3	43.08	4.0	6.0	257
California (Los Angeles)	60.6	72.5	293	63.3	6.54	0	7.8	270
California (San Francisco)	52.7	59.6	211	76.0	20.79	trace	9.3	52
Colorado (Denver)	36.3	63.5	210	55.0	16.87	83.2	8.7	5,280
Connecticut (Hartford)	33.7	64.0	165	71.0	64.55	58.2	8.5	169
Delaware (Wilmington)	41.1	76.1	181	69.5	48.13	9.5	9.1	74
Florida (Tampa)	66.5	79.8	233	75.25	42.18	0	8.7	19
Florida (Miami)	72.1	79.7	252	76.25	63.11	0	8.3	7
Florida (Orlando)	67.9	80.7	231	72.0	51.35	0	8.5	108
Georgia (Atlanta)	50.2	71.5	206	70.8	50.61	trace	9.2	1,010
Hawaii (Honolulu)	72.9	79.6	244	68.8	26.90	0	13.2	7
Idaho (Boise)	34.5	62.3	216	57.5	11.43	21.4	9.1	2,838
Illinois (Springfield)	35.3	67.8	176	74.3	32.03	26.2	11.2	588
Indiana (Indianapolis)	36.4	66.9	159	72.3	40.27	18.1	9.7	792
Iowa (Des Moines)	29.1	62.3	176	73.5	36.02	36.7	10.4	938
Kansas (Topeka)	37.7	68.4	180	69.8	31.21	26.1	9.9	877
Kentucky (Louisville)	42.4	69.5	177	69.0	49.38	10.4	9.0	477
Louisiana (New Orleans)	59.7	77.5	234	78.8	63.98	0	8.5	4
Maine (Portland)	28.6	58.1	178	74.8	48.62	123.7	9.6	43
Maryland (Baltimore)	41.8	67.7	186	69.0	52.33	13.0	8.8	148
Massachusetts (Boston)	36.5	64.3	175	68.3	53.11	40.7	11.4	15
Michigan (Detroit)	25.6	63.8	188	66.5	29.96	30.6	10.6	619
Minnesota (Duluth)	15.2	53.9	165	74.0	39.61	110.2	9.8	1,428
Mississippi (Jackson)	55.0	77.4	226	76.0	50.03	trace	7.4	310
Missouri (Kansas City)	38.7	70.6	194	66.8	27.75	15.9	10.3	1,014
Montana (Helena)	27.1	55.1	169	57.0	8.22	40.0	8.3	3,828

Table 6 (continued)

State and City	Average Temp., F		Sunny Days	Humidity, (%)	Precipitation (in.)		Average Wind (mph)	Elevation (ft)
	Winter	Summer			Rain	Snow		
Nebraska (Omaha)	32.6	66.3	185	71.8	35.56	27.1	9.8	977
Nevada (Reno)	37.0	60.8	245	48.3	5.52	trace	8.4	4,404
Nevada (Las Vegas)	52.4	80.1	297	28.8	4.85	0.4	9.5	2,162
New Hampshire (Concord)	27.7	58.8	167	77.0	42.07	100.3	7.25	342
New Jersey (Trenton)	40.2	66.8	193	70.6	47.13	17.2	6.4	56
New Mexico (Albuquerque)	44.0	69.4	271	42.3	10.11	6.4	9.7	5,311
New York (New York)	39.9	67.8	232	67.8	67.03	22.9	8.8	132
North Carolina (Raleigh)	47.8	69.1	201	70.5	51.74	4.0	8.6	434
North Dakota (Bismarck)	19.9	58.8	171	67.0	15.16	45.6	9.6	1,647
Ohio (Columbus)	36.4	63.4	151	69.8	45.60	27.1	9.7	812
Oklahoma (Oklahoma City)	45.2	74.0	226	65.5	27.63	14.6	12.8	1,285
Oregon (Portland)	44.4	63.6	156	61.0	38.82	6.5	8.1	21
Pennsylvania (Harrisburg)	38.8	66.8	191	68.0	59.27	33.4	7.5	338
Rhode Island (Providence)	35.8	63.4	179	71.0	65.06	30.4	10.5	51
South Carolina (Charleston)	56.2	74.7	226	75.5	42.86	0	9.2	40
South Dakota (Rapid City)	28.5	59.6	202	64.3	17.19	23.1	11.1	3,162
Tennessee (Nashville)	47.4	71.8	198	71.8	54.41	2.5	9.1	590
Texas (Austin)	57.9	79.0	221	67.5	26.07	trace	9.0	597
Utah (Salt Lake City)	37.5	67.2	211	51.3	15.74	76.8	9.5	4,220
Vermont (Burlington)	25.5	59.2	151	73.0	38.10	121.6	8.0	332
Virginia (Richmond)	45.9	66.8	188	73.5	59.34	14.3	7.4	164
Washington (Seattle)	42.9	69.4	151	72.5	48.36	22.2	8.6	400
West Virginia (Charleston)	42.9	66.1	128	71.3	51.15	26.5	6.1	939
Wisconsin (Madison)	25.2	60.8	163	75.5	30.96	50.2	10.0	858
Wyoming (Cheyenne)	31.8	57.6	204	53.3	12.04	48.6	13.5	6,126

SOURCE: U.S. Department of Commerce, National Oceanic and Atmospheric Administration. Based on period 1941 to 1970. Dickinson, Peter. *Retirement Edens*. Washington, D.C.: American Association of Retired Persons, 1986.

Table 7 Delirium, Medications Causing

Disorder	Medication	Common Examples
Cardiovascular conditions	Antiarrhythmics	Procainamide, propranolol, quinidine
	Antihypertensives	Clonidine, methyldopa, reserpine
	Cardiac glycosides	Digitalis
	Coronary vasodilators	Nitrates
Gastrointestinal conditions	Antidiarrheals	Atropine, belladonna, homatropine, hyoscyamine, scopolamine
	Antinauseants	Cimetidine, Cyclizine, homatropine-barbiturate preparations, phenothiazines
	Antispasmodics	Methanthelene, propantheline
Musculoskeletal conditions	Anti-inflammatory agents	Corticosteroids, indomethacin, phenylbutazone, salicylates
	Muscle relaxants	Carisoprodol, diazepam
Neurologic-psychiatric conditions	Anticonvulsants	Barbiturates, carbamazepine, diazepam, phenytoin
	Antiparkinsonism agents	Amantadine, benztropine, levopoda, trihexyphenidyl
	Hypnotics and sedatives	Barbiturates, belladonna alkaloids, bromides, chloral hydrate, ethchlorvynol, glutethimide, methaqualone
	Psychotropics	Benzodiazepines, hydroxyzines, lithium salts, meprobamate, monoamine oxidase inhibitors, neuroleptics, tricyclic antidepressants
Respiratory-allergic conditions	Antihistamines	Brompheniramine, chlorpheniramine, cyproheptadine, diphenhydramine, tripelennamine
	Antitussives	opiates, synthetic narcotics
	Decongestants and expectorants	Phenylephrine, phenylpropanolamine, potassium preparations
Miscellaneous conditions	Analgesics	Dextropropoxyphene, opiates, phenacetin, salicylates, synthetic narcotics
	Anesthetics	Lidocaine, methohexital, methoxyflurane
	Antidiabetic agents	Insulin, oral hypoglycemics
	Antineoplastics	Corticosteroids, mitomycin, procarbazine
	Antituberculosis agents	Isoniazid, rifampin

SOURCE: Brocklehurst, J. C. *Textbook of Geriatric Medicine and Gerontology.* New York: Churchill Livingstone, 1985.

Table 8 Differential Growth of Various Age Groups in Percentage, Estimated

Age Group	Proportion of Age Group in Total Population in 1950	Interperiod Growth			Proportion of Age Group in Total Population in 2025
		1950–1975	1975–2000	2000–2025	
A. The World					
0–4	13.44	59.26	21.77	4.94	8.43
5–14	21.32	75.78	28.74	11.66	16.60
15–59	56.76	55.87	63.50	37.52	61.29
60+	8.48	61.65	70.69	89.99	13.68
Total	100.00	61.02	50.47	33.92	100.00
B. More Developed Regions					
0–4	10.23	1.70	2.11	4.61	6.72
5–14	17.55	26.25	−3.20	2.00	13.22
15–59	60.85	29.45	18.26	1.54	57.16
60+	11.37	75.54	38.76	36.89	22.90
Total	100.00	31.29	16.47	8.22	100.00
C. Less Developed Regions					
0–4	15.03	78.52	25.52	5.00	8.78
5–14	23.19	94.20	36.46	13.31	17.29
15–59	54.73	70.30	82.30	47.22	62.10
60+	7.03	50.69	100.07	123.96	11.03
Total	100.00	75.69	62.96	40.62	100.00

SOURCE: Shuman, T. "The Aging of the World's Population," in Goldstein, E. C., ed. *Aging,* Vol. 2, Art. 66. Boca Raton, Fl.: Social Issues Resource Series, Inc., 1981.

Table 9 Diuretic Side-Effects

	Common Side Effects	Less Common Side Effects
General	Hypovolemia	Gastrointestinal intolerance
	Postural hypotension	Skin rashes
	Potassium imbalance	Hypersensitivity reactions
	Sodium depletion	Marrow depression
	Alkalosis	Pancreatitis
	Impaired glucose tolerance	Cholestatic jaundice
	Urinary incontinence	Hypocalemia
Specific	Frusemide ⎫ in Ethacrynic Acid ⎬ high ⎭ dose	Otoxicity
	Spironolactone	Gastrointestinal hemorrhage Gynecomastia Impotence

SOURCE: Brocklehurst, J. C. *Textbook of Geriatric Medicine and Gerontology.* New York: Churchill Livingstone, 1985.

Table 10 Drugs Whose Absorption Is Decreased When Given with Food

Ampicillin	Penicillins
Isoniazid	Rifampin
Levodopa	Tetracyclines
Lincomycin	

SOURCE: Covington, T., and Walker, J. *Current Geriatric Therapy.* Philadelphia: W. B. Saunders Co., 1984.

Table 11 Drugs Whose Absorption Is Enhanced When Given with Food

Carbamazepine	Methoxsalen
Dicumarol	Methoprolol
Erythromycin stearate	Nitrofurantion
Griseofulvin (fatty foods)	Phenytoin
Hydralazine	Propranolol
Hydrochlorothiazide	Riboflavin
Lithium	Spironolactone

SOURCE: Covington, T., and Walker, J. *Current Geriatric Therapy*. Philadelphia: W. B. Saunders Co., 1984.

Table 12 Elderly: Methods Used to Control Their Adult Children

Methods	Percent
Scream and yell	43
Pout or withdraw	47
Refuse food or medication	16
Manipulate, cry, or use physical or emotional disability	32
Hit, slap, throw objects	22
Call police or others for imagined threats	10

SOURCE: Steinmetz, S. K. "Elder Abuse," in *Aging*, Goldstein, E. C., ed. Vol. 2, Art. 3. Boca Raton, Fl.: Social Issues Resource Series, Inc., 1981.

Table 13 Fertility Rates and Expectation of Life at Birth for Major World Regions

Region and Subregion	(a) General fertility rates*				(b) Expectation of life at birth (years)			
	1950–1955	1975–1980	1995–2000	2020–2025	1950–1955	1975–1980	1995–2000	2020–2025
World	150	119	94	72	47.0	57.5	63.9	70.4
Africa	203	203	174	98	37.3	48.6	57.8	67.2
Eastern Africa	205	213	191	106	35.7	46.8	50.6	66.6
Middle Africa	191	194	174	102	35.3	44.6	54.4	64.9
Northern Africa	201	187	138	79	41.5	53.7	62.4	70.1
Southern Africa	168	167	147	89	47.3	58.8	66.6	72.2
Western Africa	218	219	192	103	34.5	46.3	56.0	66.2
Latin America	180	143	106	85	51.2	62.5	68.1	71.8
Caribbean	159	117	93	81	51.8	62.8	67.0	70.7
Middle America	209	174	114	78	50.2	63.2	69.7	72.6
Temperate South America	108	90	75	63	60.3	68.1	71.1	72.1
Tropical South America	195	146	110	92	49.9	61.3	67.1	71.1
North America	101	64	56	61	69.0	73.0	74.1	75.1
East Asia	159	87	63	56	47.5	67.6	72.7	74.8
China	170	90	62	56	46.0	67.3	72.6	74.6
Japan	92	56	58	60	64.0	75.6	77.3	77.4
Other East Asia	153	108	74	60	48.2	63.2	69.5	73.6
South Asia	196	160	106	66	39.4	50.6	59.5	68.6
Eastern South Asia	185	147	92	62	39.4	52.5	61.8	69.5
Middle South Asia	200	164	108	65	38.9	49.2	57.9	67.7
Western South Asia	199	176	132	79	44.7	57.9	65.2	71.5
Europe	77	60	54	59	65.4	72.0	74.3	75.7
Eastern Europe	89	70	59	61	63.0	70.8	73.5	75.3
Northern Europe	68	55	51	58	69.2	72.9	74.7	75.9
Southern Europe	80	66	57	59	63.3	71.1	74.2	75.6
Western Europe	69	49	49	60	67.6	73.0	74.8	76.1
Oceania	117	91	75	67	60.7	65.6	70.2	73.8
Australia–New Zealand	98	69	59	62	69.8	73.0	74.8	76.0
Melanesia	195	192	131	77	36.1	51.1	61.8	69.8
Micronesia–Polynesia	210	144	97	68	54.0	64.6	70.0	73.8
U.S.S.R.	88	70	66	66	61.7	69.6	71.5	74.6

*Annual number of live births per 1,000 women aged 15–49 years.
SOURCE: Shuman, T. "The Aging of the World's Population," in *Aging,* Goldstein, E. C., ed. Vol. 2, Art. 66. Boca Raton, Fl.: Social Issues Resource Series, Inc., 1981.

Table 14 Gastric Emptying Time, Drugs that Delay

Aluminum hydroxide
Analgesics (narcotic)
Anticholinergics
Drugs with anticholinergic activity
   Antihistamines
   Phenothiazines
   Tricyclics
Ganglionic blockers
Isoniazid
Lithium

SOURCE: Covington, T., and Walker, J. *Current Geriatric Therapy.* Philadelphia: W. B. Saunders Co., 1984.

Table 15 Global Deterioration Scale

Reisberg's scale describes how Alzheimer's disease's pattern parallels in reverse that of child development—and tells doctors and relatives what to expect next of Alzheimer's victims.

Approx. Age	Abilities Acquired	Alzheimer's Stage	Abilities Lost
12+ years	Hold a job	Borderline	Hold a job
7–12 years	Handle simple finances	Early	Handle simple finances
5–7 years	Select proper clothes	Moderate	Select proper clothes
5 years	Put on clothes	Severe	Put on clothes
4 years	Shower unaided		Shower unaided
4 years	Go to toilet unaided		Go to toilet unaided
3–4½ years	Control urine		Control urine
2–3 years	Control bowels		Control bowels
15 months	Speak five or six words	Late	Speak five or six words
1 year	Speak one word		Speak one word
1 year	Walk		Walk
6–9 months	Sit up		Sit up
2–3 months	Smile		Smile

SOURCE: Roach, M. "Reflection in a Fatal Mirror," in *Aging,* Goldstein, E. C., ed. Vol. 2, Art. 83. Boca Raton, Fl.: Social Issues Resource Series, Inc., 1981.

Table 16 Homes, Median Price, in Selected Metropolitan Areas

Area	Median Price of Homes
Albany, NY	$ 60,500
Akron, OH	52,000
Anaheim-Santa Ana, CA	135,200
Atlanta, GA	72,200
Baltimore, MD	71,900
Birmingham, AL	65,000
Boston, MA	131,000
Buffalo-Niagara Falls, NY	47,000
Chicago, IL	81,800
Cincinnati, OH	61,100
Cleveland, OH	66,400
Columbus, OH	61,400
Dallas-Ft. Worth, TX	88,100
Denver, CO	83,700
Detroit, MI	51,000
Ft. Lauderdale, FL	73,300
Hartford, CT	97,200
Houston, TX	76,200
Indianapolis, IN	55,400
Jacksonville, FL	58,800
Kansas City, MO	63,600
Los Angeles, CA	116,900
Louisville, KY	51,000
Memphis, TN	63,800
Milwaukee, WI	68,700
Minneapolis-St. Paul, MN	75,200
Nashville, TN	66,000
New York City (area)	130,000
Oklahoma City, OK	65,000
Orlando, FL	71,900
Philadelphia, PA	66,700
Phoenix, AZ	75,700
Portland, OR	60,600
Providence, RI	65,500
Rochester, NY	64,000
St. Louis, MO	65,700
Salt Lake City, UT	67,200
San Antonio, TX	68,100
San Diego, CA	104,300
San Francisco, CA	134,500

SOURCE: Dickinson, Peter. *Retirement Edens*. Glenview, Ill.: Scott, Foresman and Company, 1987.

Table 17 Hospital Costs

State	Number of Hospitals	Beds	Average Daily Semiprivate Room
California	593	111,500	$337
Alaska	25	1,750	328
Michigan	223	48,300	324
Pennsylvania	310	82,900	307
Illinois	281	57,800	296
Nevada	25	3,600	289
Hawaii	27	4,100	277
Oregon	83	11,900	276
Massachusetts	178	41,400	275
Ohio	237	62,700	275
Washington	121	15,700	275
New York	344	125,900	269
Delaware	14	4,000	257
U.S. AVERAGE			$256
Colorado	97	15,100	254
Vermont	19	2,900	253
Maine	47	6,600	251
Connecticut	65	18,200	247
Rhode Island	21	5,900	246
Montana	67	5,200	244
Idaho	52	4,000	239
New Hampshire	34	4,700	239
Arizona	80	12,100	232
New Mexico	57	6,300	230
Minnesota	182	29,300	226
Maryland	85	24,900	226

Table 17 Hospital Costs (continued)

State	Number of Hospitals	Beds	Average Daily Semiprivate Room
Missouri	169	34,200	222
Indiana	133	31,900	221
Kansas	166	18,500	221
New Jersey	131	42,400	220
Florida	253	59,600	218
Iowa	139	20,500	215
Kentucky	118	18,800	211
North Dakota	59	6,000	211
Utah	42	5,300	203
Wisconsin	163	29,000	200
Wyoming	31	2,700	199
Oklahoma	142	17,700	198
Virginia	137	31,600	197
West Virginia	76	12,900	197
Alabama	146	25,900	194
South Dakota	68	5,700	194
Texas	561	84,600	191
Louisiana	157	26,000	187
Nebraska	110	11,800	186
Georgia	191	33,000	181
Tennessee	164	31,800	170
Arkansas	97	13,600	169
South Carolina	91	17,100	168
North Carolina	159	32,500	167
Mississippi	118	17,500	137

Rates prevailing in 1986–87

SOURCE: Dickinson, Peter. *Retirement Edens*. Glenview, Ill.: Scott, Foresman and Company, 1987.

Table 18 Housing Costs in Sunbelt

State	Average Selling Price Per Square Foot Living Space
Alabama	$34.47
Arizona	$36.65
Arkansas	$38.35
California	$49.14
Florida	$32.69
Georgia	$41.37
Hawaii	$43.05
Louisiana	$31.45
Mississippi	$33.50
New Mexico	$31.45
North Carolina	$36.19
South Carolina	$35.52
Texas	$36.43

SOURCE: Dickinson, Peter. *Sunbelt Retirement*. Glenview, Ill.: Scott, Foresman and Company, 1986.

Table 19 Laxatives, Pharmacologic Properties of

Category	Site of Action	Onset of Action	Specific Drug	Usual Adult Dose
Bulk formers	Small and large intestine	12–24 hours (may take up to three days	Methylcellulose	4–6 g
			Psyllium	7 g
			Polycarbophil	1 g
Stimulants				
Castor Oil	Small intestine	3 hours	Castor oil	15–30 ml
Anthraquinones	Small intestine	6–12 hours	Senna	2 ml
			Cascara sagrada	1 ml
			Danthron	75 mg
Diphenylmethanes	Small intestine	6–12 hours	Bisacodyl	10 mg
			Phenolphthalein	10 mg
Saline	Small and large intestine	½–3 hours	Magnesium and sodium sulfates	15 mg
			Magnesium citrate	200 ml
			Sodium and potassium tartrates and phosphates	10 gm
Hyperosmotics	Colon	30 minutes	Glycerin	3 gm
			Lactulose	15–30 ml
Surfactants	Colon	24–48 hours	Dioctyl sodium and calcium sulfosuccinates	50–500 mg
Emollients	Colon	6–8 hours	Mineral oil	15–30 ml

SOURCE: Covington, T., and Walker, J. *Current Geriatric Therapy*. Philadelphia: W. B. Saunders, 1984.

Table 20 Laxatives, Precautions in Use of

Bulk formers	Contraindicated in patients with esophageal, gastric, small intestinal, and colonic obstruction.
	Do not swallow or chew tablets without water.
	Mix powder with water and drink at least eight ounces of fluid.
	Diabetics should avoid dextrose-based products.
	Patients given sodium-restricted diets should avoid sodium containing instant mix formulations.
Stimulants	Drugs most commonly associated with laxative abuse and "cathartic colon."
	Abuse of these products may lead to hypokalemia, protein-losing enteropathy, and malabsorption.
	Do not administer antacids or histamine—two antagonists with enteric coated bisacodyl—since abdominal cramping and vomiting may result.
	Phenolphthalein is associated with skin hypersensitivity in the form of a fixed drug eruption.
	If the urine is alkaline, a pink to red color will develop during phenolphthalein ingestion.
Saline	To avoid fluid loss, the patient should ingest at least eight ounces of fluid.
	Avoid magnesium containing products in patients with renal impairment.
	Phosphate laxatives contain 96.5 mEq. of sodium and should be administered cautiously to patients given sodium-restricted diets.
Hyperosmotics	Glycerin suppositories are ineffective if fecal impaction with hard dry stool is present.
Surfactants	Appear to be of little value in preventing constipation. May exacerbate gastric mucosal damage induced by aspirin.
Emollients	Avoid in elderly.
	Can cause lipid pneumonitis secondary to aspiration.
	Chronic use can decrease absorption of food and fat-soluble vitamins.
	May indirectly induce lung cancer by production of pulmonary fibrosis.

SOURCE: Covington, T., and Walker, J.: *Current Geriatric Therapy*. Philadelphia: W. B. Saunders, 1984.

Table 21 Population Aged 60 Years and Over of the World, 1950–2025

Area	Age Group	1950	1975	2000	2025
	A. *Number* (millions)				
World	60 years and over	214	346	590	1,121
	60–69	133	208	338	656
	70–79	65	106	193	354
	80+	15	32	60	111
More developed regions	60 years and over	95	166	230	315
	60–69	56	93	119	162
	70–79	31	53	81	109
	80+	8	19	30	44
Less developed regions	60 years and over	119	180	360	806
	60–69	78	115	219	494
	70–79	35	53	111	245
	80+	7	13	29	67
	B. *Percentage of population 60 years of age and over*				
World		100	100	100	100
More developed regions		44	48	39	28
Less developed regions		56	52	61	72

SOURCE: Shuman, T. ''The Aging of the World's Population,'' in *Aging*, Goldstein, E. C., ed. Vol. 2, Art. 66. Boca Raton, Fl.: Social Issues Resource Series, Inc. 1981.

Table 22 Population Age 65+ by Selected Ethnic-Minority Groups, United States, 1980[a]

Ethnic-Minority Group	All Ages	Age 65+		
		Number	Percent of All Ages	Percent Distribution by Minority Group
Hispanic[b]	14,609	709	4.9	100.0
Mexican	8,740	367	4.2	51.8
Cuban	803	97	12.1	13.7
Puerto Rican	2,014	69	3.4	9.8
Other	3,051	175	5.7	24.7
Asian/Pacific Islander	3,500	212	6.0	100.0
Chinese	806	58	7.2	27.4
Philipino[c]	775	57	7.4	27.0
Japanese	701	53	7.5	25.0
Asian Indian	362	19	5.2	8.9
Korean	355	9	2.6	4.4
Vietnamese	262	5	2.0	2.5
Hawaiian	167	9	5.1	4.0
Samoan	42	1	2.2	0.4
Guamanian	32	1	2.3	0.3
Native American	1,420	75	5.3	100.0
Indian	1,364	72	5.3	96.7
Eskimo	42	2	4.3	2.4
Aleut	14	1	4.5	0.9

SOURCE: United States Bureau of the Census, 1981 c.
[a]Numbers are in thousands and have been tallied from the separate state reports form Chapter B, Volume 1 for 100 percent data from the 1980 Census of the Population.
[b]Hispanics may be of any race.
[c]The Philipino community generally prefers "Philipino" to "Filipino."

Table 23 Population and Sex Ratios for Persons Age 60+ and 65+ by Race and Ethnicity, United States, 1980

Race and Ethnic Status	All Ages (Number)	Population Age 65 and Over			
		Number	Percent Distribution	Percent of All Ages	Sex Ratio
Total U.S. Population	226,505	25,544	100.00	11.3	67.6
White	188,341	22,944	89.82	12.2	67.2
Black	26,488	2,086	8.17	7.9	68.3
Native American	1,418	75	0.29	5.3	78.3
Asian/Pacific Islander	3,501	212	0.83	6.1	96.4
Hispanic	14,606	709	2.77	4.9	75.6

SOURCE: Manuel, R. C., "A Look at Similarities and Differences in Older Minority Populations," in *Aging*, Goldstein, E. C., ed. Vol. 2, Art. 50. Boca Raton, Fl.: Social Issues Resource Series, Inc. 1981.

Table 24 Retirement Community, Good and Bad

Good	Bad	Good	Bad
People one's own age—peer support	Age segregation		Not suitable as you grow older and more passive
Organized activities and recreational facilities	Isolation—often far from city		Widow may be out of place in couple-oriented community
Easy housing maintenance	Sameness in housing		Keeping up with "Retiree Jones"
Usually good in-community transportation	Sometimes escalating maintenance and recreation costs		Restrictions on landscaping and altering housing
Good housing value	Less civic pride and responsibility		Good hospitals often not close
Stress on active living	Lack of privacy		
Attractive surroundings	Less intellectual stimulation		

SOURCE: Dickinson, Peter. *Retirement Edens*. Glenview, Ill.: Scott, Foresman and Company, 1987.

Table 25 State Income Taxes for Retirement Decision*

State	Taxes per $1,000 of Income	State Tax Burden Ranking	State	Taxes per $1,000 of Income	State Tax Burden Ranking
Alabama	$100	45	New Jersey	117	22
Alaska	286	1	New Mexico	126	12
Arizona	120	17	New York	165	3
Arkansas	97	46	North Carolina	105	35
California	115	23	North Dakota	115	24
Colorado	106	36	Ohio	111	29
Connecticut	112	28	Oklahoma	106	37
Delaware	112	27	Oregon	124	14
Florida	95	48	Pennsylvania	114	25
Georgia	105	38	Rhode Island	121	15
Hawaii	129	8	South Carolina	108	34
Idaho	101	43	South Dakota	100	44
Illinois	113	26	Tennessee	93	51
Indiana	105	39	Texas	97	47
Iowa	119	18	Utah	129	10
Kansas	103	40	Vermont	129	11
Kentucky	102	41	Virginia	101	42
Louisiana	109	32	Washington	118	19
Maine	126	13	West Virginia	121	16
Maryland	117	21	Wisconsin	137	7
Massachusetts	117	20	Wyoming	209	2
Michigan	138	6	District of Columbia	146	4
Minnesota	114	5			
Mississippi	108	33	U.S. AVERAGE	117	
Missouri	93	49			
Montana	129	9			
Nebraska	110	31			
Nevada	111	30			
New Hampshire	93	50			

SOURCES: Tax Foundation, 1875 Connecticut Ave., N.W., Washington, D.C.; Dickinson, Peter. *Retirement Edens*. Glenview, Ill.: Scott, Foresman and Company, 1987.
*The Tax Foundation ranks states according to tax burden (the higher the number the lower the burden) and gives an average amount of taxes per $1,000.

Table 26 State Property Taxes for Retirement Decision*

State	Taxes per $1000 of Income	State Tax Burden Rating	State	Taxes per $1000 of Income	State Tax Burden Rating
Alabama	$12	51	New Jersey	48	9
Alaska	53	5	New Mexico	16	50
Arizona	34	25	New York	50	7
Arkansas	19	45	North Carolina	24	39
California	30	31	North Dakota	28	34
Colorado	35	24	Ohio	33	26
Connecticut	45	14	Oklahoma	18	47
Delaware	16	49	Oregon	53	4
Florida	31	29	Pennsylvania	30	30
Georgia	28	35	Rhode Island	48	10
Hawaii	23	41	South Carolina	26	37
Idaho	27	36	South Dakota	42	16
Illinois	42	17	Tennessee	22	42
Indiana	33	28	Texas	36	22
Iowa	46	11	Utah	36	23
Kansas	38	21	Vermont	50	8
Kentucky	18	46	Virginia	29	33
Louisiana	16	48	Washington	33	27
Maine	45	13	West Virginia	21	44
Maryland	30	32	Wisconsin	45	15
Massachusetts	40	19	Wyoming	92	1
Michigan	52	6	District of Columbia	41	18
Minnesota	39	20			
Mississippi	23	40	U.S. AVERAGE	35	
Missouri	21	43			
Montana	60	2			
Nebraska	45	12			
Nevada	24	38			
New Hampshire	56	3			

SOURCE: Dickinson, Peter. *Retirement Edens*. Glenview, Ill.: Scott, Foresman and Company, 1987.
*These are the amounts of property taxes per $1,000.00 of personal income and how the states rank in property tax burden. Figures are supplied by the Department of Commerce, the Bureau of Census, and Tax Foundation.

Table 27 Urinary Incontinence, Causes of in Old Age

Transient Incontinence
    Acute confusional disorder
    Acute cerebrovascular accident
    Acute urinary tract infection
    Environmental change
    —becoming bedfast
    Psychological
    Retention with overflow
    —faecal impaction
    —drug effect (anticholinergic)

Established Incontinence
    Unstable bladder
    Uninhibited neurogenic bladder
    —stroke
    —focal frontal lobe lesion
    —dementia
    —Parkinsonism
    —normal pressure hydrocephalus
    Reflex neurogenic bladder
    —spinal cord lesion (disc prolapse, infarct
        etc.)
    Prostatism
    Carcinoma or calculus in bladder
    Retention with overflow
    —atonic neurogenic bladder (diabetes, tabes)
    —urethral stricture
    —prostatic enlargement

NOTE: Incontinence is the inability to retain urine. It may occur in a number of otherwise healthy old people and occurs more often in the hospital. This chart is not in the order of occurrence.

SOURCE: Brocklehurst, J.C. *Textbook of Geriatric Medicine and Gerontology*. New York: Churchill Livingstone, 1985.

Table 28 Urinary pH, Foods that Alter

Alkalinizers	Acidifiers
Almonds	Bacon
Chestnuts	Breads
Coconuts	Cheese
Citrus fruits	Corn
Milk	Cranberries
Vegetables	Eggs
	Fish
	Fowl
	Lentils
	Meat
	Pasta
	Plums

SOURCE: Covington, T., and Walker, J. *Current Geriatric Therapy*. Philadelphia: W. B. Saunders, Co., 1984.

Graph 1 Age, Percentage Blacks, Hispanics, and Total Population

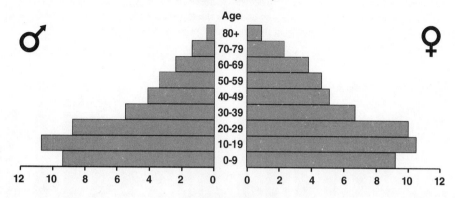

Blacks by age
(1980 / in percent)

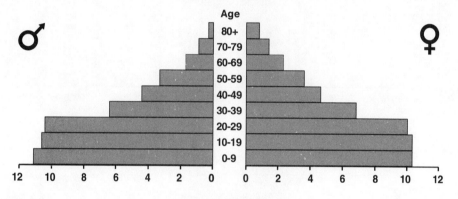

Hispanics by age
(1980 / in percent)

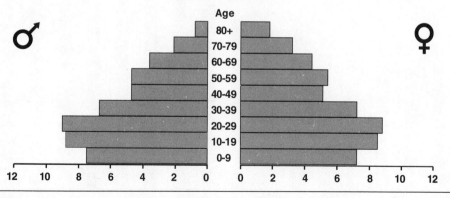

Total Population
(1980 / in percent)

SOURCE: Robey, B.: "Age In America," in *Aging,* Goldstein, E. C., ed. Vol. 2, Art. 12. Boca Raton, Fl.: Social Issues Resource Series, Inc., 1981.

Graph 2 Life Expectancy, Increase in

The rise in life expectancy between 1900 and 2050, plus the 75 million Baby Boomers born between 1946 and 1964, result in the dramatic increase in numbers of older Americans shown here. As projected by the U.S. Bureau of the Census, the chart on the top shows Americans 65 and over; chart on bottom shows the especially large jump in the number of persons 85 and older.

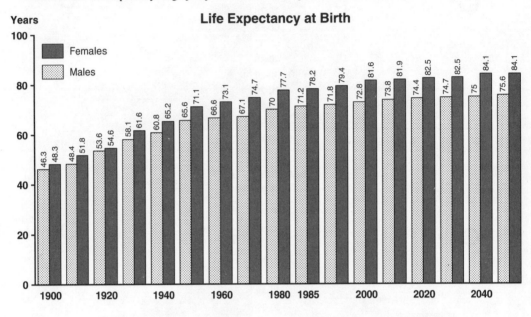

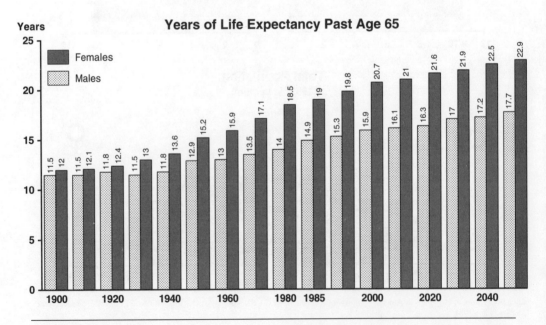

SOURCE: Whitney, E. "Golden Years Threatened By Shifts in Population," in *Aging,* Goldstein, E. C. ed. Vol 3, Art. 19. Boca Raton, Fl.: Social Issues Resource Series, Inc., 1981.

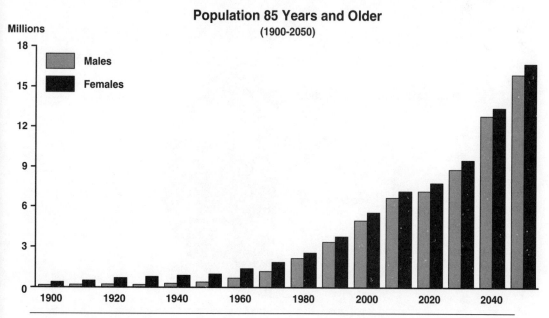

Graph 3 Living Longer

Population 65 Years and Older

(1900-2050)

Millions

- Males
- Females

Population 85 Years and Older

(1900-2050)

Millions

- Males
- Females

SOURCE: Social Security Administration.

267

Graph 4 Where the Aged Get Their Money
1950

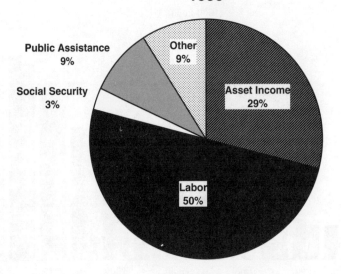

Public Assistance
9%

Other
9%

Social Security
3%

Asset Income
29%

Labor
50%

1984

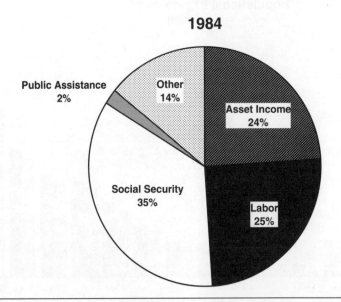

Public Assistance
2%

Other
14%

Asset Income
24%

Social Security
35%

Labor
25%

SOURCES: Urban Institute, Congressional Budget Office.

APPENDIX II
SOURCES OF INFORMATION

APPENDIX II

NATIONAL ORGANIZATION LIST

American Medical Association
535 N. Dearborn Street
Chicago, IL 60610

AARP (American Association of Retired
   Persons)
1909 K Street, N.W.
Washington, DC 20049
(202)872-4700

AARP
Consumer Affairs, Program Department
1909 K Street, N.W.
Washington, DC 20049

AARP Fulfillment
P.O. Box 2400
Long Beach, CA 90801

ACE (Active Corp of Executives)
% Small Business Administration
6th Floor
1111 18th St., N.W.
Washington, DC 20036
(202)634-4950; 205-7151

ACTION
806 Connecticut Ave, N.W.
Washington, DC 20525
(Accept written requests for lists of
   regional offices)

Administration on Aging
U.S. Dept. of Health and Human Service
Washington, DC 20201
(301)496-4000

Aging—National Council on Aging
409 Third Street, S.W.
2nd Floor
Washington, DC 20024
(202)479-1200

Alcoholism—National Council on
   Alcoholism
12 West 21st Street
New York, NY 10010
(212)206-6770

Alzheimer's Society
National Headquarters
70 East Lake Street
Suite 600
Chicago, IL 60601
(312)853-3060

Arthritis Information Clearinghouse
Box AMS
Bethesda, MD 20892
(301)468-3235

Arthritis—National Arthritis Foundation
1314 Spring Street, N.W.
#103
Atlanta, GA 30309
(404)872-7100

Better Business Bureaus, Council of
1515 Wilson Blvd
Arlington, VA 22209
(703)276-0100

Black-Aged—National Caucus and Center
   on Black Aged
Suite 500
1424 K Street, N.W.
Washington, DC 20005
(202)637-8400

Blind—American Foundation for the Blind
15 W. 16th Street
New York, NY 10011
(212)620-2000

Blind—National Society to Prevent
   Blindness
79 Madison Ave
New York, NY 10016
(212)980-2020

Blue Cross/Blue Shield Association
676 North Saint Clair
Chicago, IL 60611
(312)440-6000

Broward Senior Intervention Education
   Program
South Regional Court House
3550 Hollywood Blvd.
#100
Hollywood, FL 33021
(305)963-7500 ext. 265

Cancer—American Cancer Society
National Office
5099 Clifton Rd, N.E.
Atlanta, Ga 30329
(404)320-3333

Caring Children of Aging Parents
% Ethel Burdell
4835 East Anaheim Street
#210
Long Beach, CA 90804
(213)498-0364

Catholic Golden Age
National Headquarters
P.O. Box 3598
Scranton, PA 18505
(717)342-3294

Children of Aging Parents
1609 Woodburn St.
Levittown, PA 19057
(215)945-6900

Consumer Federation of America
1424 16th Street, N.W.
Washington, DC 20036
(202)387-6121

Consumer Product Safety Commission
Washington, DC 20207
1-800-638-CPSC

Dentistry—American Society for Geriatric
   Dentistry
1121 W. Michigan
Indianapolis, IN 46202

Diabetes—American Diabetes Association
ADA National Service Center
1660 Duke Street
Alexandria, VA 22314
1-800-232-3472

Disabled American Veterans
3725 Alexandria Pike
Cold Springs, KY 41076
(606)441-7300

Easter Seals Society
Chicago, IL 60612
(312)726-6200

Elderhostel
75 Federal St.
Boston, MA 02110
(617)426-7788

Ex-Partners of Servicemen/Women for
   Equity (EX-POSE)
P.O. Box 11191
Alexandria, VA 22312
(703)941-5844

Federal Reserve System
Board of Governors
Washington, DC 20551
(202)452-3000

Federal Trade Commission
Public Reference
6th and Pennsylvania Ave, N.W.
Washington, DC 20580
(202)326-2000

Food and Drug Administration
5600 Fishers Lane
Rockville, MD 20857
(301)443-1544

Foster Grandparent Program
% ACTION
806 Connecticut Ave, N.W.
Washington, DC 20525
(202)678-4215

Gray Panthers
3635 Chestnut Street
Philadelphia, PA 19104

Green Thumb
2000 14th St.
Suite 800
Arlington, VA 22201
(703)522-7272

Handicapped—Clearinghouse on the
   Handicapped
Switzer Bldg.
Rm. 3132
330 C Street, S.W.
Washington, DC 20202-2524
(202)732-1241

Hearing Aid—National Hearing Aid
   Society
20361 Middlebelt
Livonia, MI 48152
(313)478-2610

Health Care Financing Administration
Department of Health and Human Services
Baltimore, MD 21207
(301)966-3000

Health Insurance Association of America
1025 Connecticut Ave., N.W.
Washington, DC 20036
(202)223-7780

Heart—American National Heart
   Association
7320 Greenville Ave.
Dallas, TX 75231
(214)373-6300

High Blood Pressure Information Center
120-80 National Institutes of Health
Bethesda, MD 20892
(301)907-7790

Hispanic—National Association for
   Hispanic Elderly
1730 W. Olympic Blvd.
Suite 401
Los Angeles, CA 90015
(213)487-1922

Hospice—National Hospice Organization
1901 N. Moore St.
Suite 901
Arlington, VA 22209
(703)243-5900

Hospital—American Hospital Association
840 North Lake Shore Dr.
Chicago, IL 60611
(312)280-6000

Incontinence—Help for Incontinent People
   (HIP)
P.O. Box 8306
Spartanburg, SC 29305
(803)579-7900

Internal Medicine—American Society of
   Internal Medicine
Suite 500
1101 Vermont Ave, N.W.
Washington, DC 20005
(202)289-1700

International Association of Financial
 Planners
Suite 120C
5775 Peachtree Dunwoody Rd. N.E.
Atlanta, GA 30342

Jewish Association for Services for the
 Aged
40 West 68th Street
New York, NY 10023
(212)724-3200

Legal Counsel for the Elderly
% AARP
1909 K Street, N.W.
Washington, DC 20049

Life Insurance, American Council of
 Information Services
1850 K Street, N.W.
Washington, DC 20006

Lifeline Systems, Inc.
1 Arsenal Marketplace
Watertown, MA 02172
(617)923-4141

LIFT
East Arkansas Area Agency on Aging
311 S. Main Street
Jonesboro, AR 72401
(501)972-5980

Living Bank
P.O. Box 6725
Houston, TX 77005
(713)528-2971

Lung—American Lung Association
1740 Broadway
New York, NY 10019

National Interfaith Coalition on Aging
298 S. Hull Street
P.O. Box 1924
Athens, GA 30603
(404)353-1331

National Senior Citizens Law Center
Suite 701
2025 M Street, N.W.
Washington, DC 20036
(202)887-5280

National Support Center for Families of the
 Aging
P.O. Box 245
Swarthmore, PA 19081
(215)544-5933

National Urban League
500 East 62nd Street
New York, NY 10021
(212)544-5933

Nursing Homes—American Nursing Home
 Association
1101 17th Ave.
Washington, DC 20036

Older Women's League
1325 G Street, N.W.
Lower Level B
Washington, DC 20005
(202)783-6686

Paralyzed Veterans of America
801 18th Street, N.W.
Washington, DC 20006
(202)872-1300

PRIDE (Promote Real Independence for
 Disabled and Elderly)
1159 Poquonock Road
Groton, CT 06340

Readers Digest Fund for the Blind, Inc.
Large-Type Publications
P.O. Box 330
Mount Morris, IL 61054
(written requests accepted for list of
 available publications)

RSVP (Retired Senior Volunteer Program)
% ACTION
806 Connecticut Ave, N.W.
Washington, DC 20525

SCORE (Service Corp of Retired
   Executives)
% Small Business Administration
6th Floor
1111 18th Street, N.W.
Washington, DC 20036
(202)634-4950

Senior Companion Program
% ACTION
806 Connecticut Ave, N.W.
Washington, DC 20525

Small Business Administration
6th Floor
1111 18th Street, N.W.
Washington, DC 20036
(202)634-4950

Social Security Administration
Rm. 4-J-10 West High Rise
6401 Security Blvd.
Baltimore, MD 21235

Speech-Language-Hearing Association
10801 Rockville Pike
Dept. AP
Rockville, MD 20852

Travel Agents—American Society of
   Travel Agents
4400 MacArthur Blvd, N.W.
Washington, DC 20007
(202)965-7520

United Seniors Consumer Cooperative
Suite 500
1334 G Street, N.W.
Washington, DC 20005
(205)393-6222

U.S. Department of Labor
Pension and Welfare Benefit Programs
Office of Communications
Room N4662
200 Constitution Ave, N.W.
Washington, DC 20210

U.S. Public Health Service
Food and Drug Administration
5600 Fishers Lane
Rockville, MD 20857

Vision Foundation
2 Mount Auburn Street
Watertown, MA 02172

VISTA (Volunteers In Service To
   America)
% ACTION
806 Connecticut Ave, N.W.
Washington, DC 20525

Women's Equity Action League (WEAL)
Suite 305
1250 Eye Street, N.W.
Washington, DC 20005

STATE UNITS ON AGING

Alabama
Commission on Aging
State Capitol
Montgomery, AL 36130
(205)261-5743

Alaska
State Agency on Aging
Older Alaskans Commission
Pouch C, Mail Stop 0209
Juneau, AK 99811
(907)465-3250

Arizona
Aging and Adult Administration
P.O. Box 6123
1400 West Washington Street
Phoenix, AZ 85005
(602)255-4448

Arkansas
Arkansas State Office on Aging
Donaghey Building—Suite 1428
7th and Main Streets
Little Rock, AR 72201
(501)371-2441

California
Department on Aging
Health and Welfare Agency
1020 19th Street
Sacramento, CA 95814
(916)322-5290

Colorado
Aging and Adult Services Division
Department of Social Services
717 7th St., Box 181000
Denver, CO 80218-0899
(303)294-5913

Connecticut
Department on Aging
175 Main Street
Hartford, CT 06106
(206)566-7725

Delaware
Division on Aging
Department of Health & Social Services
1901 North Dupont Highway
New Castle, DE 19720
(302)421-6791

District of Columbia
District of Columbia Office on Aging
1424 K Street, N.W.
Second Floor
Washington, DC 20005
(202)724-5622

Florida
Program Office of Aging
Department of Health and Rehabilitation
   Services
1317 Winewood Bld.
Tallahassee, FL 32301
(904)488-8922

Georgia
Office of Aging
Department of Human Resources
878 Peachtree St. N.E., Room 632
Atlanta, GA 30309
(404)894-5333

Hawaii
Executive Office on Aging
Office to the Governor
State of Hawaii
335 Merchants St., Rm. 241
Honolulu, HI 96813
(808)548-2593

Idaho
Idaho Office on Aging
Statehouse—Room 114
Boise, ID 83720
(208)334-3833

Illinois
Department on Aging
421 East Capitol Avenue
Springfield, IL 62706
(217)785-3356

Indiana
Department on Aging and Community
   Services
115 North Penn Street, Ste. 1350
Indianapolis, IN 46204
(317)232-7006

Iowa
Commission on Aging
914 Grand Avenue
Jewett Building
Des Moines, LA 50319
(515)281-5187

Kansas
Department on Aging
610 West 10th Street
Topeka, KS 66612
(913)296-4986

Kentucky
Division for Aging Services
Bureau of Social Services
275 East Main Street
Frankfort, KY 40601
(502)564-6930

Louisiana
Office of Elderly Affairs
P.O. Box 80374
Capitol Station
Baton Rouge, LA 70898
(504)925-1700

Maine
Bureau of Maine's Elderly
Department of Human Services
State House, Station 11
Augusta, ME 04333
(207)289-2561

Maryland
Office on Aging
State Office Building
301 West Preston Street
Baltimore, MD 21201
(301)225-1100

Massachusetts
Department of Elder Affairs
38 Chauncy Street
Boston, MA 02111
(617)727-7751

Michigan
Office of Services to the Aging
300 East Michigan
P.O. Box 30026
Lansing, MI 48909
(517)373-8230

Minnesota
Board on Aging
204 Metro Square Building
7th and Robert Street
St. Paul, MN 55101
(612)296-2544

Mississippi
Council on Aging
301 West Pearl St.
Jackson, MS 39201
(601)949-2070

Missouri
Office of Aging
Department of Social Services
Broadway State Office Building
P.O. Box 570
Jefferson City, MO 65101
(314)751-3082

Montana
Community Services Division
Department of Social and Rehabilitation
    Services
P.O. Box 4210
Helena, MT 59604
(406)449-3865

Nebraska
Department on Aging
P.O. Box 85044
301 Centennial Mall South
Lincoln, NE 68509
(402)471-2306

Nevada
Division of Aging Services
Department of Human Resources
505 East King Street, Room 600
KinKead Building
Carson City, NV 89710
(702)885-4210

New Hampshire
Council on Aging
105 London Rd., Bldg. 3
Concord, NH 03301
(603)271-2751

New Jersey
Department of Community Affairs
P.O. Box 2768
363 West State Street
Trenton, NJ 08625
(609)292-4833

New Mexico
State Agency on Aging
LaVilla Rivera Building
224 East Palace Avenue
Santa Fe, NM 87501
(505)827-7640

New York
Office for the Aging
Agency Building 2
Empire State Plaza
Albany, NY 12223
(518)474-5731

North Carolina
Division on Aging
Department of Human Resources
708 Hillsborough St.
Raleigh, NC 27603
(919)733-3983

North Dakota
State Agency on Aging
Department of Human Services
State Capitol Building
Bismarck, ND 58505
(701)224-2577

Ohio
Commission on Aging
50 West Broad Street
Columbus, OH 43215
(614)466-5500

Oklahoma
Special Unit on Aging
Department of Human Services
P.O. Box 25352
Oklahoma City, OK 73125
(405)521-2281

Oregon
Senior Services Division
Human Resources Department
Room 313
Public Services Building
Salem, OR 97301
(503)378-4728

Pennsylvania
Department of Aging
213 State St.
Harrisburg, PA 17101
(717)753-1550

Rhode Island
Department of Elderly Affairs
79 Washington Street
Providence, RI 02903
(401)277-2858

South Carolina
Commission on Aging
915 Main Street
Columbia, SC 29201
(803)758-2576

South Dakota
Office of Adult Services and Aging
Division of Human Development
Richard F. Dreip Building
700 N. Illinois Street
Pierre, SD 57501
(605)773-3656

Tennessee
Commission on Aging
703 Tennessee Building
535 Church Street
Nashville, TN 37219
(615)741-2056

Texas
Department of Aging
P.O. Box 12786
Capitol Station
Austin, TX 78711
(512)475-2717

Utah
Division of Aging Services
150 West North Temple, Room 326
Salt Lake City, UT 84103
(801)533-6422

Vermont
Office on the Aging
103 Main Street
Waterbury, VT 05676
(802)241-2400

Virginia
Office on Aging
101 North 14th Street
James Monroe Bldg., 18th Floor
Richmond, VA 23219
(804)225-2271

Washington
Bureau of Aging and Adult Service
Department of Social and Health Services,
  OB-43G
Olympia, WA 98504
(206)753-2502

West Virginia
Commission on Aging
State Capitol
Charleston, WV 25305
(304)348-3317

Wisconsin
Department of Health and Social Services
1 West Wilson Street—Room 686
Madison, WI 53703
(608)266-2536

Wyoming
Commission on Aging
Hathaway Building, Room 139
Cheyenne, WY 82002
(307)777-7986

BIBLIOGRAPHY

Abrahams, E. "Let Them All Be Dammed—I'll Do As I Please." *American Heritage.* 44–57, (Sept./Oct., 1987).

Achenbaum, W. A. *Old Age in a New Land: The American Experience Since 1790.* Baltimore: The Johns Hopkins University Press, 1978.

Adult Day Care Annotated Bibliography. Washington, D.C.: National Council on the Aging, 1982.

American Association of Retired Persons. *A Guide for Long Distance Caregivers.* Glenview, Ill.: AARP, 1986.

American Society of Plastic and Reconstructive Surgeons, Inc. "Facelift." Chicago: 1984.

Anderson, H. C. *Newton's Geriatric Nursing,* 5th ed. St. Louis: C. V. Mosby Co., 1971.

Areen, J. "The Legal Status of Consent Obtained from Families of Adult Patients to Withhold or Withdraw Treatment." *JAMA.* 258: 229-235 (1987).

Asenath, L. R.; Dessonville, C., and Jarvik, L. F. "Aging and Mental Disorders," in Birren, J. E., and Schaie, K. W., eds. *Handbook of the Psychology of Aging,* 2nd ed. New York: Van Nostrand Reinhold Company, 1985.

Atchley, R. C. *Social Forces and Aging,* 4th ed. Belmont, Calif.: Wadsworth Publishing Company, 1985.

Averyt, A. C. *et al. Successful Aging.* New York: Ballantine Books, 1987.

Babson-United Investment Advisors. *United Mutual Fund Selector.* Vol. 21: 12, Issue 516 (June 30, 1989).

Background Paper on the Elderly Long Term Care System in Massachusetts. Burlington, Mass.: Massachusetts Hospital Association, July 1982.

Ballenger, J. J. *Diseases of the Nose, Throat, Ear, Head and Neck,* 13th ed. Philadelphia: Lea & Febiger, 1985.

Beck, C. M., and Phillips, L. R. "Abuse of the Elderly." *J. of Gerontological Nursing.* 9: 97–102 (1983).

de Beauvoir, Simone. *Coming of Age*. New York: Warner Books, 1973.

Begmagin, V. and Hirn, K. *Aging is a Family Affair*. New York: Thomas Y. Crowell, 1979.

Bengtson, V. L.; Reedy, M. N.; and Gordon, C. "Aging and Self-Conceptions: Personality Processes and Social Contexts," in Birren, J. E., and Schaie, K. W., eds. *Handbook of the Psychology of Aging*, 2nd ed. New York: Van Nostrand Reinhold Company, 1985.

Benjamin, B. *Are You Tense?* New York: Pantheon Books, 1981.

Berland, T. *Fitness for Life*. Glenview, Ill.: Scott, Foresman and Company, 1986.

Binstock, Robert and Shanas, E., eds. *Handbook of Aging and the Social Sciences*. New York: Van Nostrand Reinhold Co., 1985.

Birren, J. E., and Cunningham, W. R. "Research on the Psychology of Aging: Principles, Concepts, and Theory," in Birren, J. E., and Schaie, K. W., eds. *Handbook of the Psychology of Aging*, 2nd ed. New York: Van Nostrand Reinhold Company, 1985.

Bockus, H. I. *Gastroenterology*. Philadelphia: W. B. Saunders, 1985.

Boyd-Monk, H., and Steinmetz, C. G. *Nursing Care of the Eye*. Los Altos, CA: Appleton & Lange, 1987.

Breytspraak, L. *The Development of the Self in Later Life*. Boston: Little, Brown and Co., 1984.

Brocklehurst, J. C. *Textbook of Geriatric Medicine and Gerontology*. New York: Churchill Livingstone, 1985.

Brocklehurst, J. D. *Textbook of Geriatric Medicine and Gerontology*, 3rd ed. St. Louis: C. V. Mosby Co., 1982.

Brody, J. A., and Brock, D. B. "Epidemiological and Statistical Characteristics of the United States Elderly Population," in Finch, C. E. and Schneider, E. L., eds. *Handbook of the Biology of Aging*, 2nd ed. New York: Van Nostrand Reinhold Company, 1985.

Butler, Robert N., and Lewis, Myrna I. *Aging and Mental Health*, 3rd ed. St. Louis: C. V. Mosby Co., 1982.

Calkins, Evans, M.D.; Paul, J., M.D.; and Ford, Amasa, M.D. *The Practice of Geriatrics*. Philadelphia: W. B. Saunders Co., 1986.

Campion, Edward; Bang, Axel; May, Maurice. "Why Acute-Care Hospitals Must Undertake Long-Term Care." *New England Journal of Medicine*, Vol. 308 (January 13, 1983).

Cantor, M., and Little, V. "Aging and Social Care," in Binstock, R. H., and Shanas, E., eds. *Handbook of Aging and the Social Sciences,* 2nd ed. New York: Van Nostrand Reinhold Co., 1985.

Carlin, V. F., and Mansbery, R. *If I Live to Be 100: Congregate Housing for Later Life.* West Nyack, N.Y.: Parker Publishing Co., 1984.

Chasen, Nancy H. *Policy Wise.* Glenview, Ill.: Scott, Foresman and Co., 1983.

Cherlin, Andrew J. and Furstenberg, Frank F., Jr. *The New American Grandparent: A Place in the Family, A Life Apart.* New York: Basic Books, 1986.

"Closing the Gap," *AARP News Bulletin.* 28: 8–9 (1987).

Cohen, H. J., and Lyles, K. W. "Geriatics." *JAMA.* Vol. 261, No. 19 (May 1989), p. 2847–2848.

Coile, Russell C. *The New Hospital: Future Strategies for the Changing Industry.* Rockville, Md: Aspen Publishers, 1986.

Coleman, Barbara. *A Consumer Guide to Hospice Care.* Washington, D.C.: National Consumers League, 1985.

Columbia University College of Physicians & Surgeons. *Complete Home Medical Guide.* New York: Crown Publishers, 1985.

Cousins, N. *Anatomy of an Illness as Perceived by the Patient.* New York: W. W. Norton & Co., 1979.

Coverage. Blue Cross and Blue Shield of Arkansas Publication. 18: 1987.

Cox-Gedmark, J. *Coping with Physical Disability.* Philadelphia: The Westminster Press, 1982.

Covington, T., and Walker, J. *Current Geriatric Therapy.* Philadelphia: W. B. Saunders, 1984.

Crichton, J. *Age Care Sourcebook.* New York: Simon & Schuster, Inc., 1987.

Cristofalo, V. J. *Atherogenesis.* Frankfurt, Germany, New York, London, Tokyo: Springer-Verlag, 1986.

Davidson, M. B. *Diabetes Mellitus Diagnosis and Treatment.* New York: Wiley Medical Publications, 1981.

Deedy, John. *Your Aging Parents.* Chicago: The Thomas More Press, 1984.

Department of the Treasury, Internal Revenue Service. Publication #503, 1987.

Dickinson, Peter A. *Retirement Edens.* Glenview, Ill.: Scott, Foresman and Company, 1987.

————. *Sunbelt Retirement.* Glenview, Ill.: Scott, Foresman and Company, 1986.

Directory of Homemaker/Home Health-Aide Services in the United States, Puerto Rico and Virgin Islands. New York: National Homecaring Council, 1982.

Directory of Hospital Services for Older Adults. Chicago: The Hospital Research and Educational Trust, 1982.

Dychtwald, Ken. *Age Wave: Challenges and Choices for Our New Future.* New York: Bantam Books, Inc., 1990.

Dychtwald, Ken, and Zitter, Mark. *The Role of the Hospital in an Aging Society.* Emeryville, Calif.: Age Wave Publications, 1986.

Evashwick, Connie. *Hospitals and Older Adults: Current Actions and Future Trends.* Chicago: The Hospital Research and Educational Trust, 1982.

————. "Long-Term Care Becomes Major New Role for Hospitals," *Hospitals,* Vol. 56 (July 1, 1982).

Evashwick, Connie, and Hickey, Kevin. "Care of the Elderly in the USA," *World Hospitals,* Vol. 19, Nos. 1 and 2 (April 1983).

Evashwick, Connie, and Read, William. "Hospitals and LTC: Options, Alternatives, Implications." *Journal of Healthcare Financial Management* (June 1, 1985).

Evashwick, Connie; Rundall, Thomas; and Goldiamond, Betty. "Hospital Services for Seniors: Results of a National Survey," *The Gerontologist,* Vol. 25 (1985).

Evashwick, Connie, and Weiss, Lawrence. *Managing the Continuum of Care: A Practical Guide to Organization and Operations.* Rockville, Md.: Aspen Publishers, 1987.

Ferguson, Tom, M.D. *Medical Self-Care.* New York: Summit Books, 1980.

Finch, C. E. and Schneider, E. L., eds. *Handbook of the Biology of Aging.* 2nd ed. New York: Van Nostrand Reinhold Co., 1985.

Fromme, Allan, Ph.D. *Life After Work.* Glenview, Ill.: Scott, Foresman and Company, 1984.

Gallup, George, M.D., and Hill, Evan. *The Secrets of Long Life.* New York: Bernard Geis Associates, 1960.

Gilchrest, B. A. "At Last! A Medical Treatment for Skin Aging." *JAMA* 259: 569–570 (1988).

Gillies, John. *A Guide to Caring For and Coping with Aging Parents*. Nashville: Thomas Nelson Publishers, 1981.

Glasscote, R., and Gudeman, Jr. *Creative Mental Health Services for the Elderly*. Washington, D.C.: The Joint Information Service, 1977.

Goldberg, Myron D., M.D., and Rubin, Julia. *The Inside Tract*. Glenview, Ill.: Scott, Foresman and Co., 1986.

Goldstein, E. C., ed. *Aging*, Vol. 1–3. Boca Raton, Fl.: Social Issues Resources Series, Inc., 1981–1989.

Griffith, H. Winter, M.D. *Complete Guide to Symptoms, Illness, and Surgery*. Tucson: The Body Press, 1985.

Gutman, R. *The Healthy Back Book*. Chicago: Blue Cross/Blue Shield, 1986.

Haight, Barbara K. "The Therapeutic Role of a Structured Life Review Process in Home-bound Elderly Subjects." *J. of Gerontology,* Vol. 43, No. 2 (1988), 40–44.

Ham, Richard J., M.D. *Geriatric Medical Annual—1986*. Oradell, N.J.: Medical Economics Books, 1986.

———. *Geriatrics Medical Annual—1987*. Oradell, N.J.: Medical Economics Books, 1987.

Harris, L., *et al. The Myth and Reality of Aging in America*. Washington, D.C.: The National Council on Aging, 1975.

Harris, D. K., and Cole, W. E. *Sociology of Aging*. Boston: Houghton Mifflin Company, 1980.

Hartman, J. T. *The Sleep Book: Understanding and Preventing Sleep Problems in People Over 50*. Glenview, Ill.: AARP and Scott, Foresman and Company, 1987.

"Health Care for the Aged: A Special Issue." *Hospitals,* Vol. 54 (May 16, 1980). American Hospital Publishing.

Hen Chong Wei, *et al.* "Addresses to the Sino-American Workshop on Gerontology." Beijing National University, Tuesday, September 18, 1986. Unpublished.

Henig, Robin Marantz. *The Myth of Senility: The Truth About the Brain and Aging*. Glenview, Ill.: Scott, Foresman and Company, 1981.

Home Care. Washington, D.C.: National Association for Home Care, 1987.

Hooyman, N. R., and Lustbader, W. *Taking Care*. New York: The Free Press, 1986.

Horne, Jo. *Caregiving*. Glenview, Ill.: Scott, Foresman and Company, 1985.

Hospitals, Vol. 60, March 20, 1986. Special Issue on Services for the Elderly. American Hospital Publishing.

Hospitals and Older Adults: Current Actions and Future Trends. Chicago: The Hospital Research and Educational Trust, 1982.

Hospital Statistics, 1986. Chicago: American Hospital Association, 1987.

How to Select a Nursing Home. U.S. Department of Human Services. Baltimore: Health Care Financing Administration, 1980.

Hurst, J. W. *The Heart,* 6th ed. St. Louis: McGraw-Hill Book Co., 1986.

Hypothermia Bulletin. Washington, D.C.: Center for Environment Physiology, 1985.

Innovative Utilization of Older Persons in Volunteer Service Programs: Six Hospitals Report on Model Projects. Chicago: The Hospital Research and Educational Trust, 1981.

Kalish, R. A. "The Social Context of Death and Dying," in Binstock, R. H., and Shanas, E., eds. *Handbook of Aging and the Social Sciences,* 2nd ed. New York: Van Nostrand Reinhold Co., 1985.

Kamal, Asif, and Brocklehurst, J. C. *Color Atlas of Geriatric Medicine.* Oradell, N.J.: Medical Economics Books, 1984.

Kart, C. S.; Metress, E. S.; and Metress, J. F. *Aging and Health: Biologic and Social Perspectives.* Menlo Park, Calif.: Addison-Wesley, 1978.

Kastenbaum, R. A. "Dying and Death: A Life-Span Approach," in Birren, J. E., and Schaie, K. W., eds. *Handbook of the Psychology of Aging,* 2nd ed. New York: Van Nostrand Reinhold Company, 1985.

Kelly, W. E. *Alzheimer's Disease and Related Disorders.* Springfield, Ill.: Charles C. Thomas Co., 1984.

Kemp, B. "Rehabilitation and the Older Adult," in Birren, J. E., an Schaie, K. W., eds. *Handbook of the Psychology of Aging,* 2nd ed. New York: Van Nostrand Reinhold Company, 1985.

Kenny, James, and Spicer, S. *Caring for Your Aging Parents: A Practical Guide to the Challenges, the Choices.* Cincinnati: St. Anthony Messenger Press, 1984.

Kenyon, Gary, "Basic Assumptions in Theories of Human Aging," in Birren, J., and Bengtson, V. *Emergent Theories of Aging.* New York: Springer Publishing Co., 1988.

Kent, Saul. *The Life-Extension Revolution.* New York: William Morrow and Company, Inc., 1980.

Kirkwood, T. B. L. "Comparative and Evolutionary Aspects of Anatomy," in Finch, C. E., and Schneider, E. L., eds. *Handbook of the Biology of Aging,* 2nd ed. New York: Van Nostrand Reinhold Company, 1985.

Klipper, Miriam. *The Relaxation Response.* New York: Avon Books, 1975.

Kohut, Sylvester, Jr., Ph.D.; Kohut, Jeraldine, R.N. M.A., N.H.A.; and Fleishman, Joseph J., Ph.D. *Reality Orientation for the Elderly,* 3rd ed. Oradell, N.J.: Medical Economics Co., Inc., 1987.

Kornhaber, Arthur, M.D., and Woodward, Kenneth. *Grandparents, Grandchildren: The Vital Connection.* New York: Anchor Press/Doubleday, 1981.

Kübler-Ross, E. *Death: The Final Stage of Growth.* Englewood Cliffs, N.J.: Prentice-Hall, 1975.

Kuntzleman, Charles T. *The Complete Book of Walking.* New York: Simon and Schuster, 1978.

LaBuda, Dennis. *The Gadget Book.* Glenview, Ill.: Scott, Foresman and Company, 1985.

Leonard, Jon N.; Hofer, Jack L.; and Pritikin, Nathan. *Live Longer Now.* New York: Gosset and Dunlap, 1974.

Leonard, Jon N., and Taylor, Elaine A. *The Live Longer Now Cookbook.* New York: Gossett and Dunlap, 1977.

Lester, Andrew D., and Lester, Judith L. *Understanding Aging Parents.* Philadelphia: The Westminister Press, 1980.

Leibermann, Morton. *Self-Help Groups for Coping with Crisis: Origins, Members, Processes and Impact.* San Francisco: Jassey-Bass, 1979.

Lipowski, Z. J. "Delirium (Acute Confusional States)." *JAMA.* 258: 1789–1792 (1987).

Loewinsohn, Ruth Jean. *Survival Handbook for Widows.* Glenview, Ill.: Scott, Foresman and Company, 1984.

Loewinsohn, R. J. *Survival Handbook for Widows.* Washington, D.C.: AARP, 1986.

———. *Widowhood in an American City.* Cambridge, Mass.: Schenkman, 1973.

Long, Barbara C., and Phipps, Wilma J. *Essentials of Medical Surgical Nursing.* St. Louis: C. V. Mosby, Co., 1985.

Lopata, H. Z. *Women as Widows: Support Systems.* New York: Elsevier Press, 1979.

Lovenheim, B. "Katherine Hepburn at 80." *McCalls* (November 1989), 125–129.

Lynch, J. J. "Man's Best Friendly Medicine." *Creative Living* 16: 16–20 (1987).

Mace, Nancy. *The 36-Hour Day: A Family Guide to Caring for Persons with Alzheimer's Disease, Related Dementia Illnesses and Memory Loss in Later Life.* Baltimore: Johns Hopkins University Press, 1981.

Mann, G. V., *et al.* "Cardiovascular Disease in African Pygmies," *J. of Chronic Diseases* 15: 341–371 (1961).

Marmot, M. G. *Acculturation and Coronary Heart Disease in Japanese-Americans.* Ph.D. thesis. University of California, Berkeley, 1975. Unpublished.

Marmot, M. G., and Syme, S. L. "Acculturation and Coronary Heart Disease in Japanese-Americans." *Amer. J. of Epidemiology* 104: 225–247 (1976).

Massow, Rosalind. *Travel Easy.* Glenview, Ill.: Scott, Foresman and Company, 1985.

Modern Maturity. AARP, Feb., March, 1987.

Myers, G. C., "Aging and Worldwide Population Change," in Binstock, R. H., and Shanas, E., eds. *Handbook of Aging and the Social Sciences,* 2nd ed. New York: Van Nostrand Reinhold Company, 1985.

McMeekin, Betty. *Family Involvement in the Nursing Home Experience.* Denton, Tex.: North Texas State University Press, 1985.

Narrow, B. W., and Buschle, K. B. *Fundamentals of Nursing Practice,* 2nd ed. New York: John Wiley and Sons, Inc., 1987.

National Center for Health Statistics; Dawson, D. A.; and Adams, P. F. "Current Estimates from the National Health Interview Survey; United States, 1986." *Vital and Health Statistics.* DHHS Pub. No. (PHS) 87-1592. Series 10, No. 164. Public Health Service. Washington, DC: U.S. Government Printing Office, 1987.

Nauheim, Ferd. *239 Ways to Put Your Money to Work.* Glenview, Ill.: Scott, Foresman and Company, 1986.

Nelson, Eugene C., D.Sc.; Roberts, Ellen, M.P.H.; Simmons, Jeanette, D.Sc.; Tisdale, William, M.D. *Medical and Health Guide for People Over Fifty.* Glenview, Ill.: Scott, Foresman and Company, 1986.

Nelson, Thomas C. *It's Your Choice.* Glenview, Ill.: Scott, Foresman and Company, 1983.

Newell, Frank W. *Ophthalmology Principles and Concepts,* 6th ed. St. Louis: C. V. Mosby Co., 1986.

O'Brien, R., and Chafetz, M. *The Encyclopedia of Alcoholism.* New York: Facts On File, 1991.

Page, L. B., *et al.* Antecedents of Cardiovascular Disease in Six Solomon Islands Societies.'' *Circulation.* 49: 1132–1146 (1974).

Pearson, Durk, and Shaw, Sandy. *Life Extension; A Practical Scientific Approach.* New York: Warner Books, 1982.

Persico, J. E., and Sunderland, George. *Keeping Out of Crimes Way.* Glenview, Ill.: Scott, Foresman and Company, 1985.

Persily, Nancy, and Brody, Stanley. *Hospitals and the Aged: The New Old Market.* Rockville, Md.: Aspen Publishers, 1984.

Phipps, W. J., *et al. Medical Surgical Nursing.* St. Louis: C. V. Mosby Co., 1983.

Phipps, Wilma, R.N.; Long, Barbara C., R.N.; Woods, Nancy Fugate, R.N. *Medical-Surgical Nursing Concepts and Clinical Practice.* St. Louis: C. V. Mosby Co., 1983.

Pillemer, K., and Finkelhor, D. ''The Prevalence of Elder Abuse: A Random Sample Survey.'' *The Gerontologist,* Vol. 28, No. 1, 51–57 (1988).

Powell, L. S., and Courtice, K. *Alzheimer's Disease.* Reading, Mass.: Addison-Wesley Publishing Company, 1983.

Quinn, J. B. ''Saying the Big Goodbye.'' *Newsweek* (October 9, 1989).

Quinn, M., and Tomita, S. *Elder Abuse and Neglect.* New York: Springer Publishing Co., 1986.

Ralston, Jeannie. *Walking for the Health of It.* Glenview, Ill.: Scott, Foresman and Company, 1986.

Raper, Ann Trueblood. *National Continuing Care Directory.* Glenview, Ill.: Scott, Foresman and Company, 1984.

Reichel, William, M.D. *Clinical Aspects of Aging.* Baltimore: Waverly Press, 1979.

Reisberg, B., ed. *Alzheimer's Disease: The Standard Reference.* New York: The Free Press, 1983.

Rochleau, Bruce. *Hospitals and Community-Oriented Programs for the Elderly: Innovations in Health Care.* Ann Arbor: AUPHA Press, 1983.

Rogers, C. Stewart, M.D.; and McCue, Jack D., M.D., F.A.C.P. *Managing Chronic Disease.* Oradell, NJ: Medical Economics Books, 1987.

Rosenwaike, I. ''A Demographic Portrait of the Oldest Old.'' *Milbank Memorial Fund Quarterly: Health and Society,* Vol. 63: 2 (Spring 1985).

Ross, R. "The Pathogenesis of Atherosclerosis." *N. Engl. J. Med.* 314: 488 (1986).

Rossman, I. *Clinical Geriatrics,* 3rd ed. Philadelphia: J. B. Lippincott Company, 1986.

Ruff, C. D. "In the Eye of the Beholder: Views of Psychological Well-Being Among Middle-Aged and Older Adults," *Psychology and Aging,* Vol. 4, No. 2, 195–210 (1989).

Russell, C. H. *Good News About Aging.* New York: John Wiley and Sons, 1989.

Russell, C. H., and Megaard, I. *The General Social Survey, 1972–1976: The State of the American People.* New York: Springer-Verlag, 1988.

Russell, Martha, and Bantarri, Marlene, eds. *Developing Potentials for Handicaps.* Minneapolis: The Minnesota Home Economics Association, 1978.

Rzetelney, Harriet, and Mellor, Joanna. *Support Groups for Caregivers of the Aged: A Training Manual for Facilitators.* New York: Community Services Society, 1981.

Sargent, Jean. *An Easier Way: Handbook for the Elderly and Handicapped.* Ames: Iowa State University Press, 1981.

Schaefer, E. J., and Levy, R. I. "Pathogenesis and Management of Lipoprotein Disorders." *New Engl. J. Med.* 312: 1300 (1985).

Schaie, K. Warner. "The Hazards of Cognitive Aging." *The Gerontologist* 29:4, 484–493 (August 1989).

Schaie, K. W., and Willis, S. L. *Adult Development and Aging,* 2nd ed. Boston: Little, Brown and Company, 1986.

Schatz, I. J. *Orthostatic Hypotension.* Philadelphia: F. A. Davis Co., 1986.

Scheie, H. G., and Albert, D. M. *Textbook of Ophthalmology,* 10th ed. Philadelphia: W. B. Saunders, 1986.

Scheier, R. L. "Development Continues in Older Adults." *American Medical News* (Nov. 11, 1986).

Scherer, J. C. *Introductory Medical-Surgical Nursing,* 3rd ed. Philadelphia: J.B. Lippincott Company, 1983.

Schulz, J. H. *The Economics of Aging,* 4th ed. Dover, Mass.: Auburn House Publishing, 1988.

Schick, F. L. *Statistical Handbook of Aging Americans.* Phoenix: The Oryx Press, 1986.

Seskin, Jane. *Alone—Not Lonely.* Glenview, Ill.: Scott, Foresman and Company, 1985.

Shea, Timothy P., D.P.M., and Smith, Joan K. *The Over Easy Foot Care Book*. Glenview, Ill.: Scott, Foresman and Company, 1984.

Simmons, L. *The Role of the Aged in Primitive Society*. New Haven: Yale University Press, 1945.

Slatt, B. J., and Stein, H. A. *The Ophthalmic Assistant Fundamentals and Clinical Practice*, 4th ed. St. Louis: C. V. Mosby Co., 1983.

Soldo, B. J. "America's Elderly in the 1980s," *Population Bulletin*, Vol. 35, No. 4. Washington, D.C.: Population Reference Bureau, Inc., 1980.

Soled, Alex J. *The Essential Guide to Wills, Estates, Trusts and Death Taxes*. Glenview, Ill.: Scott, Foresman and Company, 1984.

"Special Issue: Long-Term Care: Challenges and Opportunities." *Hospitals*, Vol. 56 (July 1, 1982). American Hospital Publishing.

Spencer, M. E. "Truth About Aging: Guidelines for Accurate Communications." Washington, D.C.: AARP, 1984.

Springer, Dianne, and Brubaker, Timothy. *Family Caregiving and Dependent Elderly*. Beverly Hills: Sage Publications, Inc., 1984.

Steinberg, Franz U. *Care of the Geriatric Patient*. 6th ed. St. Louis: C. V. Mosby Co., 1983.

Stern, Newton S., A.B., M.D., F.A.C.P. *Rare Disease in Internal Medicine*. Springfield, Ill.: Charles C. Thomas Publisher, 1966.

Sterns, H. L.; Barrett, G. V.; and Alexander, R. A. "Accidents and the Aging Individual," in Birren, J. E., and Schaie, K. W., eds. *Handbook of the Psychology of Aging*, 2nd ed. New York: Van Nostrand Reinhold Company, 1985.

Steward, Dana, ed. *A Fine Age: Creativity as a Key to Successful Aging*. Little Rock: August House, 1984.

Stough, D. B., and Cates, J. "Contemporary Techniques of Hair Replacement." *Postgraduate Medicine*, 69 (1981).

Stough, D. B., *et al.* "Surgical Procedure for the Treatment of Baldness." *Cutis* (May 1986).

Sumichrast, Michael; Shafer, Ronald G.; and Sumichrast, Marika. *Planning Your Retirement Housing*. Glenview, Ill.: Scott, Foresman and Company, 1984.

"The Advent of the Gold-Collar Worker." *Modern Maturity*. (October–November 1986).

Tucker, E. "Annuity Fundamental." *United Retirement Bulletin* (September, 1989).

———. "How Long Must You Plan For?" *United Retirement Bulletin* (May 1988).

The Hospital's Role in Caring for the Elderly: Leadership Issues. Chicago: The Hospital Research and Educational Trust, 1983.

Uhlenberg, P., and Myers, M. A. P. "Divorce Among the Elderly." *The Gerontologist* 21, 276–282 (1981).

U.S. Bureau of the Census. *Statistical Abstract of the United States: 1989,* 109th ed. Washingont, D.C.: U.S. Government Printing Office, 1989.

U.S. Department of Commerce, National Oceanic and Atmospheric Administration. *National Weather Service Pamphlet. NOAA/PA 79018* (Rev. 8/83).

U.S. House of Representatives, Select Committee on Aging. *The Senior Community Service Program: Its History and Evolution.* Comm. Pub. No. 100–695. December 1988. Washington, D.C.: U.S. Government Printing Office, 1989.

Vogel, Ronald J., and Palmer, Hans C. *Long-Term Care: Perspectives from Research and Demonstrations.* Rockville, Md.: Aspen Publishers, 1985.

Walford, Roy L., M.D. *120 Year Diet, The.* New York: Simon & Schuster, 1987.

Walford, Roy L., M.D. *Maximum Life Span.* New York: W. W. Norton & Company, 1983.

Wallworth, J. "New Adventures for Seniors in World of Work," in *Aging,* Goldstein, E. C., ed. Vol. 1, Art. 67. Boca Raton, Fl.: Social Issues Resource Series, Inc., 1981.

Ward, R. A. *The Aging Experience,* 2nd ed. New York: Harper and Row, 1984.

Weaver, Peter, and Buchanan, Annette. *What to Do with What You've Got.* Glenview, Ill.: Scott, Foresman and Company, 1984.

Weaver, P., and Buchanan, A. *What to Do with What You've Got: The Practical Guide to Money Management in Retirement.* Washington, D.C.: AARP, 1985.

Watkin, Donald M. *Handbook of Nutrition, Health and Aging.* Park Ridge, N.J.: Noyes Publications, 1983.

Weindruch, R., and Walford, R. L. *Retardation of Aging by Dietary Restriction.* New York: Raven, 1987.

Weiss, J. S., *et al.* "Topical Tretinoin Improves Photoaged Skin." *JAMA.* 259: 5277–532 (1988).

Western, Leone Noble. *The Gold Key to Writing Your Life History.* Port Angeles, Wash.: Peninsula Publishing Inc., 1981.

What Are You? I Am Old. New York: State Communities Aid Association, 1983

Wilmer, William H. *Atlas Fundus Oculi.* New York: The MacMillan Company, 1934.

Wisnieski, C. J. "Media Guideline For Sexuality and Aging," in *Television and the Aging Audience.* San Diego: University of Southern California Press, 1980.

Wood, J. "Caregiver." *Modern Maturity* (August-September, 1987).

Zaccarelli, Herman. *The Cookbook That Tells You How: The Retirement Food and Nutrition Manual.* Boston: Cahners Publishing Company, 1972.

INDEX

Bold face numbers indicate main headings

A

abdominal pain
  cancer, pancreatic, 40
  constipation, 52
  diarrhea, 72
accidents, 1
  death, causes of, and declining
    death rates, 60–61
  falls, 89–90
  living with one's children, 149
  premature death reduction, 187
  security, advice on, 206
Accreditation Council for Graduate
  Medical Education, 101
acculturation, 1–2
acculturation rank, 2
acetaminophen
  hepatitis, drug-induced, 116
ACTION, 3, 271
  Foster Grandparent Program, 94
  RSVP, 204
  Senior Companion Program, 208
  VISTA, 231
Active Corps of Executives, 271
  SCORE, 206
activity theory, 3–4
acute pain, 175–176
acute respiratory disease (ARD), 4
Addison's disease
  depression, 70
Adenauer, Konrad, 2, 136
Administration on Aging, 271
adult children, relationships with,
  4–5
Adult Development and Education
  (K. Warner Schaie and Sherry L.
  Willis), 238
adult education
  leisure, 139
advance directives
  living wills, 148
Africa
  age, 6
  bushmen of the Kalahari, 33
  Hottentot elderly, 119
  Masai, 153
  Somali camel herdsmen, 213
African pygmy, 5
After Many a Summer Dies the Swan
  (Aldous Huxley), 142–143
Agayev, Mezhid, 125
age, 5–7
age bias in employment, 7
  hiring age, 118
age cohort, 6
Age Discrimination in Employment
  Act (1977)
  age bias in employment, 7
  gerontology, 102
  hiring age, 118

retirement age, history of, 201
ageist language, 7–8
Age Wave, 26
aging, biological theory of, 8–10
Alabama
  office of aging, 275
Alaska
  office of aging, 275
alcohol abuse, 10–11
  folic acid deficiency, 91
  longevity, rules of, 151
  National Council on Alcoholism,
    271
  pneumonia, 184
Alcoholics Anonymous, 11
allergic reactions
  drug reactions, adverse, 78
  external otitis, 88
Alzheimer's disease, 11–12
  global deterioration scale (table),
    254
  National Institute on Aging, 226
  Reisburg's global deterioration
    scale, 194–195
  treatment, 12
Alzheimer's Society, 271
amaurosis fugax, 12–13
American Academy of Family
  Physicians
  geriatrics, 101
American Association of Retired
  Persons (AARP), 13, 271
  caregiver, 42
  discounts, senior citizens', 74
  driving and old age, 77
  insurance, supplemental, 132
  taxes, 219
  volunteer work, 234
American Board of Internal Medicine
  geriatrics, 101
American Cancer Society, 272
  cancer, breast, 35
American Council of Life Insurance,
  144
American Diabetes Association, 272
American Foundation for the Blind,
  272
American Heart Association, 273
American Hospital Association, 273
  patient rights, 177–178
American Lung Association, 274
American Medical Association,
  271
American Nursing Home
  Association, 274
American Society for Geriatric
  Dentistry, 272
American Society of Internal
  Medicine, 273
American Society of Travel Agents,
  275

amphetamines
  depression, 70
anemia, 13
  arthritis, rheumatoid, 21
  cancer, stomach, 41
  chronic disease, 13–14
  epistaxis, 83
  iron deficiency, 14
  megaloblastic, 14
  multiple myeloma, 163
  polymyalgia rheumatica, 186
  ulcerative colitis, 225
  vitamin B_{12} deficiency, 232
aneurysm, 15
  abdominal, 15
  arteriosclerosis, 20
  cerebral vascular accident, 46
  congestive heart failure, 51
anger, 15–16
angina pectoris, 16–17
  anemia, 13
  arteriosclerosis, 20
anosmia, 17
  rhinitis, 203
antacids
  ulcer, peptic, 224
anti-aging diet, 17–18
anticonvulsant drugs
  seizures, 207–208
antidepressants
  depression, 70
antioxidants, 18
  free radical theory of aging, 95
anxiety, 18–19
Area Agencies on Aging
  caregiving, long-distance, 43
Aristotle, 126, 138
Arizona
  office of aging, 275
Arkansas
  office of aging, 275
  retirement states, 203
arrhythmias, cardiac, 19
arteriosclerosis, 19–20
  congestive heart failure, 51
arteritis, giant cell, 20
arthritis—*See also osteoarthritis*
  gout, 105
  infectious, 21
  National Arthritis Foundation,
    271
  rheumatoid, 13, 21–22
  sexuality, 209
Arthritis Foundation, 21–22
Arthritis Information Clearinghouse,
  271
asbestos
  cancer, lung, 37
Asia
  Chinese elderly, 46–47
  Japanese elderly, 133–134

295